Not Just
One in Eight

"Barbara Stevens's book is a must-read for every woman who has had breast cancer—and for every woman who worries about it."

—Judge Judy Sheindlin

"These important stories remind us that we women are experts at taking care of others, and the magic comes when we learn to nurture ourselves—especially during the toughest of times."

—Kay Allenbaugh
author of *Chocolate for a Woman's Soul*

"It would have been wonderful if Heather and I had been able to read *Not Just One in Eight* in 1989 when she was diagnosed. We had no resource that dealt with *real* women . . . *real* situations. It would have provided valuable information and direction as well as the comfort of listening to people who have dealt with the same situations we were facing. Only a person who has been there can know how alone you feel!"

—Sharon Farr
the mother of the late Heather Farr,
LPGA golfer

"This is an extremely valuable book for anyone facing the challenge of a breast cancer diagnosis—and that includes not only the patient but the family and friends who are also deeply affected. It is the first book to address what breast cancer survivors already know, that fighting this illness is a group effort that changes many lives in a ripple effect. The interviews in this book are compassionate, absorbing, and provide immeasurable insight into all aspects of coping with this fearsome disease."

—Jami Bernard
author, film critic for the *New York Daily News,*
columnist for *Mamm* **magazine and**
breast cancer survivor

Not Just One in Eight

Stories of
Breast Cancer Survivors
and Their Families

BARBARA F. STEVENS

Health Communications, Inc.
Deerfield Beach, Florida

www.hci-online.com

Taxol® is a registered trademark of Bristol-Myers Squibb.

Library of Congress Cataloging-in-Publication Data is
on file with the Library of Congress.

©2000 Barbara F. Stevens

ISBN 1-55874-832-6

Publisher: Health Communications, Inc.
            3201 S.W. 15th Street
            Deerfield Beach, FL 33442-8190

Cover and inside book design by Lawna Patterson Oldfield
Cover photo by Artville ©2000
Author photo ©Head Shots/Studio II

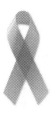

*T*his book is dedicated
to all the women and men who
have fought this disease,
and to their families.

One

Barbara Stevens

Breast Cancer Really Is a Wake-up Call!

Survivor Profile:

Age at diagnosis: forty-three (7/28/93)
Date of interview: support team 1/97, Barbara 2/2000
Type of breast cancer: infiltrating ductal
Size tumor: 1 cm; stage I
No positive lymph nodes
Surgical procedure: bilateral mastectomy (one breast prophylactic)
Reconstruction: both sides, not immediate
Estrogen receptors: borderline positive; Progesterone receptors:
   negative

Who's Who:

Barton Stevens, her husband; Betty Weiss, her friend
Stephanie Johns, her friend; Irene Rosenblum, her friend
Rosalind (Roz) Jacobs, her aunt *[see chapter 4]*
Gerald (Jerry) Jacobs, her uncle
Amy Falk, her cousin (Roz and Jerry's daughter)
Shirley Stevens, her mother-in-law
William Stevens, her father-in-law
Elyse Horvath, Betty's daughter and Barbara's friend

3

BEFORE THE BEGINNING

Barbara: At the age of forty-nine my mother was diagnosed with breast cancer. I was twenty-one. I have asked my husband, Bart over the years, "Was I a good daughter?" because I have blocked so much of her cancer experience from my mind. He reassures me I was. I am still embarrassed that never once did I call my mother during her ten-day hospital stay when she had a Halsted radical mastectomy. Nor did I visit. I am sure she was hurt, but she never said a word. I have no memories of our family discussing my mother's cancer experience other than one in which my father commented, "The skin graft goes this way. I thought it would go the opposite way." Life went on. I suppose that was how families coped in 1971.

It's odd. Even though from that point on I was followed closely by my mother's surgeon, had yearly mammograms, and lived for years with an albatross around my neck knowing it was only a matter of time before I got breast cancer, I never really stressed about it. Do I buy into the thinking that a person creates their own disease? Yes and no. I certainly did nothing to assist my body in staying healthy. I abused my body: I ate horribly, did not exercise and smoked a pack of cigarettes every day for twenty years until I quit at the age of thirty-five. By the time I decided, at the age of forty-one or forty-two to take responsibility for myself, the damage had already been done. Shortly after my forty-third birthday in July of 1993, my own cancer journey began.

Bart, her husband: Barb and I did visit her mother once in the hospital, but she just does not remember. Barb wanted to talk to her mother on the phone while she was in the hospital, but her mother wanted to be left alone. That is how she coped—by withdrawing. I won't say that I expected Barb to get cancer, but it was certainly a strong possibility with her family history and it was a concern.

THE BEGINNING

Barbara: I will state up-front that I do not believe in coincidence. I will also state that I believe I have always had guardian angels watching over me. Several months prior to finding my lump I woke up one morning and said to myself, *You need to learn how to meditate.* I found a teacher and was taught Kundalini yoga meditation which incorporates physical and breathing exercises. While rolling around on the floor as I did the physical exercises I felt a lump in my breast.

Gillian, our goddaughter whom we had not seen in several years, was coming to visit the next day. My annual mammogram had been scheduled weeks earlier and my appointment was the day following her departure. We had a wonderful time, but I was worried and could not keep my fingers off the lump. It was hard, it moved and it hurt.

Something did show on the mammogram and I was told my doctor would be in touch. I got into my car, looked toward the heavens and quietly said with no anger, "Thanks, Mom." Within hours my doctor called, "You need to see a surgeon," and she referred me to a man whom a close friend of mine had recently seen and had been very pleased with. I think as soon as he examined me and looked at the X-ray he knew. Clearly showing on the X-ray was a sun with rays shooting out of it. When I scheduled the biopsy the voice at the other end of the phone mentioned something about my having a double mastectomy. I said, "I haven't even been diagnosed yet!" I found out later the voice belonged to the surgeon's wife. She back-pedaled quickly, but of course she knew. So did I, but until it was confirmed I could still hope that it was not.

Bart, her husband: Barb had had fibrocystic breasts for years. I was genuinely concerned with this lump because it protruded from her skin. During the meeting with her surgeon he was playing middle of the road, but I could see it written all over his face. I thought it would be a miracle if she did not have breast cancer.

Betty, her friend: Bart, Barb and her father were at my house for dinner. Her father and I were doing a great job reassuring one another Barb's lump was nothing to be concerned about. We never dreamt it would be anything but fine.

LONG FACES

Barbara: I was scared. As I undressed and put on the hospital gown one of the nurses said to me, "Would you like to speak with so-and-so, one of our nurses? She had a bilateral mastectomy ten years ago." My comment was, "No thank you. I haven't even had my biopsy," as I thought to myself, *What's going on? Is someone trying to prepare me or what?*

I was awake during the biopsy. My senses were so heightened I could hear my surgeon cutting the tumor out of my body. I drifted in and out, but did hear him say to me that we should have a diagnosis in about twenty minutes. He had sent a piece of the lump to pathology for a frozen section evaluation. It seemed like only a minute before I heard the telephone ring. He answered. It was a moment frozen in time. My world turned upside down as I heard words I will *never, ever* forget. "Honey, I am so sorry. You have breast cancer." I could *hear* the blood pounding in my ears.

After I was dressed my family came in to see me. They stood around me in a horseshoe formation with faces that said, "Oh my God. She's going to die." They were all crying. Bart went to get the car. They all left with the exception of my father. He just held my hand. His face was a picture of anguish. The nightmare was beginning again. My mother had died in 1988 from ovarian cancer and now his daughter was diagnosed with breast cancer.

Bart, her husband: Not only was I worried, but Barb and I were the ones giving our family and friends moral support. When I saw her surgeon walking towards me I took one look at his eyes and I knew. We spoke privately. Then I told everyone there. They put on their "How do I act?" faces that people do who do not know how to react.

Betty, her friend: Bart is the kind of person who constantly makes jokes. When he called to tell my husband Johnny and me the news, that was the most unfunny he has ever been. He was not morbid, just factual. I felt sick, then really awful. I had told Barb she was going to be okay.

Stephanie, her friend: At the time, I was living in New York City and Barbara and Bart lived in Scottsdale, Arizona. Our relationship had been by telephone the past several years. I know many women who have had scares, but Barbara was the first to have breast cancer. Finding out was almost surreal. *How can something that is on the TV news possibly happen to someone I know?*

Amy, her cousin: I was crying hysterically. I thought she only had six months to live.

Shirley, her mother-in-law: One look at Bart's face said it all. I felt as though a hammer had hit me in the chest. It was not until my husband Bill and I left the hospital that I began to cry. All I could think about was the fact that Barbara had cancer. I know that Bill was not sleeping well. He told me he lay awake at night thinking about her, too.

THE NEXT HELLISH WEEKS

Barbara: The following day I went for the standardized tests most of us have when first diagnosed: a bone scan to determine whether the cancer has spread to the bones, chest X-ray and blood work. The day after Bart and I met with my surgeon. I was petrified. "Had the cancer spread?" It had not. My tumor was a 1-cm infiltrating ductal cancer. My decision had been made years ago. I was definitely having a lumpectomy and radiation therapy. Never in a million years had a mastectomy *ever* entered into the equation. My surgeon recommended a bilateral mastectomy. He had no objection to my wanting to get a second opinion. In fact, he encouraged it.

The next several weeks were busy as Bart and I began to do extensive research. We met with an oncologist at a very well-known medical facility within minutes of our home. Without a doubt that was the worst experience of my entire cancer journey. The oncologist was rude, insensitive and treated me as though I were not even in the room. When he spoke it was to Bart. When we questioned something he said, he became angry and cut short our meeting. I left in tears. The *only* good thing to come out of the meeting was that he, too, recommended I have a bilateral mastectomy.

It amazes me that I decided to have a bilateral mastectomy; a modified radical on the breast with the cancer, a prophylactic (preventive) on the other. My reasons were numerous. I did not want to subject my body to either radiation or chemotherapy. X-rays were very difficult to read because my breasts were so dense. I had been lucky to find my lump so early this time. Would I be that lucky next time? It would also be very difficult for a plastic surgeon to match my full-sized D breast if I only had a single mastectomy. And perhaps the key reason was, I knew I had the strength to go through it once, not twice. Many people thought my decision radical; however, to this day I am so grateful to my surgeon for making a bilateral mastectomy an option. Why don't all doctors?

Bart, her husband: I disliked the medical facility we went to for a second opinion which reminded me of "production line" medicine, and I strongly disliked the oncologist whose attitude was condescending from the moment we met. It was quite obvious he was unprepared for the meeting and had reviewed none of the records Barb had been asked to drop off days earlier.

THE DAY OF RECKONING

Barbara: I have since thought, *How odd I never said good-bye to my breasts.* It was a day of experiences and wonderful people. Two examples are: as I was being wheeled into the operating room one of the medical staff held my hand. I cannot express how comforting that was. I made terrible jokes to my medical team. Things such as never having breast pain again. The anesthesiologist who came to visit me the next day told me I had nearly given him a heart attack when I started in on Dr. Kevorkian jokes.

I was freezing when I woke up. My chest hurt terribly. Not from surgery, but from the bandage that was wrapped so tightly around me. My nurse was wonderful. She rubbed my back because it hurt. I was unable to lie on my stomach because of the surgery or my sides because of the drains. When Bart came to visit early the next morning he crawled into bed with me and we went to sleep in one another's arms. Neither of us had slept the night before. My husband is the most wonderful, gentle, caring man I have ever known.

Bart, her husband: Barb does not remember her surgeon showing us pictures of women who had undergone mastectomies so that we would be prepared. That is one of the reasons I went with her to all of her doctors' appointments. There were things both of us missed. I agreed with her decision to remove her breasts. Had she not done that she would have lived her entire life wondering, "When will I get it in my other breast?" I have no doubt she would have.

When her bandages were removed the day she was discharged from the hospital I knew the best way for me to handle it was to look directly at her scars and get used to them. You know what? I looked and thought, *No big deal!* She looked great. She just did not have breasts, and I thought, *Barb still looks sexy!* After awhile I no longer saw the scars.

Betty, her friend: It's funny how I thought I knew Barb, but I really did not. She used to make a big deal over a hangnail. I would think, *God forbid anything major were ever to happen to her.* Johnny and I thought she was a total wuss. The night before her surgery Barb, Bart, other friends Jay and Irene and Johnny and I went out to dinner. I was petrified for Barb. *How was she going to get through this?* I could not understand how she seemed to be doing better emotionally than I. Even Bart appeared to be fine, but I knew he was not. I did not show my feelings in front of anyone, but when we left the restaurant I cried the entire way home.

Neither Johnny nor I slept well the night before her surgery. We went to the hospital. I was sick to my stomach over what was about to happen to Barb. Everyone who came to support her that day gathered in her room until we were asked to leave. It was time. We gathered in the waiting room. Suddenly there she was. Sitting up on the gurney, like a queen in a parade waving to us. Smiling. I wondered, *Who is this woman? Where is she getting all this strength?* I had never seen her like that before and we have been friends since the mid-1980s. I had always thought I was the stronger one even though I cope by withdrawing when it's about me.

Jerry, her uncle: Roz and my two daughters Sheri and Amy never told Barb, but we thought, *Why is she having such drastic surgery? Is it necessary?*

THE POWER OF REIKI

Barbara: One day I said to Bart, "I want to learn Reiki" (a form of energy work that uses universal energy—like a laying on of hands). I have no idea where that came from particularly since I knew almost nothing about Reiki. I knew only that I had to learn how to do it. Several days later Bart and I sat in the audience as three women explained what it was. We signed up for the weekend workshop they were offering. A couple of months later I found my lump. Bart immediately began to do Reiki on my breast. I am convinced to this day the energy he brought forth prevented the cancer from spreading to my lymph nodes. His hands were red hot, and the sweat was running down both of us while he worked. "Your lymph nodes were slightly enlarged" is what I was told later by my surgeon. After the lump was gone the energy was no longer intense, only gentle.

TRYING TO COPE

Barbara: The telephone was ringing off the hook, and I was on it four to eight hours a day. It was exhausting to educate, console, bolster and ease everyone's fears, although they were marvelous support, which is why I never felt the need to attend a formal support group.

My terrier, Chanel, knew months before my diagnosis that I was sick. She would cling to me, literally stand on my chest and put her forehead to my forehead. Obviously she was trying to communicate. Since then I have learned to listen. When I took Chanel and our cockapoo, Odie, for walks I wore little tees. I didn't care if I looked like a boy. When we ran it was a weird feeling not to have breasts bouncing up and down. Actually I thought that was kind of cool. I am not saying I was happy not to have breasts. It was just a different experience.

Bart, her husband: Barb was the first in my family to have cancer, and the first of my generation to have a serious illness. They were shell-shocked when she was diagnosed. It's not that they handled it poorly, they just did not know what to do. Perhaps there was also a little bit of, "Thank God it isn't me." My parents were beside themselves. Barb is not a daughter-in-law, she is a daughter. Barb handled the whole thing magnificently. Even though she put on a great facade for everyone else I knew how scared she really was. It got to the point where she was on the phone so much I would take it from her hand and say, "I'm sorry. Barb has to hang up now and rest."

It's weird. I was scared, yet I wasn't. I don't know why, but I absolutely knew she was going to be okay. I was totally focused on Barb being emotionally and physically well because if she were, I would be, too. I never felt the need for any kind of moral support although I was touched

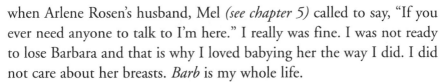

when Arlene Rosen's husband, Mel *(see chapter 5)* called to say, "If you ever need anyone to talk to I'm here." I really was fine. I was not ready to lose Barbara and that is why I loved babying her the way I did. I did not care about her breasts. *Barb* is my whole life.

Betty, her friend: I felt a little as though Bart was feeling neglected. That is why when I came to visit I always brought sweets. Not for Barb, for Bart. He needed the attention.

Stephanie, her friend: I think too often men cannot deal with anything that has to do with a women's issue. Bart was and is completely involved in her life on a level most men would never delve into because they think it has something to do with their own masculinity or some such nonsense. It is marvelous that Barbara can have a relationship with a man who has no qualms talking about a woman's body, and should not because what is happening is not a sexual thing. Bart is not talking about his wife's sexy breasts. He is now talking about something that is creating a problem with her health. Period. Bart is what every one of us would want if we had to go through something like this with a spouse.

Roz, her aunt: Of course Bart was concerned, and he was definitely stressed and worn out, but under the circumstances he seemed to be handling things well. He never talked to Jerry or me about his fears and he always reassured me when we spoke, "Barb is going to be fine."

Irene, her friend: The night the six of us went out neither Jay nor I wanted Barb to know how upset we were. Jay does not know how to deal with things like this. Maybe he felt vulnerable that it could happen to me. And I kept telling myself, *She's going to be fine.*

I went over to visit as soon as Barb got home from the hospital. The night before I was so worried. On the drive over I was very nervous. Then she opened the door and was so bubbly. She had such a good attitude it really helped me, which is so stupid because I should have been the one helping her! But I was afraid. I talked to Bart a lot. He was so concerned that Barb was overdoing it. He was like an old mom, but I think that was because he was scared and felt as though he had no control. I believe he also acted as he did because of the love he has for her. That is why he is so overprotective.

TAKING CONTROL

Barbara: Since my cancer diagnosis I have chosen to partner with my doctors. I asked lots of questions and disagreed with some of the recommendations, but I always listened to what they had to say and then did what I wanted to do. Because of my pathology and the tumor's size, my surgeon felt chemotherapy was unnecessary. I wanted to get a second opinion. He referred me to an oncologist he trusted who also did not feel that I needed to do chemotherapy. Every once in a while I wonder, *Did I make the right decision?*

Bart, her husband: Barb had some great doctors. I think a lot has to do with the patient having a positive attitude which she did. We were well read and asked the right questions. We made it clear that we wanted straight answers. Because of that her doctors spoke to us on a mature and intellectual level.

Stephanie, her friend: I am a magazine junkie. Anything I read that pertained to breast cancer I sent to Barbara. That was my way to be involved since I could not physically be there. She was never a victim, and took control from the very beginning. But that is just how she is. She quizzed and challenged her doctors and made them rise to the occasion. But then I do not think a person should ever hand over control. There were moments when I wondered if her being so upbeat and in control was how she disguised her fear. I do not know.

Barbara is the kind of person who consoles everyone even when she is sick. Neither she nor Bart ever had a "Woe is me" attitude. Everyone took their cues from them. Their attitude was: "Here are the facts. Here is what we have to do. Here is what we are going to do." With some people their illness becomes their crutch and life becomes a tragedy. Barbara took this thing and said, "You know what? I am going to do something with this. It will not control my life." And it has not. She took control when she made the decision to remove both breasts. Fear would have caused her to do as little as possible. She had the courage to do what she did because she said, "I am not going to go through this again in five years. I do not need these breasts that badly."

Roz, her aunt: None of us were ever afraid to ask Barbara questions.

She was always bringing it up, "So. What do you want to know?" She always seemed to have the answers. Her openness and willingness to talk about her illness let the family and their friends know that it was okay to talk about it. Otherwise it becomes hush, hush.

Amy, her cousin: I always wondered, *Could Barbara have had chemotherapy and not had a double mastectomy? Should she have had chemotherapy?* I thought it odd she had not had it.

A TEENAGER'S PERSPECTIVE

Elyse Horvath, Betty's daughter and Barbara's friend: I was eighteen, in college and invincible. It was not until my mother explained to me how serious breast cancer was that I became frightened. Barb always told my mom things like, "I'm fine. Let's move on and talk about life." She was totally positive which helped me to feel positive and took away some of my fear. When I saw her for the first time, she did not look unhealthy, but she did not look or act like her normal chipper self. There was something different about her. It wasn't a huge change, but she had somehow shifted. She has never gone back to how she was before this happened.

Around the age of twenty or twenty-one it finally sunk in, *This could happen to me.* Barb having had breast cancer made it more real. It was at that time that I went to my doctor and asked, "Please teach me breast self-examination. What am I looking for?" I was so cystic I never knew which were the good lumps and which were the bad. I had seen the card in the college dormitory showers that explained how to do a BSE, but it did not explain what a lump felt like. He gave me a wonderful explanation: "You are looking for a frozen pea in a bunch of cottage cheese."

SUPPORT

Bart, her husband: It was fantastic that Barb's friends all over the country were concerned, and other than one or two of them, they rose to the occasion. Knowing *who* they are I expected no less and would have been shocked if they had not. Barb deservedly got the support she did; however, I was grateful that she did and loved it that she got so much attention: the cards, flowers, gifts and their good wishes. Our friends and family would have done anything for us. They always called to see how both of us were doing. It probably would have been helpful to everyone, ourselves included had we accepted their offers to cook us meals, even clean the house but Barb always said, "No." She did not want to be an imposition. We had no right to make assumptions or decisions for anyone else. I knew it would make them feel helpful, but that was neither the time nor the place for me to start lecturing Barb.

Betty, her friend: I have told so many people that if anybody had to have a husband behind them Bart was the perfect one. He would make things lighter, although sometimes his humor went a little over the edge. An example was, "So what if she doesn't have breasts? We'll get new ones!" This was said around the time of her mastectomy surgery.

I am not sure when I made the decision to be at every one of Barb's surgeries. I would sit with her until she was physically being wheeled into the operating room. My being there turned into, "If I am not there something bad will happen." I felt as though I were her good luck charm. Perhaps I felt a little guilty: Barb has this and I don't. The least I can do is be there for her.

I truly believe she had the support she did because of her positive attitude. Had she fallen apart people might have had a tendency to stay away because then they might have felt more vulnerable or scared. Because she was so strong everyone felt comfortable around her.

Irene, her friend: When something bad happens to a person I care about I become obsessed with it. I called Barb every day to ask, "What can I do for you?" I just tried to be as supportive and good a friend as I knew how to be.

RECONSTRUCTION: EVERY WOMAN'S CHOICE

Barbara: There was never any question that I would have reconstructive surgery, but as with everything else that is a woman's *choice*. I healed remarkably quickly, and within two months my surgeon gave me the go-ahead. Networking with other women and nurses, who are a wonderful resource, I asked, "Who is the best plastic surgeon?" I interviewed four. Because I was so slender my choice was limited to using expanders that would first stretch my skin and then a later surgery would replace the expanders with permanent implants. I was fortunate in that I had a choice of using either silicone or saline. A little arm twisting by two of my doctors convinced me to use saline. I have a very high pain threshold. In my opinion, on a scale of one to ten with ten being the highest, the bilateral mastectomy was a one, reconstruction was an eleven. Each time I was filled with saline solution to expand my breast area my chest and back would spasm for days. Sleeping was miserable. There was only one position available to me and that was on my back because I had those horrid drains again. When the permanent implants were put in I had a complication. Because my surgeon did not use drains this time, fluid collected in and above my breast on the side I had had my axillary lymph nodes removed. As a result a wall of scar tissue built which caused my implant to seat crookedly and also caused (in my opinion) the lymphedema (swelling of the arm) I am plagued with today.

My surgeon had no intention of correcting the problem. I insisted that he do a third surgery as I had no intention of living with a crooked implant the rest of my life. He was not happy, but frankly I did not give a damn how he felt. Additionally I insisted that he remove fluid from both implants because I felt I was too large. We had fought about size from the beginning. He admitted, "I like big breasts." We disagreed over the color my areolas should be. I wanted a pinky/peach color, which was my natural color. He wanted brown. I always got my way, but why don't doctors listen to their patients? Even he admits the end result is fabulous.

Betty, her friend: Barb never offered to show me her scars, and truthfully I never wanted to see them. When I jokingly said to her one day, "Show me," she said, "Not on your life!" She has since told me, "I wish I had shown you." She thought it might have been helpful for me to see what a mastectomy looked like so I would not be frightened if it ever happened to me.

ADVICE FROM A HUSBAND

Bart, her husband: I am saying this as a husband, but of course it pertains to any partner, male or female. When someone you love gets sick it is a time when the man needs to rid himself of ego, selfishness and any of his own "self" issues. He needs to concentrate 110 percent on making things as comfortable and easy for his wife as possible. She should be doted on. I am sure a lot of men run off to the golf course or their business and hide. They are scared and don't know what to do, but that still does not make it right. He needs to support her. A grown man should have the maturity to face a problem and deal with it. I understand that each of us copes differently, but I think a man who runs, who does not touch his wife or does not talk to her should be ashamed of himself. It may be corny, but remember those wedding vows? "In sickness and in health." It is his responsibility to be there. If he has a problem, he should seek counseling or go to a support group. *Do something.* I think the biggest problem with men is that they do not know *how* to deal with something like this. They do not allow their feminine side—the emotional side—to emerge.

People need to be educated that they do not work for the doctor. They are paying a doctor to work *for them.* If they have a question, they should ask it. If they get a bad feeling about a doctor, they should leave and go elsewhere. The children can get involved. There is no reason they cannot pitch in with household chores. Everyone in the family should be involved.

LYMPHEDEMA

Barbara: Lymphedema is caused by the removal of lymph nodes. It can develop immediately or years later. Since mine appeared in May of 1994 I have been on a mission to cure it. Conventional medicine says it cannot be cured. I tried physical therapy. That did not work. I used a pump for over a year to try to squeeze the fluid from my arm. That was ineffectual. My arm looked sick and was becoming worse. It was quite swollen, white, and very mottled in color. I agree that conventional medicine cannot cure lymphedema; however, I believe alternative or holistic methodologies can.

In December of 1994 I began to work with a man who practices a form of acupressure called *Jin Shin Jyutsu*. Acupressure works the meridian points of the body with fingers, not needles. I asked him, "Why can't we create new pathways for the lymphatic fluid just as the heart creates new arteries when there is a blockage?" He did not think that unreasonable. Other practitioners have also assisted in this endeavor including my friend Linda, who is an extraordinary massage therapist, and another woman I have become friends with, who is now doing energy work to complete the creation of new passageways. We are all working toward a common goal, "What will turn the pump back on?" Major progress has been made. My arm is about 70 to 80 percent back to where it was before the lymphedema began. The color is normal, my arm rarely hurts and although my forearm and wrist are still swollen, the upper arm no longer is. It continues to improve. My arm is my teacher. I am certainly not happy that I have lymphedema; however, had it not occurred I would not have gotten as deeply into alternative medicine as I have. It has changed my life.

COMBINING ALTERNATIVE AND CONVENTIONAL MEDICINE

Barbara: I believe in conventional medicine. I am vigilant about getting my annual checkups (gynecological and cancer-related). My wonderful general surgeon whom I used as my "cancer doctor" recently retired, and I chose to replace him with an oncologist. I felt it was time to bring an oncologist on board. My other doctors are holistic practitioners. Other than one naturopathic physician I see on a regular basis, none of the other practitioners holds a formal degree. Many specialize in energy work. These are the ones I have chosen to help me rebuild all my bodies: physical, emotional, spiritual and etheric. I no longer run from practitioner to practitioner looking for the "magic cure." They assist me to heal myself. It has taken me a long time to realize that the healing power resides within.

Bart, her husband: For about six months to a year after her diagnosis Barb jumped on every concoction, every alternative thing imaginable because she was so scared. Although I felt as if she were grasping at straws, I thought it was a perfectly normal reaction. The point came when I finally had to tell her she was overdoing it.

Amy, her cousin: I would probably do some of the things Barbara did, but a lot of what she does is farfetched. For instance, using the pendulum, what she calls "dowsing." It is the energy work and things that are intangible that I have a problem understanding.

THE SPIRITUAL SIDE AWAKENED

Stephanie, her friend: Barbara's cancer experience took her to another level spiritually. She was a woman from the East Coast with her diamonds, her Louis Vuitton handbags and expensive cars. For her to become such a spiritual, meditating individual is quite a departure from who she was. This is not a venue her mother would have chosen for her. Her cancer experience allowed her to step outside the world she functions in and say, "You know what? I can still have all these wonderful *things* in my life, but there is a spiritual side to me, too. Let's explore that." This experience has been such a gift. It has opened so many doors to new ways of looking at the world. It has enriched not just her and Bart, but everyone who knows them. She has grown in ways she could never have imagined. We have all learned to be better people and friends because of it.

BACK TO COPING

Barbara: Bart and I are partners in business as well as being partners in marriage. One day about six to nine months after my diagnosis I walked into the office. It was early, and only Bart and I were there. I do not remember what precipitated the argument but suddenly he began to scream at me. He was like a volcano whose steam had been building and building until suddenly the cap blows off. The vein on his forehead throbbed, his face turned beet red and I was frightened beyond words that he was going to have a stroke or heart attack. The dam burst. All the feelings he had kept bottled up inside came pouring out. He began to cry. He was so scared I was killing myself because I was running so hard and so fast that I was not taking care of myself. I sat on his lap, stroked his face and told him how much I loved him. That was the moment I realized how scared Bart was. That was also a turning point for me, and I believe for Bart as well.

Bart, her husband: Barb's father and I never had any deep conversations about Barb. I know he was torn up inside. It was one thing to have to go through it with a wife, but with a daughter? I do not think he had a clue how to help either my mother-in-law or Barb. I am sure he felt helpless, but he did the best he could. He was there for support. In Barb's case I think he backed off too much, but one of his idiosyncracies was, "I am not going to intrude or interfere." My father-in-law was a man of his times.

Barb began to get involved in everyone's lives again, counseling them, allowing herself to be sucked dry. She just kept running. The phone was once again ringing off the hook. Finally I told everyone, "You have to stop calling so much. Barb needs to rest." She was so exhausted she looked ill. She had also been getting a lot of phone calls like this one. "Hi Barb. How are you doing? My sister's cousin just died of breast cancer. She went really fast. Boy, aren't you lucky!" I know that is not the way these conversations were intended, but people need to think before they speak. The last thing a person who has a serious illness wants to hear is a story about someone with the same illness who has died. It's okay to talk about the illness. Just do not tell horror stories. Barb broke down in tears one day. "Doesn't anyone ever survive?" That is one of the reasons I cracked down on her.

Maybe people thought I was being overprotective, but I just wanted her to take care of herself and she was not. That is why the incident occurred that day in the office. I was doing everything in my power to keep her well, and she was doing everything she could to exhaust and kill herself. After I vented my pent-up emotions I felt as though I had rid myself of an ocean of poison. Her actions were making me physically sick. Finally I got through. Barb has finally stopped mothering the world and is now taking care of herself.

Betty, her friend: Some people become stronger, others become bitter or resentful when they have an experience such as Barb's. Some will not use the knowledge they have gained and turn it into something positive. Barb has done everything positive. I do not think there is any-thing she did not cope well with. She amazed me, but she amazed my husband, Johnny even more. Barb was his first exposure to a strong woman in crisis. As things progressed Barb only became stronger and stronger. Before she was wrapped up in her life, her goals and not really in tune with anyone else. Now her energies are more focused and she has become a more caring, sensitive person.

Stephanie, her friend: When a woman is beautiful no one wants to know what she is all about. They just want to be around her because she is beautiful. One of the first things men in particular did with Barbara was to look at her breasts. This has allowed Barbara to become more than just her breasts. Not that she ever was only about her breasts. Even though she has always had about herself a Marilyn Monroe-ish naughty little girl aura that attracts men, she is now about the whole person.

The fact that nothing about her cancer experience was morbid is almost refreshing. I don't think that took away any of the severity of what was happening to her, but it allowed us to deal with it. I am a firm believer that it is not necessarily the disease that kills us. Rather it is the diagnosis—the belief system. I have wondered, *How would I handle something like this if it were to happen to me?* I *think* I am a strong per-son, but I hope I am never tested, because I do not know if I really am. None of us does until we are faced with our own crisis.

Irene, her friend: Barb had such positive energy and such a good out-look that it made it easier for me to deal with. I wondered several times if she was pretending or putting on an act, but I really do not think so.

My father, who is a retired physician, began to send me all kinds of articles on breast cancer. We talked about Barb, but there were times I did not understand things. No matter how stupid I thought a question was, Barb always answered it so that I did understand. How can a per-son feel comfortable if they do not understand what is going on? Sometimes ignorance can create a wedge.

THOUGHTS ABOUT DEATH AND DYING

Barbara: Arlene Rosen told me several key things early on in my diagnosis. The first was that breast cancer is *not* a death sentence. The second was that I would go through different stages. She was right. Once my breasts were removed I was almost giddy with relief that the cancer had been cut out. *What's the big deal? It's gone!* Until several weeks later I began to bolt upright in bed at two o'clock in the morning, *Oh my God. I have cancer. I'm going to die!* That lasted about two years; however I still carry a little, tiny kernel of fear that it could come back. I sought professional help one time to try to rid myself of that fear and came to the conclusion that anyone who has ever had a life-threatening illness will always carry that kernel of fear.

Several years ago I had a lump in my neck that appeared to be a swollen lymph gland, yet I had not been sick. At first I obsessed over it. *Am I having a recurrence?* I finally asked myself a hard question: *If it is cancer how do I feel about it?* I came to the conclusion I was not afraid to die because I know there is something wonderful on the other side. I do not want to die. I have too much left to accomplish and besides, I want many more years with Bart. This is an interesting and very liberating space to be in. I have come to accept that my cancer could come back, although I do not think it will. I still have that little kernel of fear, but I am okay with that now. And whatever was swollen is long gone.

Two things greatly impacted me early on in my cancer journey. The first was told to me by two women who do not know one another and who live in different states. "Why do you think you got cancer? Would anything else have gotten your attention?" The second was, "What do you think this is all about?" It took me a long time to realize I was not afraid of dying. I was afraid of living.

Bart, her husband: I was scared. No one could give me that guarantee in writing that Barb was going to be okay, but I just knew that she would. Still, there was that little twinge of, "What if?" It has now been almost four years since her diagnosis and I can honestly say that twinge is gone. When Barb tells me about someone she knows who has had a recurrence, or who has died, I cannot and do not worry that it will happen to her. I have been living with that statistic ever since her mother's diagnosis. I truly believe, "What is meant to happen will, and we will deal with it then." I meant it when I said Barb is my whole life. I would give up everything just to have her in it. But if I were to lose her I would have no regrets. We have had an incredible twenty-seven years together. I am not ready to lose her, but I would not wake up the next day and say, "Gee. I wish we would have done that, or I wish I would have said this." Because we have.

Betty, her friend: Barb had such an impact, not just on Johnny and me, but on our children as well who are now fifteen, twenty-one and twenty-five. Her experience opened our eyes that bad things can happen to people you love. I tend to stuff my feelings when something bad happens, and I admit they are still stuffed pretty deep. I did not want to show Barb any sign of weakness or fear on my part because I would have felt selfish. Besides, I did not think she needed to hear that. Maybe I should have. I am scared of getting breast cancer. That never goes away. A friend's sister died of cancer (not breast) when I was in my early twenties. She was my youth scare. Barb is my middle-age scare.

Stephanie, her friend: On a conscious level I do not think Bart believed that Barbara would do anything but come through this. He had total and complete belief in her. However, they are so close that somewhere in the back of his mind there had to be that lingering fear. I suspect he did not talk to anyone about his fears because he did not want to hear any words from anyone that might stimulate fear he did not want stimulated. It was much easier to move forward and not think about losing her. As for me, I never had any fears that Barbara was going to die, but I can't say that in the back of my mind somewhere I do not worry because of her mother's history.

Shirley, her mother-in-law: I pray for both Barbara and Bart. I want them both to be well. And I am selfish. I want my son to have his wife.

An Ending from a Friend

Stephanie, her friend: Of all the people I know who have had bad things happen, or who have gone through traumas, Barbara was the one who said, "Okay. What am I going to get out of this besides survival?"

She took this experience and made it her calling in life. This is what Barbara Stevens is all about now. She is totally dedicated to breast cancer. It has changed *everything* about her. She and I are still silly women who like to laugh and have a good time, but there is a depth to her. It is like some books have a beautiful cover, but there is no story inside. Or the story is poorly written, or has no depth. She is a beautiful book cover and the story just continues to be written. I think we have all been on this journey together. Each of us does it in our own way.

My Postscript, February 2000

I lived twenty-five hundred miles away from my parents when my mother was diagnosed with ovarian cancer. I was not there for any of her treatments, nor when she died. In February of 1994 my father was diagnosed with terminal lung cancer. Bart and I, his hospice nurse and companion were with him when he died seven months later. He gave Bart and me such a gift. He taught us how to talk about death and dying. He allowed Bart and me to share his death with him, a gift I will treasure forever. We need to teach our children not to be afraid of death. They need to know that death is but a part of living. My father is always with me. He helped me to have the courage to write this book because I had experienced through him *living* the death of a loved one. He taught me not to be afraid.

Writing this book has been the most difficult thing I have ever done. But because of it I have met the most extraordinary women, men and children. None of us wants to join this "sisterhood," but as Lolly Champion *[see chapter 16]* said, "Once we are a part of it we never want to leave. And we mourn our sisters who do." Too many of the women survivors (I do not know about the men) I interviewed have died. In my heart they are still alive. I am so thankful that I knew them. For know them I did. We shared our stories with one another. We laughed and we cried. They wanted their stories to be heard so that their experiences would help others. Even if it was only one person.

I have grown so because of my cancer experience. I am not the person I was. And I am grateful for that. My life is so much richer now. I have goals, but they are no longer what they once were. Now they are humanitarian. I walk my dogs early in the morning and look at the beautiful Arizona sunrises. And smile. I look upon my husband's face and thank God every day for allowing me one more day with him. And I look deep within myself and know that I am happy. That I am on my path and doing what I am supposed to be doing. My life has been blessed. To each and every one of you who has been and is a part of my life I say—thank you.

Two

Susan Alexander

I Thought I Had a
Good Marriage

Survivor Profile:

Age at diagnosis: forty-three (6/95)

Age at interview: forty-four (8/3/96)

Type of breast cancer: infiltrating ductal

Size tumor: 3½ cm; stage II

One positive lymph node

Surgical procedure: lumpectomy

Treatment: chemotherapy and radiation

Estrogen receptors: negative; Progesterone receptors: information
not provided

Who's Who:*

Robert Alexander, her husband

Connie Doster, her sister

Jean Hans, her mother

Charles (Charlie) Alexander, her son (age ten at diagnosis)

Matthew Alexander, her son (age six at diagnosis)

Fictitious names by request (including survivor)

BEGINNINGS

Susan: When I began to experience more than an ordinary amount of menstrual sensitivity in my breast, I confided only to my office manager with whom I'm very close: "I'm worried. Something tells me this is bad." I scheduled an appointment to have a mammogram. Something was suspicious, and while I waited the technician took more X-rays. Of course they can tell you nothing at the time; you have to wait two weeks for the results, then see your doctor.

THE DOCTOR GAME

Susan: My primary care physician was on vacation, and the physician I was referred to wouldn't see me because he'd never seen me before; in addition, my visit wasn't routine. Frustrated, I finally told my mother and sister Connie that I'd had an irregular mammogram, and was having difficulty getting in to see a doctor. They suggested that I call my gynecologist. Unbelievably, he, too, was on vacation; however, the person I spoke to referred me to a general surgeon. He was not a doctor contracted with my HMO, but at that point I did not care. When his front office person told me the earliest they could see me was in three weeks I said, "No way. If I have to call the doctor at home tonight, I will. But I am coming in this week because I have already waited three weeks." By now I was in a total panic. Maybe it was my imagination, but there was pain over my entire body. I wasn't very composed that first meeting; in fact, I was so relieved to be face to face with any doctor that I burst almost immediately into tears. After studying my X-rays he said, "There's something there. I can't say what it is, but we need to look at it."

Robert, her husband: Susan told me nothing until she already had an appointment scheduled with the surgeon. That's just how she is. I was a little shocked; maybe even a little scared.

Connie, her sister: Coincidentally, both of us had mammograms done at the same time. It was not until I told her I had gone for a mammogram that she finally told me she had, too. In my case I had felt a lump; she had not. To this day Susan says it was a sympathy lump. She had just turned forty-three; I was forty.

Jean, her mother: Ten years earlier I'd had a biopsy, and it was benign (non-cancerous); therefore, I wasn't too concerned.

AN EVENTFUL DAY

Susan: Turning my head as I lay strapped to the table, I heard a familiar voice say, "Susan, I'm so sorry this is happening to you." It was my gynecologist who apparently had just returned from vacation, and while at the hospital had seen my name on the surgical board. Rubbing my arm he reassured me, "You're in good hands." I began to cry, "I can't believe you were gone."

Not even waiting for confirmation on the frozen section evaluation from pathology, my surgeon said to me, as I lay awake, "Yup. It's cancer. We're going to have to take that out as quickly as we can." The report came back positive while we waited in the operating room, and afterwards one of the nurses told me, "He always knows before the pathologist." I was immediately scheduled for a bone scan. Not understanding anything at the time, I assumed it meant I was riddled with cancer, and I was terror-stricken.

Robert was very quiet, shocked and stunned when he came to see me in the recovery room. I don't think he was expecting this diagnosis. It was very scary for him because his sister had died at the age of fifty, several years earlier, of breast cancer. She had ignored her lump until it was too late. By the time she had a mastectomy her cancer had metastasized (spread) throughout her body. So to him breast cancer was a death sentence.

Robert, her husband: My mother-in-law, in between sobs, was trying to reassure both of us, "It's going to be okay. She's going to be fine." Before going in to see Susan I tried putting aside my fears and concerns. To be honest those feelings never completely went away. I don't remember whether it was then or a little later, but Susan kept repeating that she would be fine. I'm not quite sure she really believed it, or was just trying to reassure herself. That's not always how she reacts in a stressful situation. Knowing the importance of a positive mental attitude I encouraged that belief.

Connie, her sister: Since I was working, and truly did not believe there was anything wrong, I did not go to the hospital. I figured if there were a problem, either my mother or Robert would call. Finding out that she had cancer was scary enough; finding out she needed a bone scan caused instant panic. *My God. It could be all over her body!* Then, *How could this happen to her? What am I going to do now?* I was now even more frightened over my upcoming biopsy the following week, yet somehow was convinced that mine would be okay. At this time, though, Susan was my main concern.

After being injected with a low level of radioactive particles, Susan was told to return to the hospital in a couple of hours for the bone scan. With tears streaming down her face she said, "Let's not go home, or back to the hospital. Just take me anywhere because this really isn't happening. Let's just go away." I drove her home despite her pleas. During those few hours at her home Susan would alternately cry, then say, "I'm okay." I said, "You don't have to worry. I'm going to take care of the boys." She looked at me, then said, "You know what? Nothing is going to happen to me because nobody is going to take care of my boys but me. I'm going to be fine." At that moment she made up her mind that she was not going to die and became a fighter. I told her, "Through this experience you are going to meet people you never would have met that, for some reason, are going to be important in your life." She said, "That stinks. I don't want to meet people because I've had cancer."

Jean, her mother: I had been so positive that it was going to be nothing, so when I heard Susan had cancer I panicked. Turning to me, her surgeon said, "I did not say your daughter was dying. I told you she had cancer. We have to deal with it." That kind of reined me in a bit. I told myself, *He's right. I'm overreacting; she'll be okay.* But when I went to call Connie I was blubbering on the phone.

THE LEARNING CURVE

Susan: The day following my biopsy Robert and I had a consultation with the surgeon. He said something like, "You're a young woman, and have the potential for a long life. This is not a death sentence. My recommendation is that you have a bilateral mastectomy as there's a tendency for cancer in one breast to jump to the other breast. If I were you I'd pursue this course. You've got children to think about." I told him I was still in shock, but did want to do some research before making a decision. I wanted to see what other options were available. He was in total agreement. "Speak to as many people as you need to, so that you feel 100 percent comfortable with the choice you make." However, time was a critical element in my case. From the time I'd had my mammogram three weeks earlier, the tumor had doubled in size.

My nature is to read extensively about whatever the subject is that I'm researching, so I came home loaded with books from the library and bookstore. I began talking to countless women in the network of people Connie and I knew. "Who are the doctors out there?" "Who are the specialists?" "Who have you talked to?" Additionally, my insurance carrier provided me with names of doctors to call for a second opinion. I saw four.

Very quickly I learned that everyone has a different opinion; furthermore, doctors' ages and specialties determine what they recommend. It soon became apparent that the younger doctors, at least those I spoke with, prefer lumpectomy and radiation therapy even though my surgeon, probably around the age of fifty, didn't. A radiation oncologist was instrumental in helping me reach my decision. He told me that the research shows that survival rates are equal for either procedure. He felt that in my case, lumpectomy and radiation would be a good choice. Plainly stated, he said, "Surgeons believe in surgery. I respect your surgeon's opinion, but that doesn't mean that surgery [meaning mastectomy] is the only answer. It is to him, but I don't believe that." What he said made sense. Considering his input, what the other doctors had told me concerning survival percentages, taking into consideration my pathology as well as what I had read, I felt that I had the fundamental knowledge to make a decision. I would have a lumpectomy and radiation therapy.

Researching where to have my radiation was quite an eye-opener. When I mentioned to someone that I had gone to a particular facility for a consultation I was warned, "You need to be aware that their equipment is ten years old, which is old for technology. If you are going to have radiation, go for state-of-the-art equipment." This meant that newer equipment specifically targets where it's aimed, while older equipment may scatter the beam which could cause later cancers elsewhere in the body. I was incredulous that so many clinics are using older equipment.

Robert, her husband: The surgeon told us that anything other than a mastectomy was not an option. Personally I felt that was pretty radical, but if that was his recommendation I could live with it, and told Susan that. I was glad when she said to him, "Gee. I'm not sure I want to do that," and then began asking other questions.

Working within the HMO system is frustrating. One of the doctors Susan had been referred to was a radiation oncologist, who was also on vacation. In his place was a "floater," a doctor who fills in. What was she supposed to do? Choose a doctor she had never met? If I had been unhappy with our experience to date with HMOs, this latest incident certainly made me dead-set against them. Maybe the problems we encountered are not indicative of all HMOs, but I am not about to try another one.

I was comfortable with my brother and sister-in-law so I spoke extensively with them about what was going on. Because my brother is very analytical he is able to look at all sides of a situation. They helped me recognize that maybe there were other approaches to this situation. They would also play devil's advocate, asking, "Is that the correct choice, or is mastectomy better?"

Neither option offered a 100 percent guarantee; nevertheless, I was comfortable with and supported Susan's decision. It had nothing to do with saving her breast. It just seemed to make more sense from a self-esteem perspective and the recovery time involved. And besides, why do more surgery than is necessary? In retrospect I think her surgeon did her a disservice. I realize that he's talking from a surgeon's perspective, but I do not think he emphasized enough the fact that there are other options, and that she should talk to other doctors. It was as if he said, "Well, talk to other people if you want, but this is what you need to do. It's the only way to go. They're going to tell you this and this, but I wouldn't pay attention to what they tell you. They'll tell you that survival rates are equal, but I don't think the research has been in long

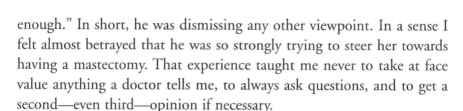

enough." In short, he was dismissing any other viewpoint. In a sense I felt almost betrayed that he was so strongly trying to steer her towards having a mastectomy. That experience taught me never to take at face value anything a doctor tells me, to always ask questions, and to get a second—even third—opinion if necessary.

Connie, her sister: Sitting on Susan's very large bed, stacks of books surrounding us, we read everything. Maybe at the time you're doing the research it might not mean much, but it helped us get through the "What's next?" step. Sometimes one, or both of us, after reading something would start to cry, "Oh my God. This is so scary," or "How could this possibly be?" Then we'd continue reading, and find out it was okay. It is the unknown that causes the fear.

A very wise woman told me, "Everyone has a different opinion, and it's going to get confusing. Whatever Susan decides to do is the right decision. Support her in that decision." My brother and younger sister were concerned that radiation would be more dangerous than having a mastectomy. In fact, my brother felt that radiation was poison; that she should do anything but radiation. Susan would say things to me like, "What do I do? This one says one thing, another says something totally different." After we became more educated it became clearer to her what she wanted to do. Not only did I support her decision, but so did everyone in our family.

Jean, her mother: From day one Connie was determined that her sister was going to beat this thing. She went to the health food store, and came back loaded with all kinds of things for Susan to take. Then she went to the library, and cleaned them out of every book she could find on breast cancer, and brought them over to her sister's.

When I read a magazine article that explained the differences between mastectomy and lumpectomy and the fact that survival percentages were equal, I was amazed because I did not know that. I always thought when a woman had breast cancer she had to have her breast removed. Up until that point I hadn't realized that a woman has a choice; nothing is cut and dried. I will admit to being a little worried because her surgeon was so insistent she have a mastectomy, and I thought, *Gosh, he knows.* But what Susan was told by the radiation oncologist also made a lot of sense.

The thing that struck me the most was that things we take as gospel, like "If your mother or grandmother never had breast cancer you don't have to worry," are really nothing more than old wives' tales. It doesn't occur to you that someone has to be first.

THE NEXT STEP

Susan: When I called my surgeon and told him my decision, he scheduled me for surgery the next day because he was so concerned about the tumor's rapid growth. Whether it was mentally induced or not, by then, I was experiencing sharp, stabbing pains in my breast. Now I could feel the tumor which felt huge. His concern was justified because it was 3½ cms, the size of a half dollar.

Robert, her husband: When we found out there were microscopic traces of cancer in one of her lymph nodes that little kernel of fear I had repressed surfaced. Pushing it back down, I expressed only optimism and confidence in whatever treatment it was that Susan would be having. Susan also had some fear, and I would reassure her that no other traces of cancer were evident anywhere else in her body, other than the one lymph node; but if there were, the chemotherapy, which was a safety precaution, would destroy it. That seemed to help.

Connie asked if I were doing okay, and told me if I ever wanted to talk about anything to let her know. She was not someone with whom I felt I could share my feelings or fears because I was concerned our conversations would get back to her sister. Only with my brother, sister-in-law and one very close friend did I feel safe; but even with them I could not talk about that little kernel of fear. I don't know why; I just did not want to let it out. It never goes away, and to this day it is still there. As optimistic as I am about her recovery, as much as I believe she'll be fine and will not have a recurrence, it is still a possibility. Maybe not in five years, maybe not even in ten. I don't know. It doesn't nag at me, but it's there because there are no 100 percent guarantees.

CHEMOTHERAPY AND RADIATION

Susan: Just the word chemotherapy conjures up words like "evil," "poisonous," "death," and "sickness." For some reason when people hear that word they think you are terminal. Right away they look at you differently. "Poor thing, she's having chemotherapy. She's almost a goner." Even my mother did that. The oncologist's office has to be *the* most depressing place on Earth next to a homeless shelter. People just sit there in a living room setup, hooked up to IVs, hair gone and looking as though they are dying. Since I didn't view myself as a dying cancer patient, and didn't want to be with them, I was always taken to a private room where I would be given an injection of methotrexate, and 5-FU that took only about two minutes to administer. For the following two weeks I would take the Cytoxan orally. Life became a blur: a month of chemotherapy, two weeks on then two weeks off, one month of radiation during which my only side effect was being tired—but I think I just felt tired in general because of all the emotional chaos I'd been through—then eight more months of chemotherapy. I was not given tamoxifen because I am estrogen-receptor negative.

Chemotherapy is awful. I felt sick, like having the flu; moreover, I felt as though I was being slowly, methodically poisoned. I would lay in the dark in my bedroom, with a towel over my head feeling very nauseated. Compazine, an antinausea medication was ineffective, because I still vomited. In fact, all it did was make me tired. The only thing that helped me was smoking a little marijuana given to me by friends. When I looked at myself in the mirror I saw a woman with dark circles under her eyes. At times my entire body felt puffy which was weird because, even though my eating habits remained constant, one week I'd be up seven pounds, the next down six. My oncologist told me, "It's just a fluctuation of body fluids."

My attention span those first two to three days was very erratic. By the fourth day I was beginning to feel good again. In the meantime, my house would be in utter chaos. Robert could not deal with my illness; consequently, he was never home. As a result my two boys, Charlie, age ten at the time, and Matt, age six would be running throughout the house, all

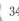

the televisions would be on, and junk food would be everywhere.

Even though I was eating smaller meals I was eating more frequently; therefore, I gained twenty-two pounds. Becoming acutely aware of what I put into my body I made an effort to educate myself on what vitamins and supplements would support it, and I also began eating organic foods. In addition, I got lots of rest, did some exercise, read spiritually uplifting books, and surrounded myself with people I liked being around. I continued to work, although there were days I did not go into the office. My staff, whom I'd told about my diagnosis from the beginning, was wonderfully supportive and picked up the slack.

Around my doctors I tried to be upbeat, and not act like doom and gloom; however, when that office door closed behind me, and I'd finally get into my car, I would just sob for about fifteen minutes; then, I'd compose myself. At first I thought I was having my own private pity party, but later realized it was my body weeping for its diminishing life essence. As the months wore on I became more tired, my concentration was really slipping away, and I had no energy for either work or my children. Not having energy to give to my children was the worst part.

As chemotherapy dragged on it became more and more difficult for me psychologically to drive myself to my oncologist's office. An overwhelming despair settled over me like a heavy cloud just knowing I had to get yet another injection. I found myself asking my mother, "Could you take me for treatment?"

I didn't think chemotherapy would trigger the onset of menopause, but it did. At first I began getting night sweats, and debilitating hot flashes. Six months after my last treatment my periods stopped; then, about six or seven months later they resumed only to permanently stop six months later. Emotionally unable to return to the doctor's office for my three-month checkup, I faxed him the results of my chest X-ray and bone scan, and we spoke on the phone. My six-month checkup is coming soon. That one I have to go to.

Connie, her sister: When I was told about Nioxin, a series of topical hair products formulated for thinning hair which includes a shampoo, scalp therapy and ointment, I immediately purchased it for Susan. Additionally I had been told that the person using Nioxin will lose only about one-third of the hair they might normally lose while going through chemotherapy. Nioxin worked. Susan did not lose her hair; it only thinned.

I went to only one chemotherapy session with my sister because she likes to do things on her own. Watching her go through it was difficult for me because I felt so helpless. She was in pain, she hurt, and there was nothing I could do to help.

A Marriage Disintegrates

Susan: Robert and I have been together twenty-two years, twenty of them married. The last five have been a challenge; this last year very rough. My getting breast cancer put more of a strain on the relationship. I think he has been in denial that I have breast cancer. It is too scary for him to comprehend, so he buries it, and escapes by going to the office. His behavior was the one big surprise throughout this whole thing. After being best friends for twenty years I did not expect him to react as he did. To this day I still don't understand his behavior, and I'm still angry. Truthfully, I don't think he understands his actions either. My mother is very old-fashioned—a stand-by-your-man kind of woman: "You can't expect them to do for you—you have to do for them." Consequently, in the beginning when I would say things to her about Robert's behavior, she had no sympathy for me. "Well, you know men. You know he loves you. That's all you need to know." However, after seeing how sick I was, that the children were left alone and we were being neglected, she herself went through a metamorphosis about our relationship. "This man is neglecting my daughter. Why is it eight o'clock at night and he's at the office? Susan's in bed sick, and her children are running around the house eating Cheese Doodles because they have not had their supper." Many times she called him at the office and said, "Robert, this is Jean. I want you to come home now," and he did. My sister went through the same metamorphosis. Finally I said to him, "If you can't help me personally or emotionally, could you at least handle the bills and paperwork for the insurance? Will you make sure claims are filed, and that the doctors get paid?" It turned out he didn't even do that, or if he did he was not very thorough. This last year has been a nightmare, and clinics and doctors are threatening to sue me.

We have made the decision to separate. I feel good about this decision because now I can move forward as I need to for myself and for my children. I am in a state of self-awareness where I am striving to be happy, and want to feel fulfilled. I don't want to live my life full of anger, resentment or hostility which is how I feel after the way he treated me. Robert is still running. Truthfully I don't think he believes my wanting a separation has anything to do with him, or his behavior. He believes I am just going through a crisis.

I explained to the boys that their father and I weren't getting along, and although children are very astute and absorb everything that's going on, they'd both say things like, "Daddy hasn't been very nice to you, but don't be mean to him because we still like him." Charlie went so far as to say, "Don't divorce him." They knew what was going on. Many times I'd hear them say things like, "Daddy shouldn't be working so much. He should be home with you," or "It's not right." So, I had to explain to them that regardless of the outcome we'd both still be involved in their lives, would never love them less, and nothing in their lives would change except for their mom and dad's relationship. Robert has taken corrective steps and is involved in their lives again.

Robert, her husband: Although our communication wasn't great, I thought our relationship had been pretty strong up until the time Susan got sick. I had gone to all her doctors' appointments including the consultation with her oncologist. I assumed we would go together to her first chemotherapy treatment. When she told me, "My mother's going with me," I not only felt as though I had been kicked, but I felt left out. A couple of other times I asked if she wanted me to come with her, and I guess she must have said no. So other than going with her to one radiation treatment, I never asked or went again. It was not until later that I found out it had affected her that I hadn't gone with her to anything, but by then it was too late. Maybe I should have asked again, or told her that I felt left out, but she should have said something as well.

We're a two-income family. Obviously, Susan's income was down. I was still building my insurance business, there were people over my head saying, "Produce or else," and marketing, sales and phone work needed to be done at night. Then there was Susan's family saying things like, "Where's Robert?" I was stuck in the middle being squeezed by everyone. I felt as though her family was judging me, and at the same time I was judging them. "Gee, can't they help, too?" There still is no solution. I'm depressed and withdrawn. By withdrawing I don't have to deal with the problem.

Not to sound like an insurance salesman, but having financial planning in place *before* something catastrophic happens, like it did to us, is essential. I didn't think about the fact that my wife probably wasn't going to be working for the next eight months or so. Having the financial burden solely on my shoulders was frightening. Nobody ever talks about that nor all the other things that have to be taken care of: picking the kids up after school, making meals, having someone come over in the evening for a few hours so that the partner can go out for a bit to do whatever. In the very beginning you don't think about the details. You think, "Okay. I'll do more." But you can't. When I asked Susan early on, "Can we ask your sister or mother to do something?" her response was, "No. I don't want to ask them." That's why I think it is a good idea to sit down with family or friends, or whoever is part of your support system, without your partner, and tell them that you need their assistance to help ease the pressure somewhat. Sometimes a spouse is uncomfortable asking for help because they're not *his* family. If that is the case maybe the family members should be the ones to take the bull by the horns and say, "Look. You're going to need help. We're here. We're your family. We know this is a difficult time for you." Sometimes you don't know how to ask for help, or you might not even know what kind of help you need. All I know is that everyone had such high expectations of me, and I was just one man. Nothing went very well—neither my business, nor my personal life. I was spread too thin. Had these kinds of things been discussed right from the beginning, perhaps some of the misunderstandings might have been prevented.

It's a little over a year now since her diagnosis. Susan's pretty well recovered, but some of that depression and withdrawal is still present. So, too, are some of the feelings of not having done all that I should have. I know she feels the same way. We haven't talked about it much, but it's there between us. I'm not sure how we're going to resolve it, and that scares me. It's frustrating having to be "the man," having to be strong. Women have certain expectations about men, and the way they think men should behave. They need to be aware that we can be just as fragile as they are. When a woman thinks a man doesn't care maybe it's just that his feelings are fragile, or he doesn't know how to deal with a situation, or even that he doesn't know how to talk about certain things. Perhaps we need to take a deep breath and tell the woman, "I'm just as fragile as you are. I know that's not how I come across. You might think I don't care, but maybe it's because I care so much and am so afraid that I run." Sometimes it's perceptions that are wrong; what they think is going on, isn't. I'm partly to blame as I should have talked more about what I was feeling. I should have told Susan that I felt left out; why I was withdrawn rather than let her think that I did not care. Sometimes I didn't talk about those kinds of things because I did not want to add to her burden. She had enough to deal with. Communication helps prevent misunderstandings which too often can create more of a problem. I would say, "Tell your partner how you're feeling because it's not just them who's going through it; you both are. Don't try to be a superman."

Connie, her sister: Because Susan's the big sister, and feels as though she has to take care of everyone else, it's been difficult for her to let her guard down. Maybe her cancer experience has shown her that it's okay to let others help. I never realized how strong she really was. My sister likes doing things on her own. I had to demand that she let me go to her oncologist with her. She was trying to *protect* us. Susan said when she introduced us, "She's here to ask you some questions because she doesn't believe what I tell her." After meeting her doctors I now understand why we're given vague answers. It's because the doctors are vague. They are merely trying to treat an immediate situation, and they have no plans for the future.

I learned to let Susan tell me how she felt, and how to listen without being judgmental. If they want to cry, and say, "Why me? How could this happen?" let them. Don't tell them, "It's going to be okay, so don't cry." It is traumatic; it is scary. I also learned to tell her how I felt.

My mother and I tried talking to Robert, but I think burying himself in work was the only way he knew how to cope. His only sister died of breast cancer, and then about a year after Susan's diagnosis his mother was also diagnosed, and had a mastectomy. He's a wonderful, sweet man, and a good father; however, I think he was overwhelmed, and that's not what my sister needed. I am angry with him for working too much and not being there for her and the boys, putting all that responsibility on her shoulders, and not caring enough to come home and take better care of her. I wanted her to rest more, and not go to work every day, but her typical response to me was, "I'm okay." There were many nights when I'd go over to check on her that I would find the boys running wild throughout the house, and Susan lying on her bed with a washcloth on her face too sick to get up. She would work herself to the very edge, and then drop. Fortunately my mother pitched in and did some of the cooking, laundry, helped with the boys, that kind of thing.

What really helped me was talking to Jan, one of the stylists in my salon who is a seventeen-year survivor of breast cancer. Every day I would remind Susan of that fact. Jan helped me with terminology, and I in turn was able to help educate not just my sister, but the entire family. She also taught me about the power of words. The importance of not owning your disease. Susan does not *have* breast cancer, she was diagnosed *with* cancer; she's a survivor of her diagnosis of cancer. It's like the surgeon telling my mother, "Excuse me. I did not say your daughter is dying from cancer. I said that she has cancer."

Jean, her mother: Susan did not want to talk about the fact that she had cancer with a lot of people, including family. If you asked her how she was, a typical response would be, "I'm fine," or "I'm wonderful." Everything with her was superficial which, I guess, is how she dealt with it.

It's been really hard to keep my mouth shut, not ask too many questions, or probe because sometimes interfering can be the worst thing you can do. I resent Robert for letting her down. She had to close her office because she lost so much momentum between surgeries and treatment. I sense that she's depressed which I'm sure is a combination of the business, what's going on with Robert, and having to take total responsibility for the boys.

Susan's told me, "I don't know what I would have done if it hadn't been for Connie." In fact, she's the one in the family Susan talks to the most, but occasionally she confided in me. Like the time I went over to her house and found her lying on her bed crying. "I'm just too sick, and my child had to fix his own supper." Robert, as usual, had not come home, and at that time her babysitter didn't know how to cook. I tried reassuring her. "Big deal. Charlie enjoyed doing it," and he piped in, "I did, Mom. It was fun." It was times like that when I had to put on a brave face, and say to myself, "She's going to get through this and be fine." I felt so badly for her I just wanted to cry. I had *assumed* he was going to be a big help.

Part of his behavior, I'm sure, was the fact that he just could not face the fact that his wife had cancer. I don't know how close he was to his sister; nonetheless, she was still his sister. My guess is that Susan's diagnosis brought it all back. Who sits in their office from eight o'clock in the morning until ten o'clock at night? That's what I consider running, and I suppose that is what he's still doing. He does not want to face the fact that their marriage is in trouble. My daughter has told him she wants out, but I think he's ignoring it because if he does maybe it will go away. She told me, "Mom, getting cancer was a wake-up call. You can drift along just so long which is what I've been doing. It's like, 'Hey, this could be the rest of your life, and if you're going to make something of it, you'd better do it.'" She just does not see a solution to this problem.

THE CHILDREN

Susan: It was scary for the boys when I came home from the hospital bandaged and with drains. Even though I explained to them what was going on, and that I was sick, I think Matt was too young to understand. He's always been a curious child; in fact, he's the kind of child who is in the bathroom with you checking everything out. Robert and I have never been very private about our bodies with the children. Matt wanted to see what was underneath the bandage, "Take it off Mom," and when I did and he saw the stitches and tremendous bruising on my breast he said, "Ooh." Charlie was never curious to see my breast, and was more interested in the mechanics of helping me clean my drain. Matt did not although he'd say things like, "It looks better," or "Now where's that hole from the tube?"

My illness worried the boys. After all, I am the life force that gets them through every day, gets them up in the morning, and puts them to bed at night. Their lives really don't function independently of me. So, it was scary for them to see me sick and in bed. You know children are worried when they are quiet. Sometimes Matt would climb into bed with me, and go to sleep for the night even if it was only six P.M. Apparently that made him feel safe, and even though I was touched, it did disturb and worry me that he did that. Charlie, on the other hand, has always been very independent and self-sufficient. He doesn't require the same one-on-one closeness and hugging that his brother does. Learning to cook simple meals and help me out a little made him feel as though he had some control, and that is how he dealt with his fears. There were times though when I'd overhear a phone conversation with their father, "Daddy, you need to come home. Mommy's very tired." Sometimes Robert did; other times he did not.

Robert, her husband: Susan did not want to tell the boys that anything was going on, and we disagreed over that. As a result all they were told was that their mother had to go in for surgery to fix something. I thought they should have been told more as it might have given them a greater understanding of what was going on. It would have made it easier for them if we had explained things up front instead of doing it after the fact, and said something like, "Okay. This is what's going to happen now; then, this will happen. . . . If you have any questions, or if anything bothers you please come ask us." I would have felt more comfortable, and it would have been better for them if we had explained in a way they would understand, that their mother had something called cancer which grows but is not supposed to be there. The doctor is going to cut it out, and she'll be having treatment to make sure that it is totally gone from her body. You don't have to go into scientific detail, and you do have to be prepared to answer their questions honestly, but at least by telling them in that way they would know that Mommy would be okay. God forbid the outcome had been different.

Kids know when you're not telling them something, and that makes them more worried. They were certainly afraid, especially Charlie because he was older and understood more. When Susan was in bed all Matt was told was, "Mommy's tired," or "Mommy just doesn't feel good." He didn't ask too many questions, at least not to me. Charlie, on the other hand, did ask me privately whether his mother was going to die. I told him, "Mommy has this illness, but I don't think she's going to die. She's going to the doctor, and they're taking care of it. It's going to take awhile, and she'll be tired for awhile, but she'll be fine." He seemed to accept that.

Connie, her sister: My daughter is the same age as Charlie; my son a couple of years older. They knew my sister had cancer; in fact, I tried discussing it with them, even got children's books out of the library, but as far as they were concerned it was kind of like getting the flu—you get over it. Maybe they would have thought it was more serious if she had lost her hair. When my daughter asked, "Does Aunt Susan still have cancer?" I told her she'd had treatment and it was gone, and she said, "That's what I thought. She only had it for a little while." Because Susan still worked, maintained her life for the most part, and wasn't in the hospital for long periods of time, I don't know how much her boys related to the seriousness of her illness. I don't think it ever dawned on my children that I could get cancer. They know I've had a lump removed, and that I have another one that needs to be removed. When they asked, "Do you have the same thing Aunt Susan does?" all I could say was, "I don't think so."

Jean, her mother: Charlie tends to fly off the handle more than he used to, and Matt is a little bit moodier. He used to be a very open, laughing child, the kind who was happy all the time. However, I don't think he is all the time now. They are both aware their parents might separate, and they cry over that. It is going to be very hard on them.

Charlie, her son: When Mom told us she had breast cancer I asked her what that was. She told me that you get a little bump in your breast, and they have to do surgery. The tube scared me. Matt and I would bring her crackers or dry toast and water because there were times she couldn't get up. Sometimes we'd lie next to her; holding her hand, giving her kisses, telling her we loved her. When I told her I was worried when she was really, really sick, she told me she would get better, and then I felt better. When I told her I was afraid she was going to die she told me that was not going to happen for a long time. Matt and I talked about what Mom was going through, and he'd ask me sometimes if she was going to die. I'd tell him "No, it isn't serious." I'd say something like, when she'd get a shot, "She's not really, really sick. She just doesn't feel good; kind of like she has a stomachache."

Matt, her son: It was kind of scary when she came home from the hospital with tubes and bandages. When she wasn't feeling well I'd get upset. I didn't want to tell my friends, or even my teachers, because I thought that would be kind of rude to my mom letting other people know she had breast cancer.

LET'S TALK ABOUT DEATH AND DYING

Susan: Some people cannot get beyond the fact that they have cancer. Once they know they have cancer their mind accepts it, expedites it and then their body dies. In my case I felt as though I were being told, "Stop—wake up!" that I was being given a second chance. Where was I in my life, and where did I want to be? I have been given an awareness of my total being—physical, mental, emotional and spiritual—and have learned to allow myself to treasure those moments that I do have. Many people fear cancer: there's a mystique about it they don't understand, particularly if you're speaking in surgical terms. It's hard for them to believe that you can get over it, survive—even get beyond it. My brother and younger sister are a perfect example. They'd call Connie or my mother to get the real scoop about how I was doing. Of course I was telling them the truth, but they had to visit frequently just to see for themselves. Both my sisters have had breast lumps. My younger sister said, "Oh my God. What's going to happen to me? Nothing has happened yet, but it will sooner or later." I'm sure she still has that mind-set. She is really, really scared.

Robert, her husband: While in college I had taken a class on death and dying. We were taught how to face death, how to help a dying person prepare themselves for death and the importance of being able to talk about it. When my sister was dying I did not cope well. I just could not do any of those things knowing that she was going to die. To be honest I just choked up. Never having really said good-bye to her has stuck with me all these years. A lot of the feelings I experienced while she was dying resurfaced when Susan was diagnosed. That cold chill I experienced when first hearing about her lump, and then again when her doctor told me she had breast cancer were suppressed memories. I was definitely fighting those feelings during the time Susan was going through everything. We had every reason to be optimistic in her recovery; however, that little kernel of doubt and fear *was* there, and once it surfaced it grew. That was something I never discussed with Susan, yet it was an internal battle I constantly fought. When my mother was diagnosed with breast cancer I thought, *What did I do to make God so angry?*

Connie, her sister: Consciously I would never consider anything but a full recovery for my sister. I do not think I am in denial, but last year I dreamt about her every single night—all the possibilities that could be. Apparently I'm afraid to think about those kinds of things while awake, so I work them out in my head while I'm asleep.

Jean, her mother: I made myself believe that she was going to be okay, but there's still that little bit of worry in the back of my mind, and I suppose it's always going to be there. Anyone who has had cancer has that little bit of fear. How could you not? Maybe in a sense that's good because it keeps you alert. This has made me so aware that we are all vulnerable. Because of Susan's experience our family has learned to say, "I love you" a little more often because nobody has any guarantees for tomorrow.

Postscript, January 2000

My husband and I were divorced following my cancer experience, but remain very close friends and devoted parents to our two sons who are now ten and fourteen. Neither boy has very much memory of the cancer/post-cancer treatment times. I have met a man with whom I have been involved for the past ten months and feel happy and alive as never before. Interestingly, his ex-wife is an OB/GYN surgeon who was personally diagnosed with fibrocystic breasts! I gave up owning my own business and went to work with a friend, and we are proud to have been chosen to produce events for many worthwhile causes including: Make a Wish Foundation, Planned Parenthood, Scratch & Sniff, Denim & Diamonds for the American Cancer Society, and more.

Robert's father was diagnosed with breast cancer in 1998 at the age of eighty-one and had a mastectomy. Both of his parents are doing well. Connie's breast lump turned out to be nothing. My health remains good.

Three

Wendy Dupont

Is Saving a Breast Worth Losing a Life?

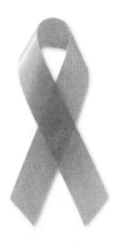

Survivor Profile:

Age at diagnosis: forty-three (4/93)

Age at interview: forty-seven (11/15/96)

Type of breast cancer: Paget's disease (nipple)

Stage III (diagnosis 10/95)

Surgical procedure: mastectomy (10/95); twelve
positive lymph nodes at time of mastectomy
(type of breast cancer: infiltrating ductal and extensive DCIS)

Treatment: alternative (holistic) medicine for more than one
year; chemotherapy (7/94); radiation; tamoxifen (6/95);
clinical trial of Taxol, Doxil (10/96)

Reconstruction: immediate, latissimus dorsi

Estrogen receptors: positive, Progesterone receptors: information
not provided

Who's Who:

Noelle Dupont, her daughter (age eight at diagnosis)

Nancy Tsuchiya, her friend

THE BEGINNING OF A LONG JOURNEY

Wendy: I knew something was wrong about a year before my diagnosis. My nipple had begun to flake and when I sought an opinion from my gynecologist she thought whatever it was looked similar to a wart; however, she suggested that I have a mammogram. There were calcifications evident on the mammogram; consequently I was sent to a surgeon. That alone was frightening, but what really scared me was when he said, "Half the time calcifications are cancerous. I think you should have a biopsy." I still cannot believe how cold this man was. He sent me home with a book about mastectomies and said, "Read it." I took one look at the picture of a woman with one breast, gasped, "Oh my God!" and made up my mind I would *never* go back to this man. I wonder sometimes, *Would I have made a different decision had it been a different kind of meeting?* I truthfully do not know. Because of that meeting, plus my strong belief system about alternative (holistic) health and medicine, I chose not to have the biopsy. I would resolve my problem holistically. The other factor that influenced my decision was my aversion to having anyone cut into my body as I have had an ileostomy (I wear a bag) since I had my colon removed as a result of ulcerative colitis at the age of twenty-one.

WHERE DO I GO? WHAT DO I DO?

Wendy: At this point I began to put vitamin E on my breast, and I also consulted with a medical doctor who integrates holistic medicine into her practice. Although she was not wholly supportive of my decision to not have a biopsy, we mapped out a program to help boost my immune system; neither of us was sure whether or not there was anything seriously wrong with me. We worked together for a year. I had two mammograms during that time. The first one showed even more calcifications in my breast, but the one taken six months later showed that there were fewer. Naturally I thought, *I must be doing something right,* so I continued doing what I was doing.

In March of 1993 my nipple was still flaking and appeared to be losing tissue. I went to a dermatologist. Imagine my shock when he said to me, "I think we should do a biopsy. How about right now?" The first thing that ran through my mind was, *He suspects cancer.*

WHAT IS PAGET'S DISEASE?

Wendy: I had Paget's disease which is not only a nipple disease, but it is also a rare form of breast cancer. Doctors are concerned about the nipple, but they are more concerned with the fact that this diagnosis usually means there is cancer elsewhere in the breast, typically in the form of tumors. The tumors can be anywhere in the breast. It is not the nipple that actually causes the problem, it is the tumors. At that point I did not have any tumors—only a flaky nipple. A mastectomy was recommended. That was the first time I knew for sure I was in trouble.

DECISION TIME

Wendy: My daughter, Noelle was eight at the time. Because she was home from school with a cold I brought her to the meeting I had scheduled with the surgeon. A different doctor from the one I had seen a year earlier began to mark my body with pens. We left and Noelle said to me, "Mom, what a jerk!" She was astounded at how cold he was. I had the mastectomy scheduled, but after having a heart-to-heart talk with myself decided instead to heal myself by going to a very well-known holistic clinic near my home.

The program I wanted to enroll in began the next day. It was very expensive—four-thousand dollars for a ten-day stay. I am a single mom, but fortunately I have a wonderful network of friends. Within a twenty-four hour period everything, including the care of Noelle, was taken care of. I put my life on hold and checked into the clinic. There, I was given the tools to help me heal myself physically, emotionally and spiritually. My day was filled with things like: meditation, massage therapy, lectures on diet and Edgar Cayce remedies to assist in my healing. I participated in group and individual therapy to help me recognize and resolve any underlying issues that might be causing me emotional pain. Perhaps some of these issues were the reason *why* this had happened. They also taught me to anchor in good memories so that those memories would be there when I needed them most. My meals were prepared for me: primarily raw vegetables and raw foods to shift my body from an acidic to an alkaline pH environment since cancer thrives on an acidic pH. I was taught the value of heated castor oil packs on my liver which help draw out the toxins.

BUT THEN YOU GO HOME!

Wendy: Most of the patients at the clinic have what I refer to as "warm and fuzzy" bodies to go home to. They have someone to pamper them, cater to them, juice the raw vegetables and make their salads so they can heal. I had only myself. Truthfully this was a very stressful time for me. I teach voice and piano. I sing. I give concerts. I am a single mom. I am only one person. I am also a type-A personality which means that I am a classic achiever and perfectionist. My day was so full that once I incorporated what I had been taught, I had no time to live. I was tied to the kitchen juicing and chopping half the day. It was very tough.

One day Noelle called while I was working at home, and I broke down into tears. My wise child said to me, "Mom, you are not a bulldozer. Take a break!" I was so strict that I would allow myself no sugars—not even one oatmeal raisin cookie. How could I? All these doctors wanted me to have a mastectomy, and I had chosen to use an alternative method that was risky.

I DO NOT WANT TO LOSE MY BREAST

Wendy: For an entire year after my diagnosis I followed strictly holistic disciplines. I gave each discipline ninety days. If I did not see results I moved on to the next one. I continued to get mammograms, and it was during this time two lumps were discovered. The ultrasound that followed showed that they had all the characteristics (smooth, round and without evidence of solid components) of being benign (non-cancerous). The discipline I was following at this particular time seemed to be working because, in my opinion, my lumps were not growing. I knew—I was feeling them constantly! In retrospect, they obviously were because they eventually grew into two meaningful tumors; one the size of a plum, the other a little smaller. Then they grew together.

I was so stubborn! I did not want to lose my breast, and I believed so strongly that there had to be something holistic that could cure this disease without being intrusive to my body. I knew so much about natural things. Everything I had ever read about allopathic (conventional) treatment was negative: cutting, chemotherapy and radiation were toxic to the body and destroyed it. Because of what I read I would say to myself, *I am not going to do that to my body.* Even after the biopsy I had in January of 1994 which showed the tumors to be malignant (cancer), I still refused to do anything about them.

I finally went to see a naturopathic physician who thought my problem was hormonal. He was correct because the biopsy had shown my tumors to be estrogen dependent. He recommended that I use progesterone cream on my breast and continued to measure my lumps telling me they were not growing. Noelle on the other hand kept saying, "Mom, they are growing and they're hard!" At the end of ninety days I knew I was in trouble. I realized the cancer was in my lymph nodes because they were swollen.

SURRENDER

Wendy: In June of 1994 I surrendered. I said to myself, *Enough is enough* and made an appointment with a breast clinic affiliated with a cancer center out of state. I was a stage IIIB. They told me the wild yam I had been using on my breast had probably aggravated the situation. By now the tumor was so large, 9 cm x 6.5 cm, and was attached to the muscle while the one in my lymph nodes was 3 cm x 4 cm [author's note: for reference, 1 inch = approximately 2½ cm], their recommendation was that I first do chemotherapy to shrink the tumor, followed by a single modified radical mastectomy, then radiation, and lastly high-dose chemotherapy with stem cell rescue (the most recent form of bone marrow transplant). I went along with their recommendation to have chemotherapy on a weekly basis instead of every three weeks. That way the overall dosage would be stronger than a "standard" treatment of having chemotherapy once every three weeks; but the weaker, weekly dose would allow me to continue to work. I found a very nice oncologist in my home city who was willing to follow the protocol that had been mapped out for me which incorporated Adriamycin and 5-FU that would be administered intravenously, and Cytoxan pills which I would take orally. I did that for three months. I never missed a day of work nor a church service even though there were days I felt lousy. I continued to teach piano and voice lessons during the day. I lost my hair, developed headaches and mouth sores, and was very fatigued. When I was able, I napped during the day. When I felt well enough, I hiked the mountain I so loved that was at the foot of my home. And I also jumped on my trampoline to keep in shape in between headaches.

GOD'S MIRACLE

Wendy: When I was first diagnosed I fell into what I refer to as the "metaphysical pit" which meant, "Oh God. Look what I did to myself." That is a terrible place to be. It is a terrible indictment and I believe metaphysics at its worst. There is a very thin line between blame and responsibility. And we, and I include myself in this, tend to blame ourselves for the bad things that happen to us and make us feel bad. I now have my own philosophy about illness and disease. I liken it to making a pot of soup with many ingredients. Some may be genetic, some may be emotional upsets which may not send a good message to the body, some may be stress, God's will and even some things that are beyond our control. There is also the "fundamental pit": "You sinned so now you pay." If a person was raised in a traditional Christian church and becomes "metaphysical" he or she is really in trouble because then they may fall into both pits. I am a Unity Christian. I do not put God or Christ into a box. It is just the way I am. It is a very dangerous thing to blame ourselves for our illness because then we are playing God. How do I, or how does anyone know what the big picture is?

One day in desperation I thumbed through the Bible looking for an answer. Did I bring this on myself? I opened to a passage in which the disciples were asking about the man born blind, "Did he sin or did his parents sin?", because that was the philosophy at the time. The answer given was, "Neither sinned. It just happened so that God's miracles can shine through. Go and be well." That really helped me realize, "Maybe I can have a miracle. Maybe I did not bring this on myself. Maybe this happened so that God's miracles can show through me!"

In November of 1994 it was time to proceed with the mastectomy. I asked my surgeon not to remove my breast if there was no cancer. There was none. He removed the tumor, but it was benign. My lymph nodes were a normal size. They kept sending tissue to the lab and the reports kept coming back negative. The cancer was gone. My surgeon did not take my breast nor any lymph nodes, but he cautioned me, "It will come back."

COMING TO TERMS

Wendy: A couple of months later my nipple began to flake again. I was back on the holistic trail and found what I thought was going to be "the cure." I continued to see my oncologist and finally began to take the tamoxifen he had been urging me to take for quite awhile in the hopes that it might help since I was estrogen-receptor positive. He knew how much I wanted to save my breast. However, in August of 1995 he said, "Wendy, I think you're in trouble. Your tissue is starting to thicken, I think there is lymph node involvement and I really think you should have a mastectomy." In October of 1995 I did. There were no tumors; however, there was infiltrating ductal and extensive intraductal cancer throughout my breast. In addition twelve out of twelve lymph nodes were positive. I believe the cancer stayed localized in my breast because of the holistic foods and supplements I continued to take to boost my immune system, such as lots of greens and chlorophyl. I had by then tailored a system to fit my life.

I think I held out as long as I did because there was something in me that I needed to address concerning my idea of sexuality and femininity. Even though I had been married a few times and had had a child, I felt as though my breasts were the only part of my "womanly" body left intact. My surrender to surgery was my realization that I was a lot more than my breast. "I am who I am. I am *not* who I am *because* of my breast." That was a tough lesson for me to learn, but when I did have the mastectomy I knew it was the right decision. Shortly after my mastectomy I sang the title song of my compact disc "Rhapsody" during one of my performances, and began to cry. The first line is: "My soul. I finally choose to liberate my soul. And I wonder *why* I waited so long." I have sung that song so many times, and it has spoken to me in many different ways. It was not until that night I realized I was so much more than my breast. I had liberated my soul in a major way and it was okay. I did what I did to live.

I STAND RELEASED FROM OLD FEARS

Wendy: I will state this very clearly. Had I thought chemotherapy and radiation were going to be healthy for me I would have chosen them earlier. However, I had such a mind-set that they would actually lessen my quality of life and take years off it that I was determined to find a cure that was healthy for me. I wanted to build my body up, not tear it down. So it wasn't only my fear of losing a breast that caused me to do what I did. There were many feelings and reasons tied to the decisions that I made. I believed that natural medicine would give me a longer, healthier life and thought my decisions were life giving, not life taking. Because of the many decisions I made and treatment options I chose, numerous people said to me, "You're crazy. You have a daughter. You need to do this." I would tell them, "It is *because* I have a daughter and *because* I want to live that I choose not to do chemotherapy and radiation. I do not want to do things that will tear me up inside." What I did not realize until I had to do it, was that it was okay to combine conventional and holistic modalities.

When I was getting my chemotherapy treatments, I would lecture patients who were also having their treatment at the same time, "Are you doing green things?" "Are you juicing?" "Are you doing things that will give your body some fight?" I was still able to function, and I did what I could to help my body detoxify. I came around the hard way, but I finally became part of a team. I combined the three components that I consider make up the braid: all the good "stuff" to build up my body, my doctors and God. That is how I got my miracle.

My oncologist and I talked about my having a bone marrow transplant, but I told him, "People die from that." Because I was responding so well to treatment he did not disagree with my decision not to have it. Through January of 1996 I had thirty radiation treatments. I really thought I was done. Unfortunately the cancer came back.

CAN I PRAY FOR ANOTHER MIRACLE?

Wendy: It was just a little bump under the skin—not a lymph node, but right near the armpit. My surgeon took it out. It was cancer. My oncologist wanted me to do radiation but I told him, "Sorry. I have plans this summer." I also did not want to get burnt like I had the last time. His comment to me was, "You have a way of line-item vetoing things."

Noelle, my sister, her daughter and I went to Ireland to celebrate. It was June of 1996. I had saved an entire year for this vacation. We had a wonderful time. I really thought, *It's small and they got it all. I'm done with this. It's out of my life!* The day we returned I began to have problems breathing. *What respiratory bug did I pick up in Ireland?* I wondered. The chest X-ray I had a month later showed my lungs to be clear, other than being scarred, which the X-ray technician attributed to the radiation I had undergone. It was at this time I decided to have further reconstructive breast surgery. At the time of my mastectomy I had the latissimus dorsi procedure (using the muscle and a flap of skin from the back to form a breast) which left my breast area flat instead of sunken like it might have been because of the extensive surgery I had had. Now I had a saline implant put in to give me a "breast." After that surgery I began to experience tingling in about one-fourth of my fingers; however, I could still play the piano. Apparently a nerve had been disturbed. I began physical therapy and was told the tingling might be the result of the radiation I had had earlier. I was still experiencing shortness of breath, and now I had some pain. When I met with my oncologist he was very concerned. He took a chest X-ray in August and one in September. There was a definite change. He suspected pleural effusion (fluid around the lungs), which could be caused by tumor activity. He suggested that I have a CAT scan. At the same time I was given neurological response tests and I flunked one of them. Because of that, and because I was now beginning to see double, he wanted me to have an MRI of the brain. I panicked.

The good news was that the MRI was negative, there was no cancer in my brain. The bad news was that there was fluid and activity in my right lung. It looked like there were a couple of nodules, but it was mostly patchiness. There was no need to have a biopsy. My oncologist was sure it was cancer given my history. I was still having problems with my vision: I had one shaded area and it was fuzzy. A nonmedical friend "diagnosed" my problem as a detached retina, so I made an appointment with an ophthalmologist having no suspicion whatsoever that this too would be cancer. "You have two tumors, one on the back of each retina. They are very small. You need to start radiation *now* because you have not yet torn anything and the fluid is intact." On top of that terrible news my arm had collapsed the night before as I reached up to turn off the light by my bed. I think my arm was just one more ingredient for me to add to "the soup." I was really panicked now. *I can't believe I'm in this again!* I immediately began radiation treatment on my retinas.

ANOTHER MIRACLE

Wendy: I felt as though I were living one of those carnival games where no sooner would I hit one of those targets with a mallet than another pops up. Every time I turned around I was being hit with more bad news. And to make matters worse now I could hardly play the piano. I felt like Job— totally stripped. I thought to myself, *How much more of this am I supposed to take?* I do not like having doubt, being depressed and living in fear. That is an awful place to be because there is no hope or faith there. Nor is there joy or love. I try not to stay in that place for very long. Instead, I continue to look for the miracles that are a part of my life.

My brother is a veterinary surgeon who combines conventional and holistic medicine in his practice. At his urging I went to a well-known cancer center only a few hours drive from my home because his philosophy is, "You have one doctor—one idea." Maybe the doctors at this cancer center would have a treatment my oncologist was unaware of. It turned out they did. When I met with the oncologist at the cancer center she smiled as she held out her hand, "Why are you here?" I said to her, "I am looking for something. Do you have anything down here I cannot find at home?" She examined me, and so subtly that I almost missed it, dropped a hint, "Maybe I do." I asked more questions and she began to tell me about a trial just beginning that involved the drugs Taxol® and Doxil. She was looking for fifteen women. This particular treatment has been highly successful in Europe with women who have advanced breast cancer. However, the treatment does not yet have FDA approval in the United States. I was accepted into the trial. I am number two. I asked her, "How do you choose people for this trial? Does attitude help?" She told me, "Yes." So it does pay to choose life and look for miracles. I look for miracles every day.

THE BATTLEGROUND

Wendy: I have just begun the protocol and have had the first of six treatments I will be getting over the next six months. This is tough stuff. The good news is that between the physical therapy I have been getting and the chemotherapy, my arm has improved. The bad news is that the drugs took away my voice in four days.

I am very fortunate in that I am rarely nauseated from chemotherapy. I never vomit. I did not when I had chemotherapy, and I have not so far this time. I did lose my hair again, but this time it was very empowering to cut it off instead of letting it fall out. I held on to the bitter end last time, and I cried when it fell out. This time I did not. In fact, Noelle just chopped it off this morning. She had a blast doing it and said to me, "Mom, it looks pretty weird now. I'll buzz it off later today." I have learned to make great turbans from scarves. In fact one of the women at my church just asked me, "Are you making a fashion statement or are you back in treatment?" Last week the inside of my mouth was raw and this week I ran a high fever and have developed a body rash. The skin on my hands is blistering. I am told the rash is a result of the Doxil which causes the skin to become very sensitive. I get really tired. My eyelashes are gone, but I have not yet completely lost my eyebrows although they have become very thin. My vanity is definitely being tested and abused. I wonder, *How am I going to get through five more treatments?* But then I think, *Maybe I am supposed to be in this trial so that I can help thousands of other women.* I feel as though I am a pioneer!

THE POWER OF PRAYER

Wendy: I started a prayer group at one of the churches where I sing around the time I was diagnosed with tumors on the retinas of my eyes. I said to some of the members, "I believe you have gifts. Let's use them." They agreed. I had my first laying on of hands the morning I had my first radiation treatment on my retinas. Six hours after that treatment I went to Noelle's school to watch her practice gymnastics. Under normal circumstances my vision is blurry. All of a sudden she was clear as crystal. From that moment on my vision has remained clear.

Once a week I attend the prayer circle. Anyone is welcome. At the end of the session we go up to the altar and hand our burdens over to God and know that it has been taken care of. That helps to remind me I am not alone. It is just one more thing that tells me that I am going to be fine. I can feel the difference when prayers are said for me. It is such a wonderful feeling. Every morning I say to myself, *I claim the power of prayer sent my way.* It is important to claim that power and be open to receive it. Prayer changes everything. This morning I opened the Bible to this scripture: "For I know the plans I have for you," says the Lord, "To give you a future and a hope." So today, right now, I am feeling physically and emotionally good. I do not know how I will feel next month. I am afraid because of how I have felt this past month.

NOELLE—MY GURU

Wendy: My daughter is a little sprite. She is wise beyond her years, yet playful as a kitty cat. She is twelve. She is a gymnast, a wonderful dancer. She is sensitive, loves to laugh, loves to tease, is a great student, is a leader, is a true friend and likes true friends. I am so proud of her. I have seen her flourish these last four years. As a parent I look at three things: Is she playing well, is she eating well and is she sleeping well? The answer to all three is, *yes*. If I do see a problem we talk about it, but in general I think she has done pretty well. Frankly I think both of us walk around with a bubble around us because we both believe in miracles. We just know that I am going to be okay. Noelle believes this because I have taught her to, or maybe she believes it because of who she is. I am not sure.

When I have been given a miracle Noelle says to me, "Oh Mom, I knew you were going to be fine." It is very healthy for me to be around her because she expects me to be healthy and well. Don't get me wrong though. My daughter is still a twelve-year-old. She becomes impatient with me when I get tired. She wants to play, and there are times I cannot. She becomes frustrated because things are not normal and are different for both of us. She can be demanding, yet I understand she only wants what any twelve-year-old child wants. However, when she stops to think about her "demands" she becomes less demanding and more under-standing and will often say to me, "Mom, I'm sorry." It's hard for her to contend with the fact that things are not normal and that there are times I have to be treated with kid gloves—physically and emotionally. I try to rest as much as I can during the day so that when I pick her up from school I have some of myself to give to her. She is such a special child. Noelle will do something out of the blue that is so kind. My having can-cer has been a blessing in one regard. It has allowed her the ability to take off those twelve-year-old blinders and see the bigger picture—what is important—and that is to enjoy the days that we do have together.

THE VOICE OF A CHILD

Noelle, her daughter: I knew something was going on because I pay attention to what my mother does, and I could see that she was talking to doctors. Mom would tell me she was trying to find out what the problem was. When she told me she had cancer I had already known something was wrong. I just did not know *what* was wrong. I may have been only eight at the time, but I knew what cancer was because I had taken science classes in school.

My mother has been very up-front with me from the beginning. Parents need to be up-front with their children regardless of their age. They could say something like, "Mommy is going to get some tests to see if she has cancer." They should tell them what is going on at all times. I think parents do their kids a big injustice when they assume that because children are young, they do not understand. Parents are actually protecting their child by telling them the truth. When they do not tell their kids things and start having "secrets," that makes us kids feel left out, uninformed and lonely. That's not right. It's like when someone at school tells a secret about me, and I don't know what that secret is. All I want is to go off into my own corner. In order to prevent me from going off into my corner I need to be brought into the picture. I do not like being left out of the loop. My teachers all knew about Mom because she has been the chorus teacher at my school for the past two years. My friends also know.

I know that what is going on with my mother is serious, but I try to treat her like a normal mom. Cancer on the one hand has not been a "normal" part of my life, yet on the other hand it is. Neither Mom nor I put our attention or emphasis on the fact that she does have cancer. It is just a part of our lives and we do not dwell on it. We try to have fun.

The first time she had chemotherapy, Mom told me she was going to lose her hair, but when it started to happen I was scared. I did not know what to expect until it all just fell out. This time I was a pro, and I cut her hair. That was fun! She was not depressed like she was the last time. My mom used to have beautiful long hair. I went with her to radiation one time, but the people there were mean. I wanted to see what it was all about, but they made me wait in the lobby. I am not a four-year-old who is attached to her mommy's hip and would push buttons I know I am not supposed to push. I never went back.

I have learned to take on a lot more responsibility. When mom comes home from the hospital I make her sandwiches, fruit salads and crackers and cheese. I love to play the piano, but I know she needs quiet and needs to rest because she doesn't feel well, so instead I will work on my computer or watch TV. Other kids need to know, "Don't be afraid." I will know when to be scared because I, like all kids, have that special instinct. We always know when something is going to happen. For now I try to live my life as normally as I can. My mom has become stronger and feistier and I think she has changed for the better because of having cancer.

WENDY'S "BLESSING OF LIFE" TALK

Wendy: My "blessing of life" talk is a combination of talk and music. Its theme is all the different ways cancer has helped me, and what I have learned from having it. I have given this talk five or six times and will give it anywhere, to anyone who wants to hear it, because I see the things that have happened because of my having cancer.

I use a lot of humor. I tell funny things Noelle has said to help lift my spirits. For instance, Noelle's offhand remark, "Just think, Mom. You can't get head lice now!" when my hair began to fall out that first time and I was having a hard time coping. Any parent who has ever lived that nightmare will know exactly what that means! Neither one of us could get rid of those lice. It took weeks! This occurred during the time I was on my holistic path and spent my days in the kitchen juicing and doing everything healthy. And here I was using bottle after bottle of extremely toxic chemicals on my head. When Noelle made that comment to me I just smiled really big because there was so much more behind that comment and I knew exactly what she meant! Then there was the time I went to the movie with a friend. I was wearing my wig for the first time and the wind outside was blowing fifty mph and here I was, frantically trying to keep my wig from being torn off my head! I wanted to cry, but all I could do was laugh.

I have learned to laugh about this whole cancer experience. What else can I do? I have looked at myself in the mirror sometimes. I have no hair, no eyelashes, no eyebrows. I am glued and Velcro-ed together. I wear my synthetic eyelashes. When I wear my wig it is held on my head by Velcro and it itches. But somehow I make it all work. I sit behind my piano and sing. Now I can't even sing well. Yet somehow my life has been blessed *because* I have cancer. This path I have been on has also blessed the lives of many people. It has helped them with their faith. Those who have helped me have helped themselves. Noelle's soul has blossomed because of this experience, and that is why I give this talk. I see the things that have happened. It's not like I want cancer, but I am on my path so it is up to me to turn lemons into lemonade.

SUPPORT

Wendy: I have friends I did not even know I had. The miracles continue. People are cooking for me, driving me to doctors' appointments even if it's two hours away from home, and are even cleaning my bathrooms. They call with, "What can I do to help?" It is really nice that people are not afraid to enter my life at this time. I try to approach each day in an uplifting way because I know no one would want to hang around me if I were living my life in fear and doubt, or if I walked around depressed. That doesn't mean I am happy every day because I'm not, particularly when I do not feel well, but . . .

I began a cabaret because I love to see "community." I gathered together everyone I knew to share their art forms so everyone could share music, poetry and other art forms. It was a joining together of old and young. Why can't ten-year-olds learn from eighty-year-olds? Now a cabaret is being put on for me next month as a fund-raiser because I can no longer work as I did before. And there have been and will be other fund-raisers. I am still working, but I have only enough energy to teach piano to my four teenage students. I have had to give up teaching the adults. I cannot give up the children. That is the reason I am here. They have special needs I think are important which are more than just music. I am helping them along their path, but they are also helping me. When I think about having to give up the children my heart cringes. God is taking care of me.

A FEW WORDS FROM NANCY

Nancy, her friend: The community Wendy and I live in is a mixture of retired folks and artists. I knew of Wendy yet I did not know her. One Sunday I attended Unity Church, the church Wendy belongs to, and at the end of the service everyone stood in a circle and we all sang. I did not know where the voice was coming from, but suddenly I heard the most beautiful, angelic, clear music I had ever heard. The voice was sound in glass. It cut without a sharp edge. "Who does that voice belong to?" I asked. Hands pointed to Wendy.

I still did not know Wendy, but circumstances brought us together and we began a friendship. She gave voice lessons to my daughter, and we hiked the mountain she so loved.

Wendy claims her voice sounds like Joe Cocker's (a blues/rock singer from the 1960s)—low and gravelly. I think she only hears her voice that way. The feedback I have heard from others is that her voice is now more soulful, just a different register. She is hearing changes she has no control over, but the beauty is not gone.

I am a strong believer in healing circle energy. For me, healing is not necessarily about getting up tomorrow and being brand new. It is living life in a way that is rich all the way to the end. I do not know whether Wendy will live or die in the short term. I do know that healing happens in any case. I told her, "You have made a new benchmark on the wall of life for me and have shown me how to live it." The courage and character Wendy has portrayed, even though she may not feel it, represents and embodies something I had never seen before. How she is living her life is a gift to everyone who knows her.

ABOUT LIFE

Wendy: Somehow my cancer experience seems to have helped the relationship between Noelle's father and me. It has allowed us to see what is important and to help each other. He helps with Noelle whenever he can during the times I normally have her. Noelle sees her father every week and loves him very much. When I asked her not too long ago, "What have you learned from this?" she told me, "Not to waste time with you or Dad." I believe she meant that when she is mad at either of us she does not stay angry for too long. She has learned that life is precious. In order for joy and love to be present she can not have all that anger.

I have unconditionally accepted that these are the cards I have been dealt for right now. I have been willing to fit cancer into my life, but I do not fit my life into cancer. Cancer is only a *part* of my life. It has been an interesting experience from a metaphysical circle. Someone patted me on the back last week, "When are you going to get it? When are you going to try to find out why your cancer keeps coming back?" That was a cruel thing to say. I told the person who said that to back off. I know he meant well, but until he walks in my shoes he cannot possibly understand. Being in my shoes changes everything.

Maybe cancer is giving me the excuse to do what I need to do. And that is to write down and create a book of visionary music that is for congregational use—solo and chorus. When I thought I had a brain tumor I panicked: What if I don't get to do that and my music is not shared? I have a tape I made eight years ago, and "Rhapsody" which is on compact disc, but I need to do this, too.

My name means "wanderer." I want to travel and see the world. I want to see more of this country. I am at my happiest when I am traveling. The year before we went to Ireland, Noelle and I went on a twenty-four hundred-mile RV trip. We called it The Adventures of Rent a Wreck. Our next trip is to Colorado. Noelle has never seen the mountains. That is planned for next summer. What else do I want? I want to fall in love.

I expect to be here for a long time, but who knows? I have told that to Noelle. I have also told her that the most important thing is that we have each other. "We can not let this illness take over our lives as though it is *the thing.* I could have a million-dollar body, do everything right and it may be my time next week. Or it could be yours. Then again, we could live for years and years. We do not know. All we can do is make the best of what we do have." I think that made sense to her. By telling her that it takes the emphasis off my illness. No one knows how long she will live. How long I am here is not necessarily dependent on whether or not I have cancer, and Noelle cannot live her life in fear thinking, "Mom may not make it because she has cancer." I have tried to put death into perspective. By reminding her that none of us knows *what* we will die from, that takes the bigness out of cancer. Cancer is just one more thing that we live with right now. I do not expect to live with cancer forever. I expect it to be gone. Cancer is only one aspect of our lives. It is not this all-encompassing thing that will determine how long I am here.

LAST THOUGHTS

Wendy: Surround yourself with positive friends. Do not put up with philosophies that make you feel bad. Eliminate people from your life if they are painful to be around. Do what brings you joy, and do not do what doesn't. If you do not have a lot of friends join a church. Find one that is loving and one that will pray for you. That is what churches are for. Find ways you can give to other people because that will make you get out of your own stuff. It's just good for the soul. Take time to enjoy nature and the people and animals that love you. Smile. Laugh when you can. And when you can't, cry. Be honest with yourself. And always believe in miracles. Just claim them as I do. I will not accept anything less than good. I am a big believer in the fact that there are things you can change, and things you cannot. My job is to know the difference. I do not know if I have any say about when I go or how long I will stay, but if I have anything to say about it I am going to do everything I can to live with faith, to live with assertion in terms of life force, and to give my life force everything I have. I may have nothing to say about how long I will be here, but I believe there is something to be said for willpower—the will to live. Maybe that's a gift we are given. If some people do not have that will to live we need to share that with them. For me, I will accept only life. Because I feel as though I am here for a reason. I need to be here for my daughter and for my own life. I believe that. I will not go gently into the night. That is the way I will continue to live my life. There is a part of me that needs to be a warrior, and a part of me that needs a little more quiet, peaceful time. I am working on that part of me now. As one of my friends so wonderfully says, *"Just be."* And see love everywhere you can.

Postscript from a daughter, January 25, 2000

It was early August, 1997. She woke up and appeared to be confused. She could not remember my name, her own daughter. I called the ambulance and had her rushed to the hospital. She spent several weeks in the hospital and was eventually moved to a nearby hospice. I had not been to the first two weeks of school because I demanded to stay by her side and spend my time with her. She mostly slept, but periodically awoke. I was always right by her side. She did not know who I was, but she could understand that I was significant. I always tried my best to hold in my tears when she was awake so I would not upset her. I held her hand and in the back of my mind I knew that these days were her last, and I pushed the tears back. The several IVs I saw drew more tears in my eyes. I looked at her and the fire in her heart was slowly dimming. Her perpetual smile was no longer there. She was not eating much anymore. It was all liquids.

The nurse called me into a room where my father and grandmother (my mother's mother) were sitting. The nurse told us that my mom's organs were shutting down and she was losing strength quickly. I instantly broke into tears. Nothing could fill the hole I felt that immediately overwhelmed my entire body and made me feel empty. I locked myself in the waiting room and curled into a small ball and cried for several hours.

I spent some time by myself with her although she was sleeping. I began to think about our infinite, wonderful memories, and I began to cry. She slowly opened her eyes, and I tried to stop crying. She looked up and asked to sit up. The remote bed slowly raised her so that she could sit up. The first words out of her mouth were, "How are you, Noelle?" My eyes opened wider, and I looked into her eyes. She had remembered my name, and she knew who I was without me telling her. We spent the next hour talking. She told me that she was hungry and I fed her some small snacks. We talked for a long time, but I was still overcome with sadness. I did not understand why she suddenly had a burst of life given to her. She told me I was her guardian angel, and she loved me more than anything. She still held my hand, and we both began to cry.

I thank God to this day for giving her one last chance to say goodbye to me. That day my prayers came true. All I asked for was one more time to talk to her and tell her good-bye, and that I know she will always be with me. I drove home that night feeling happy. That big emptiness had been filled in my heart.

I went to school the next week. I was called into the office where my grandparents were waiting. I saw them, and I began to cry harder than I have cried in my life. My entire soul felt as if it were empty and that nothing could fix it. I ran out of the office and found my closest friends, and I began to cry harder as they cried because they were also very close with my mom.

Weeks later I was still devastated, but I had time to think about everything. I realized that at my wedding I would not have a mom to help me get dressed or smile at me when I walked down the aisle. I would not have a mom when I graduate from high school, or when I get my first car. I could not cry on her shoulder, and I could not hold her hand when she needed me and I needed her.

To this day I love my mom more than anything, and I always will. She was the most beautiful, sweetest, considerate, giving person in the world. I just do not understand why she was the one who had to go.

My friend came up to me on the day of his mother's seven-year anniversary and asked me if I ever wake up crying. I nodded my head. He said he did, too. We hugged and I began to cry for both of us. He had lost his mother to cancer seven years earlier. He and I are best friends because we completely understand each other and how the emptiness can sometimes take the best of us.

Even now, just more than two years after she passed away I still think about her all the time and recall the wonderful trips we took together to Ireland and around the west coast of the United States, talks we had and music we wrote. I love her mentally and physically because I see her every day in myself and everything I am. I love her still, and I always will. I know that she will always be with me in my heart and soul, and I try to be what she wants me to be. The moment she held my hand that last time will be the moment that means more to me than any memory I will ever have.

I thank God for giving me the chance to know her and spend time with her. She has been the biggest influence in my life, and her teachings will last throughout my lifetime. I hope to pass them on to the generations to come. I also thank God for letting her go peacefully and for ending all her pain and suffering. The light burned in her eyes until she took her last breath. I know because she was strong. The chemotherapy and radiation she had throughout the six years had slowly weakened her, but she always held on. I am only sorry she had to fight so hard to live, only to lose the battle. She taught me many things, and now I can teach others how to survive and love themselves.

Her voice that sang me to sleep every night will stay in my mind forever. Every time I listen to her CD I cannot help but smile and cry just thinking about where she is now. Anyone who knew my mother knows that she was a good person and when people say, "Like mother, like daughter," I know that I will make her proud of me someday because I want to be just like her.

Someday
I'd understand,
It's better this way
And when this day came
It took all her pain
That came from the aching
Of a broken heart.

Things happen for a reason
And now I see,
That I'm here to teach others to be—
Happy.

I learn from you
My soul burns for you
I yearn to
Be with you
But that's what dreams are for.

—Noelle Dupont, Age 15

Wendy died September 2, 1997.

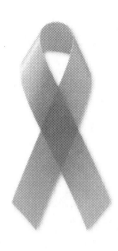

Four

Rosalind Jacobs

The Show
Must Go On

Survivor Profile:

Age at diagnosis: fifty-seven (1/10/94)

Age at interview: fifty-nine (5/1/96)

Type of breast cancer: infiltrating ductal

Size tumor: 1.2 cm: stage II

Two positive lymph nodes

Surgical procedure: lumpectomy

Treatment: chemotherapy and radiation, tamoxifen

Estrogen receptors: positive; Progesterone receptors: positive

Who's Who:

Gerald (Jerry) Jacobs, her husband

Amy Falk, her daughter (age thirty-two at time of diagnosis)

Sheri Berne, her daughter (age thirty-five at time of diagnosis)

Shirley Stevens, her sister

William (Bill) Stevens, her brother-in-law

Brad Falk, her grandson (age eight at time of diagnosis)

Brayden Falk, her grandson (age five at time of diagnosis)

Beverly Gemigniani, her friend

Barbara Stevens, her niece (author of this book)

INTRODUCING THE DANCIN' GRANNIES

Roz: Since 1991 I have been part of a nationally known troupe of twenty-five women known as the Dancin' Grannies who perform aerobic dance routines at parades and senior expositions around the country. Starting as a Parader I was invited, a year later, to be one of seven women who make up the Core Group. We perform at conventions. Beverly, who is our founder and leader (read her story in *Chicken Soup for the Woman's Soul* from Health Communications, Inc., 1996) choreographs all the dance routines which are comprised of different types of aerobic exercise: step, rubber band, and acrobatic moves such as splits, cartwheels, push-ups, somersaults and high kicks. Each show, lasting approximately thirty to forty-five minutes, consists of three to four dance routines. Then Bev teaches while we demonstrate how to work with rubber bands and how to exercise while sitting in a chair. We range in age from fifty-seven (that's me) to seventy-two. Our message is, "Health and fitness for the older woman."

LET'S NOT MAKE THIS A BIG DEAL

Roz: Five months earlier the mammogram I'd had was clear. I was not expecting to find a lump, and when I did I called my gynecologist to tell her. She immediately suggested that I have another mammogram. It, too, was clear. That is when I was referred to a surgeon who thought an ultrasound was unnecessary but did say, "There's something there. We're going to go in, see what it is, and go from there."

Jerry, her husband: Roz told me as soon as she found the lump. She had never had one before, and I just assumed it was a cyst because there was no history of cancer on her side of the family. I carried that belief with me throughout the meeting with her surgeon.

Amy, her daughter: I am always at my parents' house. One day while I was there she mentioned to me, "I found something. It's sore, and kind of feels like a lump." She was *thinking* about calling the doctor. "Don't tell me. Tell your doctor," I said to her. "There's no discussion about this. Tomorrow morning you are calling your doctor."

Sheri, her daughter: We found out afterwards that if it had not been for my cousin, Barbara's (see chapter 1) breast cancer diagnosis not even six months earlier, my mother probably would not even have been checking herself. But my cousin's diagnosis had made her nervous. Thank God. I seem to recall my mother being somewhat lackadaisical telling me she had found a lump during one of our phone conversations. My father was in total denial that it was anything other than a cyst. He would say things like, "Oh no. Not your mother. She's a Dancin' Granny." Or, "It doesn't happen in our family." He refused to listen to the surgeon who said to him, "How do you know?"

OH MY GOD—I HAVE CANCER!

Roz: As I stared out the car window on the way home I just couldn't believe this was happening to me. Jerry and I were carrying on a conversation, but I felt as though I were talking about a third person. I did not know what to think. That is how devastated I was. Frankly I was in shock for a few days. My niece, Barbara had such a positive attitude and suggested that I talk to other women. In fact, she gave me the name of a friend, Arlene Rosen (see chapter 5), who had also been diagnosed with breast cancer. When I started on this journey I did not know the kinds of questions to ask; consequently, I decided to talk to my doctor first to see what his recommendations were.

Jerry, her husband: One of the first things Roz's surgeon said to me after telling me she had breast cancer was that he knew a nurse who had had a similar type of breast cancer five years earlier, same size tumor and was doing well. Somehow that did not seem to matter to me because the first words out of my mouth were, "How long does she have to live?" I was sure this was the end. That is how little I knew about cancer. He became angry, "I don't want to hear any kind of negativity," and then walked out of the room.

Amy, her daughter: When I heard my mother had breast cancer I thought she was going to die. I was so scared I burst into tears, and could not stop crying. My father would not stop talking negatively even when the doctor said to him, "We're going to take care of this."

Sheri, her daughter: Shortly after my mother found her lump, I found one, too. Like her, if it had not been for my cousin, Barbara, I probably would not have been doing breast self-examinations either. Our biopsies were right around the same time which is why I was not there for my mother's. I don't know how I knew, but I knew mine would be fine. And it was. On the phone constantly with Amy and my parents, I did not know what to believe because I was getting different stories. Talk about being frustrated and confused!

Shirley, her sister: Feeling as though someone had thrown a bucket of cold water on my head I just could not believe that my younger sister, ten years younger than I, had breast cancer. I was stunned. It just was not possible. During the night I would lay awake replaying it over and over in my mind. Even though my daughter-in-law Barbara had breast cancer, it was different. It was in her family. There was none in ours, or so I thought until I found out much later that one of our first cousins had ovarian cancer. Apparently there is a link.

NOW WHAT DO WE DO?

Roz: Breasts were very important to me. In fact, I had breast augmentation surgery twelve years earlier because I wanted to feel more feminine, look better in clothes, and frankly feel better about myself. I was not giving them up unless I absolutely had to. My surgeon seemed to feel that my survival percentages were equal having either a lumpectomy and radiation therapy, or a mastectomy. A week later I had the lumpectomy, and he removed a 1.2-cm, pea-sized infiltrating ductal cancer along with three lymph nodes which is apparently all I had. The tumor was attached to the side of my implant.

Doing push-ups on the floor a couple of days later while at practice with the Dancin' Grannies, my leotard was suddenly soaked. My surgeon told me later that day that it was good that the pocket of fluid that had been building around the surgical site had burst through the staples he had used instead of stitches. That is when he put in a drain. Yuck!

Jerry, her husband: Even though I was scared I never said another negative word to Roz's surgeon after the day he yelled at me. Roz and I were both basketcases. As we cried and thrashed the whole thing out one night, somewhere between the biopsy and the lumpectomy, I remember thinking, *She looks so great. Now that she has cancer she won't be able to dance anymore. Her life is over, etc., etc.* Of course I did not tell that part to Roz even though we talked about our fears, about what could happen. I was so afraid of losing her. She was so afraid of dying and leaving me and the children behind. It was a very emotional night, yet was a turning point for us both. That is when we decided—no more negativity. Roz does not remember the surgeon telling her that he might have to remove her implant during surgery depending on where the cancer was, and what he found. Fortunately he did not have to. Another turning point for me was when the surgeon told me after her lumpectomy, "I think everything's going to be fine. I think she's going to do very well."

Amy, her daughter: More rational than either of my parents, even though I was still very frightened, I went to that fact-finding meeting with the surgeon specifically to take notes. It was a good thing I was there because afterwards, when the three of us talked, my parents did not remember half of what was said. My father picked out all the negatives, and my mother was not sure what she heard. She was clearly scared. "I just don't want to have to do chemotherapy." There was so much information being given that I finally asked him, "If it were you what would you suggest?"

MULTIPLE EARS ARE BETTER THAN ONE

Roz: Sheri insisted on flying out for the initial meeting with the oncologist I had been referred to. "I want to be there. You won't hear everything he's telling you." She was right. When you are that devastated you just cannot absorb it all. Both girls asked lots of questions which helped all of us understand what it was I would be going through. I was told, "We have one shot at this, so let's make it our best."

Jerry, her husband: It was a good thing both girls were there because, to be honest, neither Roz nor I were listening to the doctor. We were not thinking straight because we were so emotional, and we did not really understand what it was he was telling us.

Amy, her daughter: Our meeting with the oncologist was within a few days of my mother's biopsy, so we did not yet know whether or not any of her lymph nodes were involved. I asked him as I had her surgeon, "If it were your wife or daughter what would you do?" He also recommended the same course of treatment as her surgeon; in addition, he said that she should do chemotherapy. My father was definitely not the rock of the family. While Sheri was trying to explain to him why chemotherapy was being recommended, he was rambling on and on, "No. Absolutely not. She's not going to need chemotherapy. Everything's going to be fine," as I was thinking to myself, *Oh yes she is.* Finally able to get a word in edgewise I managed to say, "If that's what the doctor recommends and it gives her a better chance of survival she *is* going to do it." Suddenly we heard, "Excuse me. I'm right here. This is about me, so I think I ought to have a say in the matter." My mother had been sitting there almost in a daze as we talked about her as though she were not even in the room. I could tell from her tone of voice that she was quite annoyed at all of us.

Afterwards, as we rehashed what had been said, my mother had apparently made up her mind. "This is what he suggests, so I'm going to do a lumpectomy." My father was still in a dream world, and saying irrelevant things like, "But she's a Dancin' Granny."

Sheri, her daughter: By the time I came out for the meeting I had done a lot of research, even though I did not understand much of what I was reading. I had a copy of my mother's pathology report. My research indicated that for stage II breast cancer, which was her diagnosis, she would need chemotherapy. I said nothing, having decided to let the oncologist take the lead at our upcoming meeting. Amy was great. No question was too embarrassing for her to ask. She made the oncologist repeat himself, and elaborate on anything we did not understand. He, in turn, was terrific and spent a lot of time with us. My father misunderstood most of what was said at that meeting, which validates the importance of having more than one or two persons at those kinds of meetings. At that point I believe he was in total denial that my mother had cancer, plus he interpreted the recommendation that she have a lumpectomy to mean that her cancer was not as serious.

When Amy and I found out that two of her lymph nodes were positive there was no question in our minds that our mother was going to have chemotherapy. She began crying, and said only one time, "Why me?" Not as in woe is me, but more as a question. The three of us were starting to face reality at that point; my father on the other hand became irrational: "I don't want to talk about it"; "We're not going to talk about it"; "We're not telling anyone"; "People don't want to hear about these kinds of things." When my mother began to agree with him I said, "Oh no you won't. We're going to act normal, and if anyone asks we're going to talk about it. You're not going to act as though it isn't a big deal. It is. You're not going to sweep it under the carpet. If you act that way you're going to push people away." My father, probably because he did not want to deal with it, would not stop his negativity. "No. People don't want to hear; they don't understand." Reaching a breaking point Amy and I finally yelled at him, "Oh shut up!"

FOR SOME, A FEW WEEKS CAN MAKE A BIG DIFFERENCE

Roz: It did not take long for me to shift from victim to survivor mode. I had not been sleeping well and one night woke up in the middle of the night mad. I said to myself, *You know what? I'm not going to let this get the best of me or lead my life.* With that I went back to sleep.

Sheri, her daughter: It was important for my mental well-being to see my mother so I came home frequently. This particular weekend the four of us were going shopping for scarves, hats and a wig. My mother was so excited—it was going to be a fun-packed day. My father still could not accept the fact that she was going to have chemotherapy and frankly was very irritating while she was trying on wigs. "I don't like that color." "That doesn't look right." "I like your regular style better." It was apparent he was acting out his fears but even when I told him, "You're not going to lose her," he wouldn't stop. Again Amy and I yelled at him. "Just give it up! Shut up!"

TURNING CHEMOTHERAPY INTO A
POSITIVE EXPERIENCE

Roz: Because my veins roll, meaning they move all over the place and sometimes disappear, I had another surgical procedure to have a shunt inserted into my shoulder through which I would be given my drugs intravenously. Toward the end of February I began the first of six cycles of Adriamycin, Cytoxan and 5-FU. By then I had come to the realization, *This is going to help me, not hurt me,* so I was no longer frightened.

About ten days after my first treatment I knew I was about to lose my hair because my scalp became extremely sore and sensitive to the touch. Having already cut my shortish hair even shorter, it began coming out in clumps as I showered. Running my fingers through my hair as the water cascaded down my body I more or less pulled most of it out. Dressing then became a game. "How's my ensemble going to be put together today?"

Even though I was given Compazine, an antinausea drug in my IV, I learned to take more as soon as I got home from a treatment to help ease the nausea which was constant those first three months. Jerry would not let me lift a finger. Nothing was too much to ask of him. If I were tired he encouraged me to lie down. When I got up we would either go out for a bite to eat, or he would prepare a meal at home. Food smells were ghastly that first week after a treatment so I learned to eat cold foods. Tomatoes and citrus, because of their acidity, gave me mouth sores so they went on my "don't eat" list. Not unexpectedly I lost *all* of my body hair. My oncologist frightened me by saying, "If you develop a fever go directly to the hospital, and I'll meet you there. An infection could kill you." His caution remained with me throughout chemotherapy and is probably the reason why I was so paranoid about germs. When we ate out we limited my exposure to crowds by eating either a late lunch or early dinner, particularly during days eight through fourteen when my white counts were at their lowest and I was most susceptible to infection.

It was not until I had gone through one treatment that I felt ready to talk to my niece's friend, Arlene. Now I knew the questions I wanted answers to. For instance, how had she reacted to the chemotherapy? Was her experience similar to mine? What else could I expect?

During the early stages of chemotherapy Amy had videotaped one of my performances with the Dancin' Grannies at a local parade. I gave that tape, and one Beverly had made for me to the oncology nurse. Each time I had a treatment she would put them in the VCR for me to watch. As Jerry and I relaxed in the chaise lounges, me hooked up to the IV, we would chat with the other patients in the room and watch the performances. I closed my eyes and mentally did the dances in my head. That was a form of meditation for me and was how I got through chemotherapy and later on through radiation. My oncologist's office is still playing those tapes for their patients. "See what one of our patients did even while she was going through chemotherapy?" I felt they might encourage others to think, "Wow. If she can do that, there's no reason why I can't walk or do some form of mild exercise."

When I gained about twenty-five pounds my doctor said, "This is no time to go on a diet. Eat anything, anytime you want." And I did. To ease that gnawing feeling in my stomach I was on a two-hour feeding schedule including forays to the refrigerator in the middle of the night. It did not matter what I ate. Just so long as I put something, anything into my stomach. I got so heavy I began to waddle. Chemotherapy was almost always moved back a week because my counts were slow to rebound. I was not going on any road trips with the Dancin' Grannies; however, I continued to go to practice, and danced in the local performances. A couple of days after my third treatment we had a performance. We did two dances, each a minute and half long. My energy levels were not great, but I did it! By my fourth treatment I was feeling pretty wiped out. It became an effort walking from my bedroom to the kitchen, and my house is only fifteen hundred square feet. Those last three months I continued going to practice, but for the most part just watched and did not participate. That is when I developed pains in my chest, but the myriad of tests could never determine the cause. My heart was fine, and the pains went away.

Throughout my entire ordeal I kept a journal. In it, on my last day of chemotherapy I wrote, "It's over. I have such mixed emotions." I was so scared. Chemotherapy was my crutch. As I cried to the nurse, "What's going to help me now?" she reassured me that my reaction was normal. Radiation began a month later. Jerry came with me every day. As I lay on the table naked from the waist up I would close my eyes and mentally perform Dancin' Granny routines while that big machine positioned itself over me and zapped me in different places. When it was finally over, seven weeks later, my reaction this time was, "Now I can get on with my life!" Instead of fears and tears I felt great.

Jerry, her husband: Roz by now had made up her mind that she was not going to let cancer defeat her so how could I continue to be negative? Still scared, at least I was no longer thinking, *How much time does she have left?* It was not pleasant finding clumps of hair in the shower the week she lost her hair, but I knew it would happen so I was okay when it did. I had taken brochures from the oncologist's office so I had some guidelines, in addition to what he had told us about the side effects she might experience over the course of her treatment. He was very thorough. Her radiation oncologist was even more graphic. I understand *why* they do that. Still it puts ideas into your head. Thank God her implant did not get hard from the radiation!

If Roz were up to it I'd take her out to lunch after her chemotherapy treatment. We would make it like a date. I let her energy levels dictate what we did. If she wanted to go out we did; if she wanted to rest we stayed home. She was tired all the time.

Amy, her daughter: By the time my mother began losing her hair, all of us had taken a deep breath, "Okay. It's happening." We had decided to treat it like it was no big deal. Her attitude by then was very positive, which helped the rest of us deal with the fact that she had cancer. She changed her entire wardrobe and began wearing funky things such as big earrings, instead of dressing conservatively as she always had in the past. Unintentionally she became a trendsetter. People began complimenting her, "Beautiful scarf, fabulous hat." Then my father got into it. They shopped constantly. Instead of denying that she had cancer, or trying to hide the fact that she was bald, they began to dress it up, had some fun with it.

Sheri, her daughter: My mother turned a negative into a positive. What I saw was a woman making a fashion statement by the way she was dressing. Suddenly having cancer was not the tragedy my father had at first thought it to be. Her sense of humor was fabulous. One day, shortly after losing all her hair, she strutted into the living room. "Who do I look like?" she said as she whipped the towel off her head with a flourish. "Uncle Fester!" He was the bald uncle on the television show *The Addams Family.*

Shirley, her sister: What was extraordinarily difficult for me was seeing Roz with a wisp of hair here and there. It was easier for me to deal with once she was bald. She has a gorgeous face that does not need hair.

Beverly, her friend: When Roz said to me shortly after her diagnosis, "When I get better I'll come back," I knew the likelihood of that happening was slim. So I told her, "No. I don't want you to do that. In fact, I don't ever want you to leave. You're always in the Dancin' Grannies." I understood her not wanting to be around people initially because of her fear of germs, yet I knew the importance of not walling herself in because then she would not allow herself to have any fun. Fun to me is putting excitement, an energy into your body.

I made a tape of the different performances and parades Roz had been in so that while she was having her chemotherapy she would feel special. I wanted people to say to her, "You do that?" And they did, according to Roz. The tape was not just for entertainment. It accomplished several things. First, she was special within a group of people who were all hurting. Second, it was uplifting. And finally it was motivational not just to Roz, but to anyone watching.

Not sure what would motivate Roz I told her I wanted her to come to practice even if she just sat and watched while we practiced. I would say things to her like, "You'd better look at this move because you'll be doing it in two months." Or, "Do you understand the feel I'm looking for?" because each move has its own interpretation, and we are really actresses or should be. That helped take her mind off, "I'm a sick person"; in addition, it got her to use her brain and look to the future. I always made sure she knew of all our upcoming trips even if she could not be with us. Roz hung in there, and only occasionally was she feeling so ill that Jerry had to come get her and take her home.

ALTERNATIVE MEDICINE— IS IT FOR EVERYONE?

Roz: In addition to the meditation tapes Bev gave me she also came over several times a week to do Reiki on me, which is a laying on of hands. That was very effective and helped me to feel stronger. I also began using crystals and would hold them in my hands during chemotherapy.

Jerry, her husband: In my opinion Roz went overboard with vitamins, herbs and things like shark cartilage, but if she felt it helped, then it really did not matter what I thought. Since she has been taking those things she has not had any colds or sore throats. Obviously something is working. I am even taking some of them, and I have not been sick either.

Amy, her daughter: At first I thought, *What the heck is she taking now?* Then it was, *I don't care what she's taking if it's helping her. It's helping to give her a positive attitude.* Now I find myself writing down what she takes so I can pass on the information to other women who have been diagnosed with breast cancer.

TAMOXIFEN

Roz: The first thing my doctor did when I was diagnosed was to take me off hormones; the first thing he did when I finished chemotherapy was to put me on tamoxifen. Hot flashes were nothing new. I had been cooling off in the walk-in refrigerator in the restaurant we had owned for years. What is making me crazy is the weight gain. No matter how much I exercise I cannot get it off!

Jerry, her husband: I would never tell Roz not to take tamoxifen and I know it is something she has to take, but I want to know, "Why does she have to keep taking it?" because in my mind, she is fine.

Her weight does not bother me. I have been through all kinds of sizes in our thirty-nine years of wedded bliss.

WE ALL COPE DIFFERENTLY

Roz: I am not glad my niece had breast cancer, but her having had it helped me in so many different ways. Probably the most important was her emphasizing to me, "There is life after cancer." The second was the importance of maintaining a positive mental attitude. Even today people tell me what an inspiration I was. I still get phone calls, "Can you call so-and-so, and tell them what you went through?" I do and truthfully feel energized after we speak. It does not just have to be breast cancer. I'll talk to anyone who is going through a cancer experience. My niece did not go through chemotherapy; however, it is because of her that I was able to handle it as well as I did.

Before I became ill I would feel very uncomfortable when someone told me she or he had cancer. A typical response would be to either evade the subject or walk away. I would think anyone going through chemotherapy was on death's door. Now I walk right up to them. "How are you doing?" I offer them encouragement. "You'll get through this whether it's six weeks or six months from now."

Jerry, her husband: If Barbara had not gone through it first and explained things the way she did, and answered our many questions once Roz knew what to ask, a lot of things might have been handled differently. I was just as hungry for information as Roz, so when she called Arlene I was listening on the other end.

Roz and I react to each other. Not necessarily negatively, just emotionally. Under normal circumstances Roz is an emotional person. She remained emotional throughout her ordeal, but overall I would have to say she was coping okay once she made up her mind she was not going to let cancer defeat her. I would not let her quit the Dancin' Grannies and said to her, "Just go and watch if you can't participate." Sometimes I would have to walk away when I saw her just sitting there unable to perform. I never told her how much that upset me.

Amy, her daughter: When I used to hear that someone had cancer my first thought was, *They're probably going to die.* I am still a worrywart, but as a result of my mother's and cousin's experience, my attitude has changed and I find myself encouraging others. "Think positive." I'll show them my mother's picture: "Can you believe two years ago she had no hair? Look how beautiful she is now. She even continued to perform during chemotherapy." All my father remembers is that he did not want to tell anyone my mother had chemotherapy because he did not want people to feel sorry for her. He was as much a patient psychologically as she was those first few days. Once he got over the hump and realized that no one wanted to hear his negativity, or see him moping around, he was fine and back to his normal self.

Sheri, her daughter: It was not until later that I started remembering things I apparently blocked. For instance, I do not remember my mother telling me she found a lump although she insists she did.

It is really tragic the way so many people react when they find out someone has cancer, or that something bad has happened in a person's life. They don't know what to say nor how to say it. Sometimes they even avoid talking about it because they don't know and wonder, *Will they want to talk about it?* Or, *How are they going to react if I bring it up?* My mother's attitude was fantastic. Instead of avoiding questions such as, "How are you?" she might answer, "Yesterday was a bad day, but today's a good one." She talked about cancer as though it were an everyday normal occurrence, and showed them that she did not mind talking about it. Her openness helped make people feel comfortable. You could almost feel that sigh of relief, "Oh, okay."

On the other hand, my father's initial reaction was, "If we don't talk about it people don't have to worry." He did not want people to treat them differently, or feel as though they had to walk on eggshells once they found out my mother had cancer. In addition he did not want her getting hurt. He probably remembered people's reactions all those years ago when his sister was diagnosed with breast cancer. "What do I say?" "How do I act?" That is the reason I told him they had to talk about it so that people would not disappear from their lives.

Shirley, her sister: All I remember thinking was, *How did my kid sister get this, and it bypassed me?* and *Why? She doesn't deserve this.* In a sense I felt guilty that it was her and not me who had gotten breast cancer. If any of us had questions we asked my daughter-in-law, Barbara or our son, Bart, her husband. Who better to ask than the two of them who had already been through it? They offered only encouragement.

Bill, her brother-in-law: Jerry put up a good front never revealing his feelings. He maintained that great outlook he is known for—always smiling and joking. I was not going to probe because if he had broken down

I would have felt terrible; however, I was there if he wanted to talk. Shirley and I talked with one another, and she told me what was going on. As long as I knew things were under control I had some peace of mind although I did toss and turn at night.

Beverly, her friend: By nature Roz is a worrier, so the sale of their restaurant shortly before her diagnosis was a good stroke of fortune because it allowed Jerry to be by her side throughout all of her treatment. He is so positive. Wherever he is there is laughter, and it is bound to be action-packed. Roz called to tell me she had cancer. At the time it sounded as though she was handling it okay. But those were just words because she had not yet walked the distance. She had her niece whom she used as her role model as well as her family who did not have a boohoo-type attitude. Instead of sitting back and acting like a victim she began working through the process: buying hats, scarves and wigs before she lost her hair.

The whole concept of cancer was overwhelming to Roz in the beginning. I watched her attitude shift from initial fear, pulling back, tightening inward, to when she made the decision to move forward. Instead of asking a person, "How do you feel?" I read body language. Does that shoulder go forward just a little bit? Is that smile real? I look into a person's eyes. That is where I'll see the truth. Telephones serve a purpose, but I can't *see* when I talk on them. I think I hear, but is it the truth?

I would rather tell someone good news than buy them a plant or send a card. My good news for Roz would be fun things such as, "We got a call. We're going to be on television." Or, "We're going to be doing a photo shoot for such-and-such magazine. I know you'll be better, so you'll be able to do this." Then, knowing what a worrier she is, "Don't worry about your hair. We'll see how your wig is."

Not sure whether Roz would be able to perform the day the Dancin' Grannies performed outside in the 100-degree heat I did have some guilt. Disliking the connotation of the words, "Are you okay?" I probably asked her, "Do you still want to do this?" or, "Do you feel up to this?" I tend to ask only once because I expect my performers to know their own bodies. But I did watch her nonetheless. When we perform we are dancing hard and we perspire. Afterwards each of us tells the audience a little about ourselves. Roz never liked being in the limelight, but now, no matter where we perform, she walks up to that microphone with confidence and a strength in her voice, proud, "Look what I've accomplished." Not pushy, not egotistical; just Roz—a little shy, still with that sweetness she has about her. "I'm a two-year survivor of breast cancer, and I have a support team. I keep active." Then she will ad lib a little. Imagine how that group felt the day she performed when she told them she was in the middle of chemotherapy. Women always come up to Roz after a performance. "They just discovered my cancer, and it scared me. I'm so grateful for what you said." "What did you do?" "How did you feel when you did this?" "I'm just going through chemotherapy now. How do you feel now?" "My daughter has it. How can I help her?" What helps them, more so than her words, is seeing this vivacious beauty—a survivor—perform.

I love watching women of my generation walk down the path because I do not get to see it very often. Roz had to go through the trauma, but all the pieces were in place and she maneuvered right through it.

WHERE DID WE FIND SUPPORT?

Roz: Besides my family and friends, my support group was really the Dancin' Grannies. My close friends in the group would come over to the house and visit. We would laugh, talk, even cry. The tears were cleansing. Bev gave me a book, *You Can't Afford the Luxury of a Negative Thought* by Roger and Peter McWilliams, which had a tremendous impact on me.

Jerry, her husband: A lot of our friends did not know how to react. They did not call as frequently as they used to probably because they did not know what to say to Roz. We did not see them as often because we had stopped most of our socializing. I was more hurt by their actions than Roz and when I did finally talk to them they said, "If we told Roz we were going out to lunch and she couldn't join us because she wasn't feeling well, or she was tired, or her counts were too low and she couldn't chance being around us, then she might feel sorry for herself. We don't know what to do; therefore, we just haven't called." Halfway through chemotherapy Roz began to resume more of a normal life and that is when people stopped looking at her as being so sick. She was easy to be around which of course helped make them feel comfortable. That is when the phone began ringing again.

Amy, her daughter: I guess my father went through one of those "stages" you hear about—initial shock, then denial and finally he was back to normal. It seemed as though all of a sudden my mother was becoming a support for other people. Even her oncologist asked if she would be willing to talk to some of his patients about her experience. She did.

Sheri, her daughter: Becoming a Dancin' Granny was the best thing that could have happened to my mother. The camaraderie was incredible. It did not matter if she could not practice or dance with them. She was still a part of the group. They said prayers for her, they called her from the road to see how she was doing, and they did not ostracize her.

MY ONE REMAINING SIDE EFFECT —LYMPHEDEMA

Roz: Shortly after I finished radiation my forearm began to swell. For about three months I used a sequential pump to help squeeze the fluid out of my arm. You hook up the hoses, put your hand and arm into a plastic sleeve, and let the pump do the work. It did help except that my arm felt as if I hit my funny bone. Because my HMO would not pay for this equipment I stopped using it. The glove I was told would help control the swelling in my hand made it worse, so now I just live with it. It is pretty much gone except for some residual swelling in my wrist and a few fingers.

GRANDMA IS SICK— WHAT DO THE CHILDREN THINK?

Amy, her daughter: I told my boys Brad, eight, and Brayden, five, that their grandmother was sick and that for the next couple of months she would not be feeling well, so they would have to be on their best behavior when they saw her. "Try not to fight. Don't ask her to do a lot for you. Don't go near her if you don't feel well." Brayden cared only about playing; however, Brad wanted to know things like, "Can we catch it?" "Is Grandma going to die?" I explained to both of them that we were doing everything that we could. My mother talked to them about germs. "When you go to the bathroom, or sneeze you need to wash your hands." Brad became almost compulsive; in fact, he still is to this day and it has been almost two and a half years. Brayden washed them only when he remembered, or when Grandma reminded him to. He was really too young to understand. She told them there would be certain days during the month when she could not see them because that was when she would be the most susceptible to catching germs. Brad would call her just to see how she was doing.

I had mixed feelings about the children being around my mother. One part of me thought, *Keep them away from her,* while the other part thought that having the kids around her would be great therapy. They would keep both my parents busy so that they would not be sitting around feeling sorry for themselves; in addition, they would help keep their minds off what my mother was going through. Disregarding that little voice I kept hearing, *Gosh, that's asking a lot,* I asked if they would watch the children four half days a week. It worked out great for everyone. I guess the bottom line is that instead of second-guessing what they will say, ask and give them the choice. Do not assume.

Brad, her grandson: When Mom came home that day she was crying. When Brayden and I asked why she was crying she told us our grandma had breast cancer and that, "She's going to try to fight through this." Mom told me how scared she was and in the beginning cried a lot, but she kept reassuring me, "Grandma's going to be okay." I knew my mom was having a hard time dealing with it so I tried not to ask her to do so many things for me and would even make myself simple meals. She was over at my grandma's a lot, and didn't work that much during that time.

Both of my parents explained things to us like what it was, how they were going to fight it, and what her treatment was going to be, but I asked Mom more questions than I did Dad because she was with Grandma more. I knew how sick she was, but Brayden was too young. He knew she was sick, but he did not understand how sick.

Mom told us our grandma would lose her hair, and that she was getting a wig. "Don't make fun of her." Once I went into her bedroom to say hi. She never saw me standing there watching her putting on her wig. I did not want to make her feel bad and never told her I saw her doing that. I understand the treatment she had, but I just cannot figure out *how* she got cancer in the first place. I was afraid she would die, and talked to my mom about my fears a little bit, but not too much because I knew that would upset her. Grandma told me they found a lump in her breast, and that they had taken it out and she would be fine, but I asked Mom questions like, "When will she be better?" "Will she be able to play with us again?" "Is breast cancer contagious?" "How did it start?" "Can Grandpa get it since they're always together?" I did not ask Grandma or Grandpa questions because I do not like to bring things up that make others feel bad.

LIFE GOES ON

Roz: Jerry and I cried together in the beginning. I thought a lot about dying; in fact, I dwelled on it the entire time I was going through chemotherapy. I try not to think about it, but the possibility of a recurrence is always there in the back of my mind. I do not worry about it, but it is there. Brayden said to me not too long ago, "Grandma, are you still sick?" I told him, "No, honey. I'm better now."

I'm living my life the way I always have. I'm not going to spend my days worrying about dying because if it is going to happen it will. We all die. It is just a matter of when. I believe in miracles. I truly believe that God intended for me to get this disease so that I could help others. My niece was right: There is life after breast cancer.

Jerry, her husband: When my sister, Lil, was diagnosed at the age of fifty with breast cancer in 1969 the big "C" was not talked about. In fact, it was kept a secret. Ten years later, as a last-ditch effort, she went to Mexico for laetrile treatments but died shortly after beginning treatment. I suppose that is why I thought when Roz got breast cancer that it was a death sentence. At first I was angry in general, and at God. Why did you let this happen? It's been two years since her diagnosis. I am still scared, but I try not to think about it. Roz and I made a pact. We do not allow ourselves to be depressed. Now I wake up in the morning and

I feel great. I try not to be a mother hen when she gets an ache or a pain, but the fear is still there. Is it coming back?

Amy, her daughter: I'd wake up in the middle of the night and think, *Will she die?* but I did not discuss my fears with my parents. Why burden them? Besides we are a very superstitious family. What happened is like a bad dream, but I still worry about her. All those supplements she takes seem to be helping her, but I just hope the cancer does not come back someplace else. See? I'm just a natural worrywart. And my mother is so cute. Every time something good happens she'll say, "I'm so glad to be alive."

Sheri, her daughter: We did not know what was wrong, but my mother's physical looks changed during chemotherapy and she began aging. That really scared us because it brought up the issue of mortality. Now she is more beautiful than ever.

After that first year I did the blocking thing again. I put her having had cancer out of my mind. Truthfully I think my attitude was pure denial. Then about six months ago a young girl in my office who had had breast cancer five years earlier had a recurrence. I was horrified, "Oh no. Not again!" It never entered my mind that my mother could get it again. That is when I began remembering things like her oncologist telling us, "There's a 50 percent chance of recurrence after five years." I still feel as though she will be okay, but there is that other part of me that now worries. It is no longer stuffed down there. I had not given any thought to the fact that I could get breast cancer until then. Now I am fatalistic. I could. If I do, I only hope that I handle it with the same grace and dignity as my mother. I never knew how strong she was; moreover, I am not so sure she did either. Amy and I talked about whether we would want to know if we carried the breast cancer gene. She wants to know. I do not.

Shirley, her sister: When Roz called to tell me she was going to the doctor because she had pain in her back, and then called me later on so excited, "It's only arthritis," I laughed. See, it is all a matter of perspective.

Postscript, January 2000

Life is good, and my health is excellent. After being on tamoxifen for five years I was taken off of it this past October. The Dancin' Grannies have disbanded because Beverly moved to another state. I'm still exercising with an instructor. Three days a week I do aerobics, and two days a week I do stretching. In addition I walk on the treadmill. Family is still the most important thing to me, and I'm so grateful for each day that I can be with them.

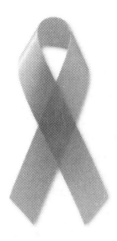

Five

Arlene Rosen

How Post-Traumatic
Stress Syndrome Almost
Cost Me My Life

Survivor Profile:

Age at diagnosis: forty-five (7/92)

Age at interview: forty-nine (5/14/96)

Type of breast cancer: infiltrating ductal

Size tumor: ¹/₂ cm; stage II

One positive lymph node

Surgical procedure: lumpectomy

Treatment: chemotherapy and radiation

Estrogen receptors: positive; progesterone receptors: negative

Who's Who:*

Mel Rosen, her husband

Ellen Rosen, her daughter (age twenty-one at time of diagnosis)

Beth Linke, her friend (age eighteen at time of diagnosis)

Pamela Fried, her mother (age seventy-one at time of diagnosis)

Fictitious names by request (including survivor)

FROM THE TOP

Arlene: In July of 1992 my husband, Mel, and I were excitedly making plans for our long-awaited dream trip to France that coming September. With thoughts still on the conversation I'd just had with a friend living in France, I went into the bedroom to give myself a breast self-examination—something I'd been doing for twenty years. Being intimately acquainted with my own very small, fibrocystic breasts, I was startled to find a lump that hadn't been there the month before. To be sure it wasn't just my imagination I asked Mel to see if he could feel it. When he said he could I knew I had cancer.

Even though Mel felt the lump was nothing to be concerned about, he suggested that I call our internist. But I felt differently. My mother had been diagnosed only three months earlier with breast cancer, the first in our family. I resolved to call sooner rather than later, and Mel and I saw my doctor the following day.

FASTER THAN A SPEEDING BULLET

Arlene: After examining my breast the doctor told me, "I'm 95 percent certain this lump isn't anything dangerous; however, I'd like you to see a surgeon." I went directly to a radiology lab for a mammogram, but when my lump didn't appear on the X-ray, I became uncharacteristically assertive and insisted that they do an ultrasound. They balked. Unable to repress my screaming instincts I turned to Mel for support, and he gave it, insisting that the ultrasound be given. I was lying on the table making idle chitchat with the doctor who thought I was overreacting, all of us watching the screen, when suddenly what looked like a sun sending rays of light across the horizon was clearly visible. It was a moment frozen in time, broken only when I heard the doctor's voice on the phone saying to my internist, "Get the surgeon to your office immediately—there is a lump and it has irregular edges."

When Mel and I returned to my doctor's office the surgeon was already there. Perhaps he was well meaning, but his patronizing tone, "Don't worry your pretty little head, I'll take care of everything" annoyed me. He did a needle biopsy which proved inconclusive, and since the lump was highly suspicious, I was scheduled for a surgical biopsy the next day, Saturday, at the hospital.

IGNORANCE IS BLISS

Arlene: The night before surgery, Mel and I went out to dinner. He tried to reassure me, "Don't worry—it's not cancer." Was he in denial or just trying to offer hope? I wanted him to face the likelihood with me that it was cancer, and talk about how were we going to deal with it. I knew once the words "You have cancer" were uttered, our life would be shattered. As bright as I am, I wasn't afraid because I did not make the connection that cancer kills—maybe I didn't want to. There was a simple solution: Remove the lump, and the problem is gone. End of story.

My children, David and Ellen, knew nothing at this point since it seemed pointless to upset them over an unknown. David was home from college for the summer. Ellen, also in college, remained on the East Coast.

Mel and I went to the hospital. My teddy bear, called Psycho for the psychologist who had given him to me, came along for security. Reassuring Mel that I would be fine, I sent him off to do his Saturday errands, and thought to myself, *Boy are you in for a surprise.* I wasn't frightened. Not really. I was too stupid to know any differently and, to be honest, was secure in my ignorance. That was how *I* coped.

When I awakened from surgery, Mel was by my side, and the surgeon brushed the hair off my forehead as though I were his child. I knew that the surgeon was trying to tell me that I had cancer. So I did it for him by saying, "I'm sorry to inform you, but you have cancer." He simply said, "Yes."

DECISIONS, DECISIONS

Arlene: Critical decisions needed to be made quickly because my infiltrating ductal cancer was aggressive. It was very confusing seeing so many doctors but not knowing *who* my team captain was. Additionally, I was irritated because this was taking time away from my very busy work schedule.

Mel had to remind me that, without treatment and doctors, I wouldn't have a busy schedule! After both of us had researched my options, Mel was in favor of my having a lumpectomy as it was more conservative than a mastectomy. We discussed all the what ifs, but ultimately, the decision was mine. I based my decision on what my internist had to say. "Every woman has a psychological profile. Given that survival rates are equal, only you know what you can comfortably live with. Some women don't ever want to worry again; therefore, they remove their breast. Others may have other issues they're dealing with, and feel they need to be more conservative. I'm not going to make a recommendation other than to say, you alone know what your psychological profile is." I trusted him and felt he had saved my life. My profile said that I wanted to keep my breast.

How Did We Cope?

Arlene: During the past six months I had faced one medical crisis after another. It was an extraordinary sequence of events: My dog died of cancer in December, my father died of cancer in February, three months later my mother was diagnosed with cancer, and then finally, so was I. Shortly after my surgery, Mel's sister had a hysterectomy, and within weeks of that, my older brother's wife, Felicia was diagnosed with colon cancer. Cancer, it seemed, was as common as the cold.

I was not in the mood or frame of mind to tell anyone, including my children, about me. If I didn't actually say the words, I could deny I had cancer; furthermore, I did not want to be treated differently *because* I had cancer. Only because Mel insisted that our family had a right to know, did I allow him to tell them, but he had to do it alone because I couldn't deal with their tears.

Ellen wanted to come home, but Mel said not to. It didn't seem to register with my son that I had cancer. My mother, although coping with her own cancer, called my two brothers in hysterics. The three of us had a wonderful conference call—they joked, and we laughed as we had always done, which helped me to feel normal. Our family has always used humor to cope with life's woes. If there is something to laugh about, we will find it—even at funerals.

I barely heard a word any of the doctors said to me so, consequently, they spoke to Mel. Emotionally I was trying to adjust to my new status as "cancer patient." Conversely my mind was on other important matters. I thought, *Why are we even here? My cancer's gone. They cut it out!* Even when Mel tried explaining things to me, I tuned him out, too.

Ellen, her daughter: It was highly unusual for me to get a phone call from home because Sally, my partner and the woman with whom I lived, did not get along with my parents. Any interaction with my family caused additional tensions between us in an already tense and troublesome relationship. By the tone of my father's voice it was immediately apparent that something was seriously wrong, and after what our family had recently been through my first words were, "Who's dead now?" When he said, "Your mother has cancer," I was stunned—it was so inconceivable. I did not know how to react.

THE DREAM CRUMBLES

Arlene: Exactly one week after my lumpectomy, I returned to the hospital to have my lymph nodes removed. Because I had researched this aspect of the treatment, I had a good understanding of the procedure, and the reasons why it was being done. Since my lump had been tiny, it was shocking to both my surgeon and me that one of the fourteen nodes they had removed was positive. The phone call in which I was told I would need chemotherapy shattered any last hope of a simple cure. My ordeal was not over and for the first time I cried. *What a waste of time,* I thought. I wondered if I would be able to attend my brother Howard's wedding the following month. Then I got mad when I realized our trip to France would have to be postponed.

Mel, her husband: I don't know why Arlene was surprised that she needed chemotherapy. We had been told that she would because of the aggressiveness of her cancer. She apparently chose not to hear that. All I could do was to be encouraging and reinforce to her that chemotherapy would help prevent a recurrence.

SOMETIMES ANTICIPATION IS WORSE THAN THE TREATMENT ITSELF

Arlene: Chemotherapy has this "reputation," and I was scared to death. When I met with the oncologist, I instructed him to tell me nothing about possible side effects because if he did, they might become a self-fulfilling prophecy. Only after I left that meeting did he discuss them with Mel.

When Mel drove me to my first treatment, I became increasingly withdrawn. At the office, passing open door after open door of patients getting their chemotherapy by IV (intravenously) I became unnerved. I had been promised mine was to be by injection; *they had lied.* By the time I reached my treatment room, I could no longer contain my fears. As I curled into a fetal position on the floor I began sobbing uncontrollably, "I am not going through with this." Only when I heard my doctor say they would have to postpone treatment did something snap and I screamed, "Just do it." The will to survive is strong.

They hadn't lied; the injection of methotrexate and 5-FU I was given in my hand was fast and painless. This was followed by two weeks of Cytoxan pills, and then two weeks of rest which completed the first of my six cycles. I never missed work.

I did make it to Howard's wedding shortly before my second chemotherapy treatment, and I felt like a celebrity. My hair, more than halfway down my back, was my pride and joy. But that evening when I took off my makeup I looked down, and there, on the bathroom floor, was half my hair. Who cared? *We* had made it through the wedding!

Helping me to cope during this difficult passage of my life were the visualization skills I had learned many years earlier. In this visualization I picked up the little "C" cells—the bad guys—and carried them off to wherever it is little "C" cells go. I did this frequently, not only during the treatment itself, but several times each day. Consequently, chemotherapy became routine and simply a place I had to be every four weeks. In the years since my treatment, I have spoken with many women and made light of chemotherapy because for me, I had neutralized it. Although many of the side effects were uncomfortable, they were not debilitating or unbearable, and my lifestyle was barely affected. Like many, in addition to hair loss I had moments of nausea and vomiting. Around the sixth month, I lost my fingernails and their beds, developed deep, dark circles under my eyes, and the elasticity of my skin changed, leaving me less youthful-looking. Having established the parameters with my oncologist that I not be told what to expect, I was taken by surprise when my periods stopped after the first month of treatment and never returned, and the hot flashes which plagued me began. As I approached my last chemotherapy cycle I was tired from the drugs' cumulative effects; nevertheless, I found myself, most times, supercharged. The ease with which I breezed through everything concerned my oncologist, and he was waiting for me to crash.

Food has never held much interest for me, and it held even less for me during this period. A nutritionist suggested I not eat foods I really enjoyed because chemotherapy has a tendency to affect one's sense of smell as well as taste. As a result, I gave up my much-loved chocolate, although to Mel's annoyance I continued to drink coffee and smoke cigarettes. By the time I had finished my six cycles, I could feel food in my mouth, but could no longer taste it. Poor Mel. Because I was nauseated by the smell of food, he had to cook his own meals and eat by himself. Additionally, because I wasn't eating, I lost almost 25 percent of my body weight, and looked anorexic at eighty pounds.

Radiation immediately followed chemotherapy. It seemed an impossibly long time—three, four-hour sessions—to get the coordinates right. Treatment was a snap: three thirty-second blasts take only fifteen minutes. Being treated as a breast and not a person was harder, but by this time I had taken back control of my life. When I asked why they were doing weekly blood draws, which I detest, I was given a "Because" answer by the doctor. I suggested he read my chart. Never during my months of chemotherapy had my numbers dropped out of normal range. When he said, "I won't treat you if you don't have weekly blood tests," I stood up, looked him in the eye and informed him that I would advise his front office where they could send my chart. With that he backed down, and I never had another blood draw.

Radiation was the more difficult treatment of the two because it physically drained all energy. All I wanted to do after a treatment was to go home, crawl into a ball and go to sleep. Consequently, my sessions were scheduled for the end of the day. Even though I am not fair-skinned, I was badly burned from the radiation. My breast is scarred, and I have a dime-sized indentation on my back as a result of a third-degree burn I received.

Mel, her husband: Even though I was with Arlene at all but one of her chemotherapy treatments I felt helpless. It bothered me that she wasn't eating, and that I had to cook my own meals, but I understood it was part of the process. There were always people at our home; things were constantly going on. When I tried to get her to slow down she snapped at me, "It's my life, so shut up." In hindsight I realize that her being hyperactive was a side effect of the antinausea drugs she was taking, but at the time I became resentful and frustrated with her.

Part of Arlene's problem was that she refused to realize that cancer could kill her. As a result she wondered, "Why am I doing this?" Perhaps she might have coped better had she been aware that chemotherapy destroys any microscopic cancer cells that are left.

Arlene also was prone to massive mouth infections which started before her cancer. After two separate one-week delays because of these infections, she didn't tell her oncologist about the third one. That may have been unwise, but she did not want any more holdups. Taking her last pill was a day of celebration for both of us. We felt as though a massive weight had been lifted from our shoulders. To me, radiation therapy was anticlimatic. I didn't feel that she needed my support for that.

Beth, her friend: Arlene is like my second mom. The night before I was leaving for my freshman year of college, Arlene called and asked me to come over. Casually, almost nonchalantly, she told me she had cancer and that I wasn't to be concerned; she would be fine. I cried more than she did. When I next saw her, over Thanksgiving, she was flying high and sailing through life. I wanted to talk about how she was, which we did a little, but she kept changing the subject.

Ellen, her daughter: Over Sally's objections, I went to Uncle Howard's wedding that August which was the first time I had seen my mother since her diagnosis. I needed to see her, to touch her. Just talking to her on the telephone was not enough. I started to cry when I saw her because now the cancer was real. My mother normally looks frail because she is so slender, but now she looked even more frail than usual, and her hair had started to thin.

I did not see her again until winter break, when Sally and I went home to visit. Instead of waiting up for me, like she had in the past, I found her in the bedroom sleeping; she looked so vulnerable. Smoothing back the few remaining white wisps of hair on her head I wondered, *What will I do if you die?* My mother is *the* most important person in my life. Sally insisted that it was time to go back to our home on the East Coast, but I wanted to extend our visit. I felt as though I was put in the position of having to choose between my girlfriend and my family. Leaving when we did was the most difficult thing I have ever had to do, and to this day I feel I made a bad decision. Shortly thereafter, my mother started to withdraw.

HUMOROUS MOMENTS

Arlene: I don't think David, my son, was ever in denial about my having cancer; I just don't think it ever registered with him that I had it. His attitude was, "Why worry? You'll be fine." I was conscientious that no one, including my children, see me without makeup or my wig because, without either, I looked ghastly. Feeling safe at six in the morning, I ventured into the kitchen to make myself a pot of coffee, looking *au naturel.* Little wisps of hair were sticking out all over my head. David, who has *never* seen this time of day, walked into the kitchen to get a glass of water, turned around and said, "Bad hair day, Mom?" To this day he thinks it was a bad dream.

BEWARE THE DANGERS OF POST-TRAUMATIC STRESS SYNDROME

Arlene: Perhaps my depression started during radiation because I felt as though I were on a short leash, having to be someplace, every day— for weeks on end. Maybe it insidiously sneaked in when treatment was finished. I felt let down, and I wondered, *Why did I go through all of that? Who cares?* The psychologist, whom I'd been seeing almost from the beginning of my diagnosis, felt *any* of the medical crises in my family could have been the trigger. I'd been running from one crisis to another and hadn't grieved for anyone, including myself. Frankly, it never occurred to me to ask for help; I was unaware that I was even suppressing my emotions. After all, I was the oldest of the siblings and it was expected of *me* to take care of things. Maybe the real truth is that it was all of the above, plus some. This later brought home another truth. Sometimes our actions communicate the wrong message to our children; I have not taught my own children how to ask for help.

I'd been depressed, feeling really blue, for about a year after I finished radiation. Mel was extremely supportive, but I became so nasty, was so emotionally abusive and impossible to live with, that he eventually withdrew from me—as I did from him. Our marriage suffered, although divorce or separation was never an issue. He didn't know, when he arrived home from work, whether he would find me manic or depressive. I accused him of being nonsupportive, and blamed him for everything—including the death of our dog. How rational was that? He had been with me every step of the way; nursing me, loving me, holding me every single night in bed, telling me, "If I could trade places with you, I would." What made this even worse was that I was fully conscious of everything I was saying and doing to him. I cut off my friends completely, refusing to return even their phone calls. My doctor kept suggesting that I take an antidepressant, and became frantic when I kept refusing. Finally, fearing for my life, he called Mel and said, "If something isn't done soon, we're going to have to institutionalize her." I was becoming suicidal—I felt so lost.

It was at this time a woman I hadn't seen in many years reappeared in my life. She, too, had been through her own breast cancer experience, including a bone marrow transplant. In desperation I asked whether she had suffered from depression. Laughingly she said she had been *so bad,* her husband wanted to kill her. She explained the direct relationship between serotonin levels and depression; the lower the level, the greater the depression. Once she began taking Zoloft, an antidepressant, she felt like a new person. As a result of this revelation, I, too, took Zoloft and began my emotional recovery.

I have spent a lot of time apologizing to Mel, and it has taken a long time to repair the damage my behavior caused. The self-imposed isolation I experienced is one of the symptoms of post-traumatic stress syndrome. With shaking hands I picked up the phone to call a close friend I'd not spoken to in eighteen months, not knowing whether or not she was still my friend. When she heard my voice she said, "I am so glad to hear from you. I have missed you and have so much to tell you."

During the worst part of my depression Ellen had graduated from college, broken up with Sally and moved back home. With her I can talk about my deepest feelings, something I have always had problems doing. I have counseled many women, but have never shared my feelings, or my emotions with any of them. By mutual consent, Ellen came with me to the psychologist. That was beneficial because she kept me honest. She was able to put her spin on things I wasn't able to articulate exactly right because the hardest words for me in the English language are, *I feel.*

I have come to realize that for me, the issue wasn't my treatment or the cancer—it was post-traumatic stress syndrome. And I have cautioned many women to be aware of its onset.

Mel, her husband: I have blocked out so much of this period in my life because it was painful. Arlene was functioning, but why was she so depressed? I didn't think it had anything to do with me. It made no sense. Obviously it was a chemical imbalance because once she took Zoloft, her mood swings evened out and her depression eventually disappeared.

This "syndrome" is real and dangerous; it is a major side effect the doctors do not discuss and they should. If a person *should* be happy but they're not, look to see if there is a medical cause for the mental depression. Arlene might take Zoloft for the rest of her life because within months of going off it, her depression returns.

Beth, her friend: Arlene had shut me out of her life which hurt. Reluctantly, she saw me the following summer which was the first time I had seen her since Thanksgiving, and I found her close-mouthed and depressed. All she would say was that she and Mel were having problems, and that her work was not going well. She explained about her depression, but it was still frustrating that she wouldn't let me help her, and I felt helpless. We did not see one another until the following spring, by which time she was almost back to the old Arlene. Our relationship is back to where it was before.

Ellen, her daughter: My parents came to my graduation in the spring of 1993. I had not seen my mother since Christmas and she looked on the verge of a breakdown: reed thin and emotionally strung out, near tears; a drowning person. It's not that my father was oblivious to what was going on, but he saw her on a daily basis whereas I was seeing her from an outsider's perspective. My perception was that he did not know how to help her and felt helpless.

With prodding, she finally told me about her depression and that she was emotionally in trouble. It crossed my mind that my mother wouldn't die from cancer, but from this depression that seemed to be eating her from the inside out. Truthfully, I do not think she would have minded dying. Her will to live was dwindling.

Since I remained on the East Coast after I graduated, my only communication with my parents was by phone, other than one short visit from them. Distance allowed me to *see* how she was—with my ears. The tone of her voice could not disguise the emotional fatigue. It was obvious to me that her "superwoman" routine was a sham. Despite her problems, she was able to help me sort through my messy relationship problems with Sally which were going from bad to worse. Besides, she claimed that my problems helped her to focus on someone other than herself.

When I finally moved back home, my mother was still a mess. Work seemed to be the only thing that kept her going. I would tell my father in various ways that mom was in bigger trouble than he realized. He has never been "Mr. Communicative" and that has been frustrating for me. Thank God I was getting help from my own therapist. It was to her I turned, in tears, when my mother confided to me one day, "I want to die." I wanted to know what would make her want to live again. Both of our lives turned around when we went on antidepressants. In my case, it was Prozac.

When someone you care about experiences any kind of crisis, watch for signs to see if they need professional help. Someone saying, "I want to die" is a *big* sign. The person in trouble needs to be able to talk with someone who is impartial; someone he or she can confide in guiltlessly—

a person who will not take offense at what is being said. It is also help-ful to accompany that person to the therapist, if he or she is willing. Not only did it help my mother, but it helped me. I only wish my father had gone for counseling—it might have helped him to cope.

Too many doctors are missing the mind/body connection. Cancer *is* a biologically based medical problem, but there are psychological problems that go with it. As research is proving, emotions do affect the physical body and its ability to recover.

SUPPORT IS A TWO-WAY STREET

Arlene: Bernie Siegel, the author and physician, made abundantly clear the power of a support system; the power of believing. Another author wrote about the power of laughter. Within eight weeks of my own diagnosis, I found myself helping other newly diagnosed women and their families, answering their "What's next?" questions. Not everyone can do what I do, and I have counseled many women that it is okay to be selfish and that there should be no feelings of guilt if they do not want to talk to others. If someone says something they don't want to hear, they can speak up by saying, "I'm sorry, but understand that what you're say-ing doesn't help me." I have repeatedly advised women who have been the recipient of thoughtlessly told horror stories, "That's their story, not yours—and it does not have to be yours. There are too many survivors."

Some women have no support system, and that is tragic. Sitting in the tiny dressing room I had just returned to after receiving my radiation treatment one afternoon, was a woman I had never seen before. She was still in her dressing gown, and sat staring at the floor with tears stream-ing down her face. I got down on my knees and asked if she wanted to talk. It was clear that she had only one breast. Words tumbling from her mouth, she told me that her boyfriend had deserted her, she had lost her job, and felt as though her world were imploding. Nobody had taken one minute—not one minute, to talk with her. The foundations of her life had crumbled, and she had nowhere to turn, no one to talk to.

Mel, her husband: Not having anyone to talk to made me aware of the importance of offering support to the caregiver (the person who's providing the care). Even if they don't want to talk, make the effort to let them know you are there if they want your help.

MOTHERS AND DAUGHTERS

Arlene: Because my mother didn't seem concerned with her cancer, it didn't dawn on me that she could be in any danger. Her cancer had not yet broken out of the duct (called intraductal or DCIS), so she was comfortable with the decision she had made to have a lumpectomy and radiation therapy. My mother breezed through everything with no complications and said her only complaint was being on a short leash for six weeks of treatment. Because of tamoxifen's side effects, she elected not to take it. At that time, we did not know its benefits like we do today. For my mother, who was seventy-one when diagnosed, breast cancer was just one more thing in her aging process.

Perhaps it was coincidental that we both got breast cancer. I will admit that I was frightened for Ellen when I was diagnosed. With time, my fear has decreased, but the concern is still there. It may be naivete on my part, but I feel the BRCA1/BRCA2 gene testing offers us an early warning system. The trouble is, she changes the subject whenever I bring it up. I probably wouldn't want to think about it either, if I were only twenty-four. Will I get tested? Maybe.

Ellen, her daughter: It seems pretty obvious that breast cancer runs in the family, and that my chances of getting it are pretty high. It's not like I think I can't get it, I just choose not to focus on it. I am more careful about what I eat, but I'm still not that careful—I want to *live* my life. As for gene testing, I truthfully don't know what I will do if my mother does get tested.

Pamela, her mother: A year and a half before I was diagnosed, a mammogram detected microcalcifications in my breast which a biopsy determined to be precancerous. At the time, my husband became very ill, and I was too busy taking care of him to take care of myself. By the time I'd had that long-overdue mammogram after he died, that suspicious lump had become cancer. Frankly, I was not surprised—I had been given ample warning. What shocked me was my daughter's cancer. What concerned me greatly was her state of mind.

SURVIVOR'S GUILT

Arlene: Within six months of completing treatment, I discovered another lump in the same breast. Neither Mel nor I panicked. When I immediately went to see my surgeon he berated me, "You should have cut them off," which infuriated me. How dare he treat me like a three-year-old and not respect the decision *I* had made! Storming out of his office, I immediately went over to Mel's office. While I was ranting and raving, my brother called to tell us that Felicia's cancer had returned and that she had just been given a terminal diagnosis. That stopped me dead in my tracks. I have never wanted to admit it, but I think this is what triggered my depression.

Until now, I had done almost no reading on cancer. With this news, I focused solely on Felicia and read everything I could get my hands on. Again, this is how I coped. All that could be done for her with conventional medicine was being done, so I pursued holistic avenues. Even then, I made no connection between her situation and mine. My cancer was gone—it had been cut out! Fortunately, this new lump turned out to be nothing.

Felicia was a remarkable mother and wife. Even while undergoing hellish treatment for her cancer, she remained active in her three children's (ages six, eight and ten) lives, continued as president of the PTA, and managed dinner parties for eighty with ease. This period was an insurance nightmare for them because my brother was unemployed at the time. Distance was between us—I in Phoenix, she in New York. All I could do was offer support by writing and talking on the phone as we had been doing since the beginning stages of both our cancers. With one another we could drop all pretenses. I was okay until I realized we were no longer in the same boat; I was recovering and she was dying. My own denial that cancer kills remained with me until the day Felicia died. She was only forty-two. Shortly thereafter, I discovered a third breast lump (same breast). And again, I was lucky.

I still suffer from survivor's guilt. My children are grown; hers aren't. *What would they do without a mother?* Brianna went through puberty at the age of nine, just like her mom. Only she did not have a mom to talk to. I would say to my brother, "Don't try to be both Mom and Dad."

When he would respond, "I don't know what to do with Brianna. She needs a female role model, she's having trouble in school, and has gained too much weight; Alex is withdrawn; Ben's out of control; and I want my wife," my heart broke. I have to come to terms with the fact that she's dead, and I'm alive. I miss her so!

COPING WITH DEATH AND DYING

Arlene: Irrational or not, the further out from diagnosis I get, the more frightened I become. Always, about a week before my oncology examination, the fear starts building; I am petrified they will find something. When they do not, I feel as though I have been given a reprieve. Fear still remains that, while doing my monthly BSE, I will find another lump, particularly in the breast that didn't have cancer.

Even before my getting cancer, Ellen's biggest fear has always been about losing me. This is an issue we have been working on for a long time, so my getting cancer only exacerbated her fears.

I am still driven as far as my work goes, but my goals have changed. I do not feel quite the sense of urgency to get things done. I have not quite come to terms with my mortality, but I do know now that cancer kills.

Mel, her husband: I was never in denial, yet my initial reaction to Arlene's finding the lump was that it could not be cancer. When it turned out that it was, I just wanted to know, "What do we do to get through this?" Concerning my accounting practice, I functioned by doing only what absolutely had to be done as I wanted to spend as much time as possible with Arlene. Truthfully, I didn't think she would die, but recurrence was a concern, particularly during those first two years.

It concerned me that Arlene was doing too much then, and even today she tends to take on more than I think is healthy for her. Maybe she feels there will not be enough time, but I remind her of the other side—*if* there isn't going to be enough time, don't forget to take time out and smell the roses.

Do I worry about Ellen getting cancer? No—well, maybe; I don't know. Maybe it's wishful thinking that she won't; maybe it's denial. I suppose that I'm hopeful that twenty years from now breast cancer will not be a major problem.

Beth, her friend: As a result of Arlene's reassurances in the beginning that breast cancer wasn't a big deal, to me it wasn't—until she became depressed. It is my fault for not telling her how hurt I was by her silence, but given her state of mind it probably would not have made a difference, except I would have felt better if I had said something. I realized that cancer kills, but chose not to dwell on it. However, I started to worry about my mom getting it, and if she did, how would I deal with it?

Then, as today, I still feel as though Arlene is putting up a front concerning her breast cancer experience. *Then,* because she wouldn't talk about *her* experience; *today,* when she says, "Everything's fine—nothing happened—no big deal."

I had my own scary incident when I, too, discovered a breast lump. Arlene's positive attitude and support was fabulous, but I was scared; I knew too much. At the insistence of my mother and sister that I seek a second opinion after my pediatrician said, "Don't worry, it's only a cyst," I sought out a surgeon. Arlene lent me Psycho, and he was in my arms comforting me, as I was wheeled into the operating room. It was a happy ending—it was only a fibroadenoma (a common, nonmalignant lump that's smooth, round and hard).

Ellen, her daughter: Distance has its pros and cons, and intellectually I know that my mother was trying to protect me by hiding her depression. However, she should have allowed me to make my own decision on how involved I wanted to become. Mothers need to let their daughters into their lives. Basically my mother is the same person she has always been, yet she seems to grab hold of life more than she did before. My father, on the other hand, seems more emotionally available these days, and I have a lot of respect for him.

Pamela, her mother: I felt alone when I was diagnosed; I was a widow, and all my friends were married. None of them had gone through breast cancer, and as a result it just wasn't a topic you discussed other than casually. As we age, death and dealing with illness become a part of our daily lives, so we tend to shy away from these subjects. My 101-year-old mother-in-law, with whom I'm close, never did find out

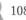

about me. What would have been the point in telling her? I did eventually find a woman I knew who'd also had breast cancer, and we did talk a little. But it was my psychiatrist, whom I'd been seeing on and off for years, who was the biggest help to me.

Shortly after Arlene had finished her treatment, I asked her to call the daughter of a friend who had just had a breast cancer recurrence. In hindsight I should not have done that because I believe it made her feel vulnerable. To this day I don't know whether she ever made that call.

As a result of Arlene's cancer, I think some of her wonderful qualities are even better. She has the ability to really *listen* to people, and she cares about them. You know that when she speaks, she's coming from something she herself experienced.

It's been five years since my diagnosis. Am I out of the woods? It's still not behind me—a couple of days ago I felt a pain and I wondered . . . *I did not have a checkup when I should have. Last time I waited, look what happened.*

Postscript, January 2000

Mel and I just celebrated our thirtieth anniversary. Ellen has found a wonderful significant other, and they have been together five years. My son David was married in 1998 to a wonderful woman and the following year we were blessed with a granddaughter who is the absolute center of our universe. My health is excellent, and I am smelling the roses. A sad note is that my mother died of kidney cancer in 1998.

Whenever I am informed of yet another woman facing breast cancer, I send Psycho to her with the following note: "This is Psycho. She is an expert in hospital routine and will help through the days ahead. The prayers and wishes for your full and speedy recovery from dozens of women come with her for she has kept vigil for them as she will for you. Keep her as long as you need her. And when you are ready, return her to me so that she can be ready for whomever needs her next." At the moment, she is back with me, packed and ready to go if she is needed. But our prayers are for the day that she need never accompany another woman to the hospital.

READER/CUSTOMER CARE SURVEY

If you are enjoying this book, please help us serve you better and meet your changing needs by taking a few minutes to complete this survey. Please fold it and drop it in the mail.

As a special **"Thank You"** we'll send you news about new books and a valuable **Gift Certificate!**

PLEASE PRINT   C8C

NAME:_____

ADDRESS:_____

_____

TELEPHONE NUMBER:_____

FAX NUMBER:_____

E-MAIL:_____

WEBSITE:_____

(1) Gender: 1)_____Female 2)_____Male

(2) Age:
1)_____12 or under   5)_____30-39
2)_____13-15   6)_____40-49
3)_____16-19   7)_____50-59
4)_____20-29   8)_____60+

(3) Your Children's Age(s):
Check all that apply.
1)_____6 or Under   3)_____11-14
2)_____7-10   4)_____15-18

(7) Marital Status:
1)_____Married
2)_____Single
3)_____Divorced/Wid.

(8) Was this book
1)_____Purchased for yourself?
2)_____Received as a gift?

(9) How many books do you read a month?
1)_____1   3)_____3
2)_____2   4)_____4+

(10) How did you find out about this book?
Please check ONE.
1)_____Personal Recommendation
2)_____Store Display
3)_____TV/Radio Program
4)_____Bestseller List
5)_____Website
6)_____Advertisement/Article or Book Review
7)_____Catalog or mailing
8)_____Other_____

(11) What FIVE subject areas do you enjoy reading about most?
Rank: 1 (favorite) through 5 (least favorite)
A)_____ Self Development
B)_____ New Age/Alternative Healing
C)_____ Storytelling
D)_____ Spirituality/Inspiration
E)_____ Family and Relationships
F)_____ Health and Nutrition
G)_____ Recovery
H)_____ Business/Professional
I)_____ Entertainment
J)_____ Teen Issues
K)_____ Pets

(16) Where do you purchase most of your books?
Check the top TWO locations.
A)_____ General Bookstore
B)_____ Religious Bookstore
C)_____ Warehouse/Price Club
D)_____ Discount or Other Retail Store
E)_____ Website
F)_____ Book Club/Mail Order

(18) Did you enjoy the stories in this book?
1)_____Almost All
2)_____Few
3)_____Some

(19) What type of magazine do you SUBSCRIBE to?
Check up to FIVE subscription categories.
A)_____ General Inspiration
B)_____ Religious/Devotional
C)_____ Business/Professional
D)_____ World News/Current Events
E)_____ Entertainment
F)_____ Homemaking, Cooking, Crafts
G)_____ Women's Issues
H)_____ Other (please specify) _____

(24) Please indicate your income level
1)_____Student/Retired-fixed income
2)_____Under $25,000
3)_____$25,000-$50,000
4)_____$50,001-$75,000
5)_____$75,001-$100,000
6)_____Over $100,000

FOLD HERE

((25) Do you attend seminars?

1)_____Yes   2)_____No

(26) If you answered yes, what type?

Check all that apply.

1)_____Business/Financial

2)_____Motivational

3)_____Religious/Spiritual

4)_____Job-related

5)_____Family/Relationship issues

(31) Are you:

1) A Parent?_____

2) A Grandparent?_____

Additional comments you would like to make:

_____

_____

_____

_____

N-CS

C8C

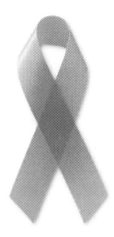

Six

Betty Fine

How Could a Trained Radiologist Miss My Lump?

Survivor Profile:

Age at diagnosis: fifty-seven (7/93)

Age at interview: fifty-nine (5/30/96)

Type of breast cancer: infiltrating ductal

Size tumor: breast 3–7 cm, axilla (underarm) 9 cm, tumors on superclavical and internal mammary chain; stage III

Eight positive lymph nodes

Surgical procedure: mastectomy

Treatment: chemotherapy and radiation, tamoxifen, Taxol, Megace

Reconstruction: no

Estrogen receptors: positive; Progesterone receptors: negative

Who's Who:*

Don Fine, her husband

Julie, her friend

Noreen, her friend

Fictitious last names by request (including survivor)

EVEN WHEN YOU DO ALL THE RIGHT STUFF

Betty: My body was bent over using free weights for arm exercises when I felt this really big lump under my arm and thought, *What the heck is that?* Since I was scheduled for my annual gynecological examination within a few weeks, I decided to wait and have it checked out then. When my gynecologist felt it, she said it needed to be biopsied and referred me to a surgeon. He did the biopsy and of course it came back malignant. That was in July of 1993. The mammogram I'd had done the previous November was negative.

Don, her husband: When Betty told me about finding a lump I didn't think much about it. I didn't know that a lump under the arm was significant. When you think about breast cancer you think of a lump in the breast. Now I know better!

We had planned a five-day trip, and decided not to cancel it. Betty scheduled her biopsy for the day after we returned. We worried the entire time and didn't enjoy ourselves. When we finally had our meeting with the surgeon, he told us it was probably cancer because there were two lumps.

Noreen, her friend: My husband and I have been friends with Don and Betty for years. They had already moved to Arizona; we hadn't—yet. Every year the four of us go to a concert festival. Don called my husband and said, "We're not going to be able to go." He started to cry and couldn't finish the call. Betty had to get on the phone and tell us that she had just been diagnosed with breast cancer. I started to swear (something I do frequently), and then we all started to cry.

AS CHANCE WOULD HAVE IT

Betty: A cousin of mine is Dean of Nursing at a hospital. I called her immediately and she recommended that I go to a particular National Institutes of Health (NIH) cancer center where other cousins of mine (one a doctor) work. We went a few days later. What we saw was simply overwhelming. The facility was huge, and cancer patients in various stages of health were everywhere. I had now joined the ranks.

It was requested that I bring with me my last two mammograms as well as the pathology slides from the biopsy. I was given numerous tests: CAT scans, bone scans, ultrasounds, different staging tests, even a dental examination because of probable mouth and gum problems I might develop as a result of treatment. When all the tests were done, a team of doctors had a tumor conference in which a strategy for treatment is planned and recommendations are made.

Because my cousin was involved in my case, she was part of the conference. As a result I got the "inside track" when the conference was concluded. We met privately. Her first words were, "I have some good news and some bad. Your bone scan is clear, but the tumors are clearly visible on the November mammogram." There were times I cried, but overall I had been fairly calm throughout my ordeal. Upon hearing this though, I was devastated and broke down. I thought, *My God. I've done everything I'm supposed to. I'm depending on the medical community to keep me well and they've just let me down.*

At the official meeting the next day which included Don, me, and both cousins, the oncologist laid everything out. He was very frank. The news was not good. I was a stage IIIB. The tumor in my breast was 3 to 7 cm and the one in my axilla (under my arm) was 9 cm. For a reference point, 5 cm equals 2 inches. In addition to those, I also had tumors on the superclavical (near the collarbone) and the internal mammary chain. My chances of recurrence were 40 to 60 percent.

WHEN THINGS MOVE SO FAST

Betty: I was the one who called everyone to let them know I had cancer because I wanted them to hear it from me, not through the grapevine. Throughout the phone calls I cried.

When we returned home from the medical center I called my parents. They were unaware of my diagnosis because I was trying to shield them. My mother was totally involved in caring for my dying father, and I didn't want to burden them with this. However, my father, who thought our two- and one-half-week trip had been for pleasure, kept asking how our vacation was. I couldn't lie. He was overwhelmed by emotion, but we got through that. Fortunately, my brother was living with my parents at this time, so I didn't have that burden.

Don, her husband: It was the initial shock of hearing that Betty had cancer that was the worst and most emotional time for me. I was never in denial; in fact, I was very realistic about everything that was going on. In my opinion, denial tends to eat away at your subconscious and is, therefore, unhealthy. Betty and I both tend to jump right in and face any situation, plot a course, and then follow it to wherever it leads us. That was fine and good; however, my mind was in constant turmoil, and initially I had problems sleeping.

As much as I wanted to, and as much as Betty wanted me to, I was unable to call our family and friends to tell them about her. Every time I picked up the telephone I got a lump in my throat. On the other hand, she actually liked talking about what was happening, and there were constant discussions between her and our family and friends. I wouldn't have minded talking about it, but no one really talked to me. It seemed I was invisible.

Being part of the process at the medical center was good for both of us because it kept our minds occupied. While she was being tested I found a quiet corner and read a book. Once we knew when she would be starting chemotherapy and that her portacath (a venous access catheter) had been surgically implanted I felt as though we were moving forward. I became emotionally calmer. That's when I began to feel that her cancer was not going to be deadly.

Julie, her friend: Betty's nickname is "the great, unflappable Betty Fine." That's because when she, Don, Noreen, Rick, my husband and I were traveling together in Spain and became totally lost, Betty calmly and unflappably figured out how to get us to where we needed to go. This is a woman who can face calamity.

A LARGE TUMOR PUTS YOU IN
A WHOLE DIFFERENT CLASS

Betty: Before we went to the medical center my expectation was that I would be having an immediate mastectomy. That was ruled out because the tumors were so large, and the doctors wanted to shrink them first. I did ask about the feasibility of a lumpectomy, but because of the size of the tumors was told that option was totally out of the question.

I started my first cycle of Cytoxan, Adriamycin and 5-FU (CAF) during my two- and one-half-week stay at the medical center. For forty-eight hours I wore a pump which continually fed the Adriamycin and an antinausea drug through the port into my body. I finished the balance of my cycles at a medical facility in my hometown using the same drugs. Don and I were taught how to keep the port sterile. I knew the importance of that because a friend of mine had died, not from her cancer, but from an infection caused by her port. Don isn't really good with medical things, and he was the one who had to clean my port. In hindsight I wish I had videotaped his first attempt. As he put his left hand into the right-hand glove, I broke out in a cold sweat. Not from pain, but from anxiety. I wondered, *Is he going to come through this? Is he doing it right?* He might have been a little shaky that first time, but he became quite adept at cleaning it!

Three months after my initial cycle I returned to the medical center for my first evaluation. They were astounded—the internal mammary and superclavical tumors had disappeared. Although the one in my breast and under my arm were still there, they were significantly smaller. But I still wasn't ready for a mastectomy as the tumors were still too big. That is when I learned that breast tissue extends beyond the breast. It encompasses the whole chest and even part of the back. So it is a misconception that having a mastectomy removes *all* of your breast tissue. Chemotherapy continued and finally, after having it every three weeks for six months, I had a single modified radical mastectomy.

Throughout my entire experience with chemotherapy I was never nauseated. My biggest problems were mouth and tongue sores. Nothing alleviated that pain. Bone loss is another side effect, and as a result, my periodontal problems were exacerbated and I lost two teeth. I was postmenopausal, but my ovaries were apparently still producing some estrogen because my migraines, which I knew were hormonal, stopped once I started treatment. And I was having hot flashes. My nails, which developed a bluish cast to them from the Adriamycin, returned to their normal color within four months of stopping the drugs. Like many others, I lost my hair, eyelashes, pubic hair, hair on my arms, but not all of my eyebrows. Food smelled and tasted fine; I gained only about ten pounds. I was a little panicky when my foot became itchy and very red. It looked awful. That was cellulitis—a skin infection which did go away.

Wigs were an experience. I was very sensitive about losing my hair and bought a really good wig. Opening the oven door one night, I was hit with a blast of hot air and singed my bangs. I bought another expensive wig. Wouldn't you think I had learned my lesson? Nope. I did the same thing again. The third time was the charm. I mail-ordered an inexpensive wig which was the most natural-looking one I'd had.

Don and I continued to live our lives as we'd always done—going out frequently to plays and concerts. I felt fine physically and emotionally, and ignored the doctor's warnings to stay away from crowds because of the risk of an infection. I never had a problem.

About a year or two prior to my diagnosis my shoulder became frozen. Even after eight months of physical therapy I still did not have full range of motion. As a result I needed an additional month of physical therapy to make it flexible enough so I could begin six and a half weeks of radiation therapy. Without the therapy my arm would not be in the correct position for them to irradiate my axilla.

Don, her husband: We were on such a high. Betty's progress was fabulous—her tumors were shrinking as a result of the chemotherapy. I had expected that she would be cured after her mastectomy because her doctor had been so positive. She'd said, "Oh, we're going for a cure. Betty's going to be hit by a bus crossing the street when she's ninety-four." So my optimism was shattered when the surgeon told me the cancer was in Betty's lymph nodes and she might want to consider massive doses of chemotherapy. I cried. Later when the doctor told Betty the news, we cried together. My sleep patterns were disturbed again, but not as badly as the first time. Betty, on the other hand, never had a problem sleeping. Not even when she slept sitting up in one of those chairs with arms that you can put on the bed because it was too uncomfortable for her to lie flat.

Noreen, her friend: I try to make people laugh and look at the humor in everyday things. Betty told me that the worst day of her life was when she lost her hair. She said, "I was sitting on the patio. My hair was blowing in the wind. I ran my fingers through it, and it came out in clumps." So, we would joke about her hair, and she would be okay.

LOTS OF POSITIVE LYMPH NODES

Betty: Like Don, I thought that after all the chemotherapy I had had, my cancer would be gone. To say I was shocked when I was told that eight out of seventeen lymph nodes were positive is an understatement. That is when my oncologist at the medical center recommended a bone marrow transplant. I could be part of a trial currently in progress at the center, but there were no guarantees I would actually get a transplant. I might be part of the control group that got regular chemotherapy. Those were odds I was not willing to take. That, and the knowledge that there's a 5 to 10 percent mortality rate among women receiving the transplant, convinced me not to participate. Besides, I was aware that the immune system becomes terribly compromised. If I had the transplant outside of the trial, the cost would have been astronomical—$150,000 to $200,000. When Don checked with our insurance carrier it wasn't (at the time) a covered expense.

When we discussed this with my oncologist at home, he suggested that we go to a different NIH cancer center for a second opinion. This center also had a transplant trial in progress, but I was ineligible. It was only for women with ten or more positive lymph nodes. However, the doctors we consulted felt that I had responded so well to conventional treatment that I should continue with it.

Don, her husband: I was not unhappy that Betty did not want to participate in any trials. In fact, when the second center made their recommendation, we went out to lunch to celebrate the good news.

TAXOL AND TAMOXIFEN

Betty: Part of the conventional treatment that had been recommended was Taxol (a derivative from the bark of the yew tree). Taxol does not shrink tumors, it goes after any loose cells and prevents further cell growth. In a sense it is a chemotherapeutic agent. Once primarily given to women with ovarian cancer, it is now being given to women with breast cancer. For me, it was a lifesaver.

Like the CAF, Taxol was given to me through an IV into my port. They were long sessions—six hours. Because some people are allergic to the yew tree, I had to take allergy pills the evening and early morning before a treatment as a precaution. With chemotherapy I had never been nauseated—I was with Taxol. My blood counts were down now when they hadn't been before. And I experienced terrible joint pain three days later, in my knees, ankles and feet. It was so painful that I could barely walk. Not only did I experience tingling in my fingertips, but I also lost sensation in them. The first time that happened I was shocked and wondered, *What is this?* Just as with chemotherapy I lost my hair—again. This time though I was not as devastated.

In July of 1994 I received my fourth and final dose of Taxol. I was finished. I have heard other women say that they feel cast adrift when treatment is over; that their lifeline is gone. Not having that kind of personality, I did not feel that way. It just felt great not having blood tests every week. It was great knowing that I did not have to go every day here or there. Truthfully, I felt relieved that it was over.

Tamoxifen followed Taxol. It was not known then whether tamoxifen was safe or effective to take for longer than five years. Many women bad-mouth tamoxifen because of its side effects, but it's kept me free and clear of cancer.

Because I was still having hot flashes, and none of the herbal remedies I tried alleviated my symptoms, I was given clonidine (a conventional drug used mostly for high blood pressure), which seemed to help. Megace, another hormonal drug like tamoxifen usually given to anorexic women to stimulate an appetite, has also been effective in controlling them.

Don, her husband: Sterilizing Betty's portacath was traumatic for me. So was giving her shots of Neupogen (white cell growth factor) in her abdomen to bring her blood counts up while she was on Taxol. I had to do this seven days in a row following each treatment. When the doctor first showed me how to give Betty the shot he used himself as the guinea pig. He said to me, "Oh Don, there is nothing to it." So when he jabbed the needle into his thigh and blood started spurting out, I became slightly anxious. It was nerve-wracking giving her the shots, particularly that first time!

THE POWER OF PRAYER

Betty: Even though I was raised as a Catholic, I am not religious and do not think I believe in God. I would not even say that I am spiritual— I just do not believe in something beyond myself. However, an aunt called to tell me that she had signed me into a prayer book at her monastery. One day while sitting quietly reading a book, I suddenly felt this kind of infusion come over me. I thought, *Boy, this is a funny feeling* and suddenly realized, *Today is the day they are praying for me.* Maybe it was just a chill, but it was such a funny kind of chill. I never asked my aunt the actual time that they prayed for me. I just chose to think that is what it was. I do know that people who are prayed for, whether they are aware of it or not, do better in their recovery than those people who are not prayed for.

MY THOUGHTS ON BREAST SELF-EXAMINATION

Betty: I did routine breast self-examination, so it is hard to believe that I never felt the lump in my breast. Dr. Susan Love says that it is cruel for women to do them because they do not know *how* to do them, and they do not know what they are looking for. I am a perfect example. I always thought a lump would be hard and round. In my case it was a flat, slightly raised area. I have since been taught to put my arm over my head when I am doing an examination.

MEDICAL MALPRACTICE —DO YOU HAVE RECOURSE?

Betty: The day following the tumor conference, when I met with my oncologist at the medical center, I asked how it was possible for my tumors to have gotten so large in the six months since my "negative" November mammogram. That is when he disclosed, "They were already there." I am not so sure, if I had not had the inside track or posed my question the way I did, whether he would have volunteered that information.

When my oncologist was a resident he worked as a researcher for a law firm specializing in medical malpractice. It was his job to determine whether the defendant had a valid claim. Suing the doctor who had misread my mammogram had never entered my mind until he said, "You obviously have a lawsuit. When you go back home you need to talk to somebody." The attorney we hired felt I had a case. I am not permitted to discuss the case, but suffice it to say that the radiologist settled out of court.

During the deposition I saw the radiologist for the first time—a young, very mild-looking man. It took all of my willpower not to leap across the table and strangle him with my bare hands. That's how furious I was. At one point I had to leave the room because I physically couldn't stand the sight of his face. After admitting that the tumors were visible on the X-rays, he had the audacity to say, like a child with an excuse, "I must have dictated the report incorrectly." My attorney received an anonymous phone call suggesting that he look into who was actually reading the mammogram. He was told, "It is oftentimes the technician."

None of my personal physicians would testify in my behalf. It was that unspoken code—doctors protecting doctors. As a result I had to find outside experts. The turning point occurred when my oncologist at the center had a change of heart and testified. At the settlement hearing the radiologist never said he was sorry. It infuriates me when I see his ad in the local paper: "Professional, competent mammogram readings."

I'm a breast cancer hotline volunteer. One of my calls was from a woman diagnosed with inflammatory breast cancer who asked me for the name of an attorney because she felt she'd been misdiagnosed. For an entire year her doctor had put off treatment, even though she had had seepage from her breast. She confided, "I kept thinking—*they are doctors!* They know best. What do I know?" It's maddening. You think you've done everything right, gone to the right doctor and then, in retrospect, you think, *Oh my God. I was so stupid! Why did I not see this? Why did I not do that?* Unfortunately, that comes at the end, not the beginning. Sometimes I think that women put too much trust in their doctors, and too often that gets them into trouble.

Don, her husband: After the tumor conference Betty was told that what happened with her mammogram is "tragically not uncommon." In fact, it is the number-one cause of misdiagnosis. We were then stunned to find out that the mammogram she had done the year prior to the "misdiagnosed" one was, quite literally, unreadable. When I asked the doctor, "Wouldn't it have been proper for the technician to have taken another one?" his response was, "You would think so, wouldn't you." Betty did have them check the mammogram done prior to that one, and it was clear.

Noreen, her friend: When we moved to Arizona I called an 800 number which gives a list of all the accredited mammography sites. Guess what? The facility where Betty was "misdiagnosed" is still accredited. Isn't that cold comfort! Apparently accreditation is given based on the equipment, not the people reading the X-rays. Who is to say that a technician is not reading your X-ray? So when people buy into the idea that they are safe because a site is accredited . . .

SUPPORT AND SUPPORT GROUPS

Betty: Shortly after my mastectomy I attended a Y-ME breast cancer support group meeting, primarily to gather information. I enjoyed myself, continued to go to meetings and eventually was recruited to serve on their board of directors. Later on I decided to become a hotline volunteer. It is a good feeling to know that you're able to help others through their crises.

The flip side in becoming involved with a support group is that sometimes you can become too involved. By that I mean that cancer is at the forefront of your mind too much of the time. I have seen the ebb and flow. Women become involved for awhile because it seems to take care of their needs, and then they withdraw. Sometimes I think they leave because they do not want to think or be reminded of their disease.

Being involved in community events and the hotline has been an eye-opener—the things you see and hear. Many women who should see a doctor do not because they are too frightened.

One of our volunteers was asked by a woman whether she could get breast cancer if her husband touched her breast. And then there was the call I received in which I was asked to call a woman at work because her husband would not allow us to talk to her at home.

Don, her husband: Maybe it is a masculine thing, but I have never felt the need for a support group. I just did what had to be done and felt whatever happened, happened. What good is talking about it going to do? I know that women benefit from talking to other women, and that they can discuss really personal things with a good girlfriend. Like most men I tend to be more closed.

Julie, her friend: My husband and I have been through cancer many times; his father, and my mother and sister. As a result of my exposure to it, I never felt uncomfortable talking to Betty about hers. My nature is to just put everything aside and listen if someone wants to talk about something. And that is what I did with Betty. I might not be knowledgeable about a particular topic, but at least I can offer emotional support. Starting with that first phone call from her, I always asked lots of questions.

LYMPHEDEMA

Betty: Shortly after I had finished radiation I noticed that my hand was becoming puffy and my arm was swollen—about half again as large as the other one. The physical therapy which involved certain exercises and massage wasn't working. Using a special pump to squeeze the fluid out of my arm seemed to help, but who has three hours a day to just sit around while their arm is immobile? It was suggested that I try a compression sleeve which looks almost like a one-piece ace bandage. That has helped control the swelling. Fortunately I haven't needed to wear a compression glove. The sleeve seems to work the best. It's not painful and I take it off at night. It was also suggested that at night I loosely wrap an ace bandage around my arm up to my fingers, but that did not work because when I awoke in the morning my hand was very swollen.

RECONSTRUCTION

Betty: From the moment I knew I was going to have a mastectomy, I chose not to be reconstructed. Surgery can be dangerous. A doctor friend of mine has avoided his own surgery because he says, "I know what goes on in surgery!" I know women who have lost their implants as a result of infection. Others have talked about the pain. Some even say that a reconstructed breast does not feel like your own breast. Why should I put myself through that? And Don's comment was, "A breast is not that important to me." For all those reasons I have chosen to wear a prosthesis. I have heard comments about women feeling unbalanced as a result of the prosthesis, but I have not had that problem.

COPING WITH FEARS OF DEATH

Betty: Too many people think that cancer is a death sentence, but it's not. At least not for me. There is life after cancer—you do not have to stop doing things. I read something that said cancer should not take over your life. You should take on the cancer. And that had an effect on me. It has taught me that you can't say you will do something next year because you don't know if there will even be a next year.

I am a "reality-based" individual and read whatever I can to keep up to date with this disease that I have had. But I also believe there is a strong mind/body connection even though I do not understand how it works. I would sit in the window seat in my bedroom listening to relaxation tapes, saying affirmations like, "I am going to be fine," or "I deserve to be healthy." For me, doing that was helpful. I dislike hearing others say that I am responsible for my cancer. What I think or what I do, emotionally or spiritually, did not cause my cancer. That kind of thinking places a terrible burden on a woman, and it is wrong. My reality is that cancer is caused by external factors such as environment, what we eat, even hormones. I have no scientific basis for saying this, but I believe my cancer was a result of taking estrogen replacement therapy three to four years before my diagnosis. I did not blindly take hormones; I researched the pros and cons. My medical experts provided scientific evidence that hormones help stop hot flashes and prevent osteoporosis, etc. That is what swayed me. It was wonderful when the hot flashes stopped. However, they are discovering that some breast cancers are fueled by estrogen.

My brother is somewhat in denial concerning cancer. Although several cousins have prostate cancer, one younger than he is, he continues to smoke, will not see doctors, or have a PSA test. We do not discuss the fact that I have had cancer. He will ask me general questions about how I am, but nothing in-depth.

One of Don's cousins, who has prostate cancer, and I were chatting one day. Both of us were saying how there are moments when you think, "I am okay *now,* but am I really going to get through this? Will my body betray me again? After all I've done to it and for it, it would not dare!" But I never feel totally safe. I do not dwell on it, but the thought is always in the back of my mind: *It could come back.* Five years is nice, but that does not mean I'm out of the woods. I never thought I would die from it, but I will admit to feeling vulnerable. Especially when I talk to someone who is terminal. You think it cannot happen to you, but it can.

Don, her husband: I guess I should have been prepared for her diagnosis because the doctor did try to warn us. It took awhile for me to adjust to the fact that Betty did have cancer. I had always assumed, since I am five years older than Betty and men statistically die at an earlier age than women, that I would die first. But in the beginning I did think she was going to die. We talked about that a little. There is a tendency to take your partner for granted, but when something like this happens you become aware that maybe they will not always be there.

Now that she has had cancer I am not cancer phobic about myself like I used to be. Actually, I just do not worry about it for myself. My thinking is, *Well, if Betty has it, what is the difference if I have it?* Besides, I am supposed to die first! *[Author's note: Don was diagnosed with early-stage prostate cancer in July 1998.]* A little cancer has taught me not to get bogged down in the small, mundane things! Do I worry about her having a recurrence? Yes. But as the months and years pass, I am slightly less nervous. That is because her oncologist said that her survival dramatically increased once she got past the three-year mark. And she is now past that. I always make it a point not to say that I know her checkups are going to be fine, because I do not know that. What I do know is that her cancer has brought us closer together.

Julie, her friend: I wish that Noreen and I did not have to say that her cancer has brought all of us closer together, but it has. Something like cancer forces you into an intimacy you did not have before; like wiping your friend's lips with a washrag because she cannot.

We all get nervous when it is time for her checkup because we know how shattering it would be for Betty to hear those words again. Our fear is focused on her having a recurrence rather than death itself. From my perception she's been through the trials of Job. Yet Betty has always kept a stiff upper lip, never lost her sense of humor, her sense of graciousness, nor her courage. Somehow, she kept this from overwhelming her. Me? I think I would have gone into a cocoon and disappeared for awhile. I can be strong and get through things as they are happening, but then I fall apart when it is over.

After my mother died from breast cancer I started to read the obituaries. Why? To prove to myself that she lived a long life. Because to me, eighty-three just did not seem that old. Betty's cancer put a whole new fear into me. If it happened to her . . .

I'm not "a Betty," but she taught me to deal with the facts, and to keep focused on what can be done. I have seen how much she has been able to accomplish. She did not give up. She did not fold her tent. I will always remember that. No matter what I go through.

Noreen, her friend: Don was fabulous—like the Rock of Gibraltar. And Betty, if asked, would say the glass is half full; I would say half empty. I am a worrier, and have a tendency to be pessimistic. My husband has always said that I am stronger than I think I am. I say that I might shut myself in a closet if something really bad happened to me, but in reality I don't think that is true.

Too often, people tend to be in awe of their doctors—they think they're God. That is starting to change. People need to ask questions, make their own decisions, take control of their lives.

Sometimes I feel as if I know too much. There is some validity to the expression, "Ignorance is bliss." The more I know, the more frightened I become. I try to take care of my body, but then—look at what happened to Betty!

Postscript, December 1999

My health is quite good. I am no longer on tamoxifen, which I had been on for five years this past July although I remain on Megace. Having recently been diagnosed with osteoporosis I am now taking Evista (raloxifene). My marriage to Don is as wonderful as ever, and he is doing quite well. Unbelievable that both of us had cancer! My friends and family have remained supportive. I continue with great satisfaction my volunteer work with Y-ME of Arizona because it is very important to me to be able to help other women through their experience with breast cancer. My anger at the radiologist has diminished, but I can never forgive him for putting my life in jeopardy. I often think how different my life would be now if I had been diagnosed earlier. Although I am in remission, I never get over the fear of the possibility of a recurrence, yet I don't dwell on it. I am grateful for each day.

Seven

Theresa Coleman

Voluntary Breast Removal:
The Prophylactic Bilateral
Mastectomy Controversy

Survivor Profile:

Age when prophylactic bilateral mastectomy done:
forty-seven (1/97)

Date of interview: 1/23/97

Reconstruction: Yes (not immediate)

Who's Who:

Catherine Morris, her sister

Mel Coleman, her husband
(not interviewed)

Jake Coleman, her son
(age eleven at time of surgery, not interviewed)

A Different Kind of Fear: Familial Breast Cancer

Theresa: There is a very strong history of breast cancer in my family. In fact, the only females on both sides of the family that haven't had it are me, my sister Cathy who's three years older than I, her daughter and my paternal grandmother.

At the age of thirty-three my maternal grandmother died from breast cancer, and her daughter (my mother) was diagnosed when she was forty-nine. For two years she walked around with inverted nipples, a clear sign that there was a problem. It is unbelievable that as a nurse she did not seek medical attention, but nurses tend not to do that. Apparently neither she nor the doctor she had seen for her annual work physical were concerned. When she did finally seek medical attention from a different doctor he expressed concern, immediately scheduling a mammogram and biopsy. The mammogram revealed nothing, yet she came out of surgery minus both breasts. They had done a Halsted radical mastectomy on one side, a modified radical on the other. In 1975 women signed a consent form permitting a surgeon to do one-step biopsies, i.e., immediate removal of the breast if cancer was present. In her case not only were both breasts totally infiltrated with cancer, but all of her lymph nodes were positive. Although given six months to live, she survived for fifteen years; cancer free well over five years. When she died it was not *from* the breast cancer. Adriamycin, the chemotherapeutic drug she'd taken when first diagnosed, had weakened her heart, resulting years later in congestive heart failure. Mother's older sister was diagnosed about fifteen years ago and is still alive at the age of eighty. My father's sister (my aunt) died of breast cancer, and her daughter (my cousin) was diagnosed at the age of thirty-nine. She is doing fine. Her breast cancer was actually in the lymph nodes, not the breast itself.

Cathy, her sister: Everyone thinks breast cancer is a female thing, that it is passed down only on the maternal side, and that only women can get it. That is simply not true. Men do get breast cancer; moreover, their breast cancer easily gets missed because doctors just don't think about it. A male friend of mine died from it at the age of forty-three. The lump in his shoulder turned out to be a metastasized (spread) breast cancer, and he had never even had a lump in his breast. Breast tissue encompasses more than just the breast itself, so you need to be aware of that.

WHAT ABOUT THE NEXT GENERATION?

Cathy, her sister: According to statistics, familial breast cancer accounts for about 8 percent of all diagnosed cases, yet I disagree and feel the percentage is much higher. That low a percentage tends to give families, even those with a history, a false sense of security. Why worry when it's *only* 8 percent? Theresa and I worry about our children. We both have sons, and I also have a daughter who is twenty-five. She is a strong-willed, strong-headed woman of the X generation. Nobody can tell her anything. I don't think she is scared of getting breast cancer, but maybe she would be if someone she knew died from it. Since the age of sixteen I have told her that she needs to check her breasts every month like I do.

Some people want to know whether they carry the BRCA1/BRCA2 gene, and that's their prerogative. I have mixed emotions about the test because what if you knew you had a predisposition, that you had the gene? What's really going to cause it to evolve into cancer? It is not clearly definitive, "Yes, you will get cancer if you carry the gene," so why put any more dark clouds over your head? That kind of information isn't necessarily constructive with some personalities, particularly if they are the type who tend to be obsessive.

WHY WOULD ANYONE VOLUNTARILY REMOVE THEIR BREASTS?

Theresa: Around the age of thirty I discovered a hard, somewhat moveable lump. Needless to say I was frightened. When I called my mother, she immediately spoke with her surgeon and scheduled an appointment for me. It turned out to be a fibroadenoma (a benign, fibrous tumor). That was the first of many biopsies I had over the years because from then on my breasts became very cystic.

A couple of years later I met and married Mel and we moved to Canada, his native country. Unlike the United States, Canada has socialized medicine, and I learned from personal experience that this type of health care is great only if you need it for everyday things. It could take months to get in to see a specialist of any type: cardiologist, neurologist, orthopedic surgeon, etc. Those stories you hear about people dying waiting for bypass surgery are true. Luckily I found an excellent family physician, who after hearing my family history, referred me to a breast center several hours' drive from my house. That is when I began to be monitored so closely.

Because I have dense breasts it was difficult to read my mammograms. During that first visit the female physician I met aspirated (drained) some cysts then shocked me by saying, "If you were my daughter I'd have those taken off right away." That was the first time I had ever heard of a prophylactic bilateral mastectomy. She kept telling me that all you could see on my X-rays was white. When I got home I did discuss it with Mel, but frankly her recommendation just did not sink in at the time. Maybe I considered it, but I'd have to say only on a very superficial level.

A couple of years later I became pregnant with Jake and forgot all about my breasts. After he was born I had another fibroadenoma. My memory is blurred because over the years I was constantly having my breasts checked, cysts drained and lumps biopsied. Because we lived in a small, rural community, whenever I'd hear of someone getting breast cancer, I would think, *Oh God. That's probably going to be me in a few years.* It was not a question of *if,* but *when.* I was not obsessed with getting breast cancer, but the thought was always there even though I pushed it to the back of my mind.

In 1990 we moved to Arizona. Once again I was fortunate to be referred to an excellent doctor, a general surgeon, whose practice consists largely of women with breast problems. Little did I realize what an impact this man would have on my life years later. He, too, was very concerned about my family history, and like the doctor in Canada also suggested that I consider having a prophylactic bilateral mastectomy. Would my mother still be alive today if her doctor had been concerned about her family history?

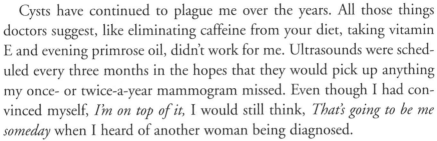

Cysts have continued to plague me over the years. All those things doctors suggest, like eliminating caffeine from your diet, taking vitamin E and evening primrose oil, didn't work for me. Ultrasounds were scheduled every three months in the hopes that they would pick up anything my once- or twice-a-year mammogram missed. Even though I had convinced myself, *I'm on top of it,* I would still think, *That's going to be me someday* when I heard of another woman being diagnosed.

In 1996 there were some major changes in my breasts; both now showed calcifications. My doctor told me, "If the biopsy shows *atypia* [irregular cells—a danger signal for increased breast cancer risk when combined with a family history of breast cancer], I'm going to recommend that you have your breasts removed. If it's not, I won't tell you to do that, but it's still an option." A wire localization biopsy was scheduled at the hospital. (Guided by X-ray images, the radiologist puts a small wire into the breast to guide the surgeon where to cut.) That part of the procedure, which took an hour, was a horrible experience as the radiologist was uncaring, insensitive and had no regard whatsoever for my emotional or physical comfort. Not once did he ask how I was doing. By the time I was in surgery I was a wreck. The biopsy itself, during which I was awake, took about forty-five minutes.

It turned out that the calcifications were *sclerosing adenosis,* a form of abnormal precancerous cells. My cancer risk was now one in two. Still I did nothing. That fall I had another huge cyst, and more calcifications were showing on my mammogram. When my doctor and I discussed the possibility of having another biopsy he said, "I don't think that is going to help. I'm afraid we are going to miss something." While examining my breasts he was muttering to himself, "I'm not going to be able to feel anything until it's too late. By the time it shows on a mammogram it will probably have spread." Even I could no longer differentiate what was what because I was so lumpy, and I hated doing breast self-examinations for that reason.

Cathy and I probably discussed this subject more than I did with Mel just because she is so knowledgeable. I never talked to him seriously about it because, deep down, I'd never really considered having this surgery. Our conversations were always on a superficial level like, "Oh maybe I should be thinking about this," and his typical response would be, "You have to do what is best for your health." What really has affected me over the last few years has been to constantly hear about young women getting breast cancer. My first thought has been, *Oh, that's going to be me,* followed by, *I don't think I could handle that,* if their cancer had spread. Then, I'd try to convince myself, *But I'm on top of it.*

My doctor never told me point blank to have a prophylactic bilateral mastectomy, but I know that's what he always thought I should do. It was always positioned as, "It's a big decision and yours to make, but it is an option." On the other hand, he never told me not to do it. I felt as though I were a walking time bomb. Although he never used that particular word, he insinuated it. That day in his office was the turning point for me because I knew one day it would be my turn and I'd hear, "Yes, it is cancer." That evening I told Mel how my doctor kept saying, "I'm afraid we're going to miss it." I also told him, "He believes I should have this done." I knew I would have his support, and that he'd never say, "Don't do it." That's just not his way.

Insurance and Preventive Mastectomies

Theresa: My doctor had told me that day in his office, "You might have a fight with your insurance company. I don't know what they're going to say, but you do have abnormal cells, and a family history." I'm somewhat of a religious person; not a Holy Roller, but I have a real faith, a belief in a higher source. Even though I had told Mel about the meeting with my doctor the day before, no one knew that I had made the decision to proceed with the surgery *if* it would be covered by insurance. So I prayed and said to God, "I'm going to give this to you. It's time to call my insurance company and get some feedback." With that I totally let go, picked up the phone and spoke with a nurse reviewer. After a forty-five minute conversation, in which I told her everything including my family history, she said to me, "If I were you I'd do it, but I've got to get approval from my supervisor. It might take me a couple of days to get back to you." Within half an hour I received a call advising me

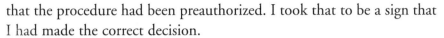

that the procedure had been preauthorized. I took that to be a sign that I had made the correct decision.

A slight hitch developed when my insurance company merged with another one. Despite that, and having to speak with a different nurse reviewer and get preauthorization all over again, things went smoothly. Surgery was scheduled for early January 1997.

WHAT DID OTHER PEOPLE THINK?

Theresa: Cathy's initial reaction when we spoke on the telephone was, "You need to think about this." Not in the sense of, "Don't do it"; rather "Just think long and hard about your decision." Later on she called back saying, "I think this is right for you."

"Oh my God, isn't that kind of drastic?" was my cousin's first response. She had had a lumpectomy, radiation therapy and chemotherapy. Yet, after we spoke, she, too, believed that I did the right thing.

Mel's family has been great. His mother has known all along about the problems I've had with my breasts, and the fact that a prophylactic bilateral mastectomy had been recommended years ago. I called to let her know that there had been changes in my breasts, and that next time I might not be so lucky.

I called anyone that cared about me. Sheri, my doctor's nurse, encouraged me to do that by saying, "Tell your friends. Tell people that care about you. You need all the support you can get." Now Mel, on the other hand, thought I should have been more closed-mouthed about telling people my intentions. He is very private about personal things, and thinks this should have been kept in the family. Mel would talk to me about it, but only if I brought it up. Being a realist he tends to see things in black and white. His philosophy is, "We'll deal with a situation if and when it happens." Yet he is also an optimist, and doesn't worry about things, particularly the small stuff.

Cathy, her sister: When Theresa elected not to have a prophylactic bilateral mastectomy ten years ago, I was glad. This time, even though initially I thought the surgery might be overkill in that it is such a drastic measure to take, I supported her 100 percent and told her, "Okay, I'm here for you.

Let's go forward." I knew what an emotional burden this had been for her. I'm really proud of her for having the *chutzpah* to do it. This was a good decision for her because it is going to bring her peace; in addition, she will be a better mom, a better wife, a better person. She already is.

My cousin thought Theresa was nuts at first. She wanted to talk her out of having the procedure, but I told her this was Theresa's decision and for her, it was the right one. Maybe my cousin had never considered this as being an option for herself because she then went to her doctor, told him what Theresa was doing, and asked, "Should I be doing this?" He told her, "No."

WAS IT THE RIGHT DECISION?

Theresa: After I had scheduled surgery I kept telling myself, *You're doing the right thing.* Nevertheless, it was almost like I was trying to talk myself into doing it. Even though I knew I would handle this better than a cancer diagnosis, or having to go through chemotherapy, I would have thoughts like, *What am I doing?* During the night I would wake up in a cold sweat. Unintentionally I lost weight which I couldn't really afford to lose because I was already slender. Deep down I was scared. This may have been a preventive surgery, but my doctor had warned me, "I don't know what I'm going to find." There were no guarantees that I didn't already have cancer. He softened his statement somewhat by also saying, "If I do find something, it'll be minute, and we'll have caught it early."

Cathy flew in to be with me for the surgery. Not only did I want her support as a sister, but she's also, literally, a great nurse. We had a wonderful evening together fixing dinner, laughing. Humor and good times have always been important to our family, even during adversity. When I woke up the next morning I was so calm. Instinctively I knew I was doing the right thing, and just felt that it was out of my hands. On the way to the hospital I was almost giddy; Mel was quiet, yet supportive. In pre-op, even without being sedated, I was so relaxed. Mel held my hand without saying much which is how he gets when he's emotional. I think he was trying not to make this too big a deal. As it was going to be a three- to four-hour procedure, he left to go back to work for an hour or so once I was taken into surgery. Mel looks like a big, tough guy until it comes to medical things. He doesn't do well in hospital settings.

Now that it is over I know that I did the right thing in more ways than one. *Sclerosing adenosis* was throughout both of my breasts. Even the pathologist, knowing nothing about my family history or the reasons for the surgery, told my doctor how fortunate I was to have done what I did. I've told very few people, other than those closest to me, how the pathology report justified my actions. Emotionally I feel tremendous relief that I did not have cancer.

My doctor is sometimes criticized as, "that surgeon who cuts off everyone's breasts." If he hadn't followed me as closely as he did, and if I didn't know how good he is, maybe I wouldn't have pursued what I did as quickly as I did. For me this was the right decision, but it might not be for someone else. Many doctors feel that what I did was very drastic and would never recommend it to their patients.

OTHER ALTERNATIVES FOR OTHER PEOPLE

Theresa: Even though Cathy has also been diagnosed with *atypia* she's emphatically told me, "I will never have my breasts removed." I'm not really sure why she feels this way, but I don't think it is because her breasts are that important to her. This is a personal choice, and it is not for me to say that what she's doing is wrong. Cathy says she's doing what is right for her; what I did was right for me. She's also told me that if she does get breast cancer it will not be a big deal because she feels that she'll be on top of it.

Cathy, her sister: Although my doctor has recommended that I consider having a prophylactic bilateral mastectomy, and Theresa's begged me to do it because she doesn't want me to die, it's not an option for me. Theresa and I have approached this whole breast cancer issue from different perspectives. She's always thought about it in terms of *when* I get breast cancer; whereas my attitude has always been *if* I get breast cancer. *If* I do, I will deal with it then, but I have already made the decision that I'll have a lumpectomy, radiation therapy and chemotherapy. Even if I didn't need chemotherapy I'd still do it because that, in combination with radiation, gives you the best outcome. To me, it is just an inconvenience you have to go through. Studies have shown that from a survival standpoint, results are equal for either a lumpectomy or mastectomy, so why put your body through all that trauma? As a nurse I've seen the disfigurement resulting from mastectomies, and think that such drastic surgery is unnecessary.

For close to the past five years I have participated in the Breast Cancer Prevention Trial. Not just anyone can be a participant; you have to qualify. Qualifying events for me were things such as having a family history, but more specifically immediate family (mother or sister), breast biopsies and any type of precancerous changes (lobular cancer in-situ or atypical hyperplasia).

When I first entered the trial I was given a battery of tests, and then checked every three to four months. Once a year I have a mammogram and a Pap smear. A uterine biopsy was added as part of the annual regimen when it was discovered that tamoxifen increases a woman's risk of endometrial cancer. That procedure is a piece of cake. We were told that there was a risk of liver problems in lab animals. As a result, when they draw blood, they also check our liver enzymes to make sure it is functioning normally. I've started taking an herb, milk thistle, to help detoxify my liver. That's my doing, not theirs.

Tamoxifen put me into menopause. I've only had one period a year for the past two years. They've told me that I am getting close to my last bottle (you can only participate for five years), and that scares me because I'm afraid that my hormone levels will increase, and I know that my mother's breast cancer was estrogen dependent. Right now I am talking to my doctor about remaining on tamoxifen. Being on tamoxifen is not as harsh a treatment as what Theresa did, and I feel as though it's giving me an edge in fighting my familial cancer.

My cousin figured she only had five years to live when she was diagnosed, and spent those years living under a cloud. Once she got beyond five years she started to live. In fact, she rewarded herself with a mink coat. It has been nine years now for her, and I believe strongly that her being on tamoxifen all these years is the reason she has not had a recurrence. She has every intention of remaining on it.

Theresa wasn't interested in participating in the tamoxifen trial even though it had been another option recommended by her doctor. She did not feel that she could emotionally deal with being thrown into menopause; in addition, she did not want to put Mel or Jake through more roller coasters.

THE CHILDREN

Theresa: Jake is an intuitive, sensitive and extremely gifted child who acts at times as though he is eleven going on thirty. Once I had made my decision to proceed with the surgery I was very up-front with him, explaining what I was going to do and why I was doing it. At the time Jake didn't get upset, yet the morning of the surgery he began to cry and said to me, "I don't want anything to happen to you." I reassured him that I would be fine. When Cathy asked if he'd like to come to the hospital with us he said, "Oh, please, please."

Cathy told me later that he was antsy, and a little nervous when they first got to the waiting room, and didn't know what to do with himself. Providence smiled on them because there was a new Monopoly game there, and they played the entire time I was in surgery. That helped to calm Jake.

Jake and I are very close. He has never been sheltered from anything I've done; in fact, he has shared just about every aspect of my life, except the bedroom. When I showed him my scars he studied them to see how even I was. He has even helped me to change the dressing on the drains. Jake knows that I plan on having reconstructive surgery once I am completely healed, and he cracked me up by saying, "Mom's going to have a new car [I'd just gotten one] to go along with her new boobies."

I DIDN'T HAVE BREAST CANCER, BUT IT WAS HARD FOR ME, TOO!

Theresa: I've tried explaining to Mel that I don't think that I grieved as much as some people over the loss of their breasts because this was *my* decision. However, it has still been tough on me emotionally and physically. That first time, when I looked at myself in the mirror, I thought, *What have I done? I'm deformed!* I looked like a little waif.

Even though surgery was easier than I had anticipated, it certainly was not a piece of cake. My chest feels tight, a nerve is bothering me and is affecting my elbow which is sore and feels like carpal tunnel, and these drains are driving me nuts! For me, I think the drains have been the worst part of this entire ordeal. I just can't find a comfortable position for sleeping. Sleeping on my stomach is obviously out, I can't sleep on my side because the drains are in the way, so that leaves sleeping on my back which is darned uncomfortable. I've taken to sleeping in my chair, and I'm just exhausted. When I told my doctor about the emotional highs and lows I was experiencing he told me that was normal. Apparently your adrenaline really picks up after surgery, and then drops afterwards. The lows might also be attributed to the effects of the anesthesia. When I felt depressed those first few days I had to keep reinforcing to myself the fact that I did something very positive, and that I really did not have a choice.

Overall though, I have done extremely well. When my in-laws came to visit from Canada shortly after surgery they called home saying, "You won't believe it. She's up and doing whatever she wants." In fact, we went out to dinner three nights after my surgery. Even Mel has told me, "You've done a lot better than I thought you would." I might have had a major surgery, but I feel on top of the world for doing it.

What I've found interesting is that until now, I have never noticed women's breasts. Now, everywhere I go, that's all I notice. Even though I didn't care about breasts before, despite being so small-breasted, I can't wait until I begin reconstruction. You know what? Now I'm not going to look like a flat pancake; I want nice breasts with cleavage!

Cathy, her sister: It was such a relief when I saw that Theresa did not have a lot of bruising or distortion from her mastectomies. I remember the horrible disfigurement my mother suffered as a result of hers. Theresa's scars, which are only about three to four inches long, were beautiful; her surgeon did a fabulous job. She didn't want to look at herself when the bandages first came off, but when she did she wasn't overwhelmed.

What really improved her mental health was being taken out of the patient role immediately, and getting back into her routine as quickly as possible because that made her feel better about herself. Five days after surgery she took me to the airport. I'd been telling her how radiant she looked, and she called later to tell me that a man had tried to pick her up when she stopped at Starbuck's to have a cup of coffee. That really helped boost her confidence.

THERE'S SUPPORT, AND SOMETIMES THERE ISN'T

Theresa: Without the support that I had, including my doctor, I don't think I could have reached the decision I made. My friends, family and boss made me feel special; in fact, like a little princess. There has been a whirlwind of attention; people constantly coming over, bringing dinner, praying for me. I was lucky to have that, but unfortunately there are some women who don't have that kind of support.

When a friend of mine called asking for the name and phone number of my surgeon, my antennae went up. A woman she knew had been diagnosed, and her surgeon had informed her that her cancer was worse than he had originally thought. She needed to have chemotherapy. This man offered no options; moreover, all he did was to give her a list of oncologists, and left her to fend for herself. This poor woman is absolutely clueless, has not seen anyone yet, and is a wreck.

Then another friend called to tell me about a friend of hers who was recently diagnosed. This woman's doctor recommended that she have a mastectomy because her tumor was sizeable, but her husband emphatically told her no because he needs her breasts. She is going to please her husband. That amazed me, and is what caused me to ask Mel, "Do you find me disgusting?" Yet, he never flinched when he saw me.

DRAWING STRENGTH FROM LIFE'S EXPERIENCES

Theresa: Knowing nothing about the problems my mother had been having with her breasts, probably because she herself wasn't concerned,

I just sobbed when she was diagnosed because I was so afraid that she was going to die. All I had was Cathy and my mom. My dad had been killed years earlier in a hunting accident. Cathy was married, so my mom was everything to me.

My mother has been a wonderful role model for me, and I've drawn such strength from seeing what she went through. She had such a strong faith, and leaned on it. Throughout her ordeal she never complained, always had a positive attitude, and took the best out of every day that she had. I have an eleven-year-old son, and I want to raise him. I don't want to go through what my mother went through. That's why I did what I did.

All I can say is *know your family history*. Don't ignore it even if you are not having any problems.

Postscript, January, 2000

Approximately two months after my surgery Mel left me for a woman he'd apparently been having an affair with. Besides losing my breasts I lost what I had thought to be one of the most important parts of my life—my partner of almost twenty years—fifteen of them married. What I thought was concern and caring was nothing but deceit and lies. My faith, reading, support groups, and most importantly family and friends, are what helped me get through this traumatic time. While I was trying to get my life back together again I met a wonderful man. We later began dating, and exactly one year after my bilateral mastectomy I began reconstruction. By now I was divorced. My new reconstructed breasts (saline implants) are beautiful. What a positive experience! December 24, 1998 I became Mrs. Jeffrey Wencel. My son Jake, now fifteen, is thrilled. He and Jeff are extremely close. This past year I had precancerous cells in my cervix which necessitated a few surgical procedures. Everything appears to be fine, but once again I will be followed closely. All in all the past several years have been a roller coaster ride of emotions; however, I feel as though I've not only been blessed, but have been given a second chance. Cathy is also doing well and has stopped taking tamoxifen.

Eight

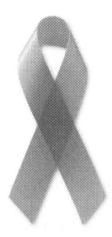

Elaine Packwood

Just Because You're Young Doesn't Mean You Can't Get Breast Cancer

Survivor Profile:

Age at diagnosis: twenty-nine (3/15/90)

Age at interview: thirty-six (8/96); Additional interview: thirty-eight

Type of breast cancer: infiltrating ductal

Size tumor: 7 cm; stage III

Three positive lymph nodes

Surgical procedure: bilateral mastectomy (one breast prophylactic)

Treatment: chemotherapy and radiation, tamoxifen

Reconstruction: immediate; defective implant replaced; then latissimus dorsi

Estrogen receptors: positive; Progesterone receptors: negative

Who's Who:

George Packwood, her husband

Brandon Packwood, her son (age five at time of diagnosis)

Ashton Packwood, her son (eleven months at time of diagnosis)

Joanne Brill, her mother

Donald Brill, her stepfather

Tara Brownlee, her friend

139

A Misdiagnosis

Elaine: While doing my monthly breast self-examination I felt a lump, and made an appointment with my primary care physician. After an examination, a negative mammogram and a needle aspiration in which he was unsuccessful in drawing fluid from the lump, I was told, "Don't worry. It's nothing; only a fibrous tumor."

Suspecting that I was pregnant, I returned to my PCP three months later. My biggest concern was now, "Will this lump have any affect on breast-feeding?" He reassured me, "It will not." So I focused on my pregnancy, not on the lump which I *knew* couldn't be cancer because two doctors, the latest being my Ob/Gyn, had said it was not. Seventeen days before my second child was born, my husband's insurance was changed. To choose a new obstetrician, I needed to see all three doctors in the practice because it was unknown which one would deliver my son. By April 1989 when Ashton was born, I'd now had the lump for almost two years, but had been consistently reassured by each of the five doctors that my lump was nothing to be concerned about.

It wasn't until the fourth month of nursing that I noticed my lump had grown from the size of a quarter to that of a silver dollar. By the time Ashton was weaned less than two months later, my periods had resumed and the lump had drastically grown into a mass the size of my fist, encompassing one-third of my breast.

George, my husband, and I had become socially friendly with a family practice physician, an osteopath (D.O.), whom I decided to see professionally. I didn't know what this lump was, but it was driving me crazy, and I could not keep my hands off of it. Although he told me he had never seen breast cancer in a twenty-nine-year-old, he nevertheless sent me to a surgeon who said, "Even though it doesn't look like cancer, doesn't act like cancer, and I don't think it's cancer, let's do a biopsy."

George, her husband: I thought that a doctor's, "No, it isn't cancer" was gospel, so I wasn't concerned about her lump.

Joanne, her mother: When I asked what the doctor's next step was going to be after the needle aspiration Elaine said, "I don't know Mother, but he said there's nothing to worry about. I have fibrocystic breasts."

Her stepfather and I happened to be visiting when she told us that she was having a biopsy. A family trip had been planned to the Grand Canyon, and Elaine, not seeming terribly concerned said, "Let's not change our plans. I'll have the biopsy, they can put a Band-Aid on it, and we'll be on our way."

Don, her stepfather: Elaine is a beautiful woman, and has the kind of breasts men drool over. I've often wondered how uncomfortable those breasts made her male doctors feel. Was it awkward for them to do an effective examination? Would a female physician have been more objective?

CANCER? I'M ONLY TWENTY-NINE!

Elaine: I just could *not* believe hearing, "I'm sorry, but you have cancer" as I awakened from surgery. Thank God my mother is a registered nurse because she immediately took charge of the medical side of things. On the way home from the hospital, she insisted that we pick up my medical records from the first doctor I had seen. Then we went to see the doctor I was friends with because I wanted some answers. Why didn't the first doctor tell me to have a biopsy in 1987? Should he have? What was his reasoning for not doing so? When he started protecting the other doctor I became infuriated, stormed out of his office, and never saw him again.

George, her husband: Elaine having cancer was like the end of the world for me.

Joanne, her mother: Hearing, "I have terrible news for you" caught me totally off guard because Elaine's surgeon had told me, "I'm sure it's nothing. Cancer doesn't run in your family." Those words changed my life. I've wondered whether the drug, DES, that I took to prevent a miscarriage had any bearing on Elaine's cancer. Studies have linked it to cervical and other types of cancer.

Don, her stepfather: All along I had been reassuring Joanne, "It's nothing. Let's not even think about it until we have some reason to be alarmed." Finding out that my vibrant stepdaughter had cancer hit me like a sledgehammer, and I cried, but not in front of her.

WHAT DO YOU TELL A FIVE-YEAR-OLD?

Elaine: Brandon is a very mature, bright child, and I knew that he could handle the truth. Not wanting to take a chance on him hearing something like, "My grandfather died of cancer" when he told the kids at school about me, I was pretty straightforward with him. He didn't want to know what breast cancer was, nor did he ask a lot of questions. Even when I told him that I had to have my breast removed, and would be given medicine that would make me sick he said very little. Losing my hair was the part he didn't understand, and that is when he started gravitating toward George. At the time though, I didn't notice because he is not a particularly affectionate child. Perhaps he felt safer with his father. Ashton, on the other hand, is a cuddlebug. Maybe that's because I clung to him. He was my lifeline, and gave me a lot of fight.

George, her husband: As soon as I got home from the hospital I told Brandon that Mom had cancer, but should get better from the treatment she would be having. It was going to be tough going for a long time, and I needed him to pitch in and help out because the house would be in turmoil. He needed to know what would be going on and seemed to handle it well.

NOW WHAT?

Elaine: Because the lump had been so large it had not been removed, and the surgeon was recommending a mastectomy and immediate reconstruction, followed only by radiation therapy. My mother, who tends to be domineering, was insisting that I fly home to Maryland with them and have my treatment done at a cancer center there. Understanding that she had my best interest at heart, I told her, "I have a long road ahead of me, and I am not going home with you to fight this battle. My family needs me here."

Don obtained a referral to a cancer center within hours of where I live, and suggested, "Let's go see them, and find out what they have to say." Armed with all my medical records and X-rays, George, my mother, and I (Don babysat the children) went, and met with a team of doctors. Pointing out the dimpling and the orange peel texture of my breast that was red and irritated, the doctor told me, "That's the cancer." I hadn't noticed until then. An aggressive course of treatment was recommended: four rounds of chemotherapy comprised of Adriamycin, 5-FU and Cytoxan to shrink the tumor, followed by a mastectomy, four more rounds of chemotherapy (same drugs), and possible radiation. Being told by these doctors, "We're going to slam you with everything we've got, but we can cure you" was the first time I had been given hope that I was not going to die. At this point I began talking with other women and started comparing my situation to theirs.

George, her husband: It was a blessing having her mother and Don with us. Knowing that I could not let my emotions get in the way, and that there would be time afterwards to let down, I tried to remain focused and figure out what we needed to do as quickly as possible. The contradictions in treatment options made that task difficult. Because of the cancer center's reputation we decided to go along with their recommendations.

Joanne, her mother: The pathology report was scary. Elaine was stage III, with an aggressive infiltrating ductal cancer. Believing that I was going to lose her, I went into a terrible depression. I couldn't understand how something like this had happened. She had seen so many doctors! Prozac, an antidepressant that I'm still taking, helped me deal with my depression. I told Elaine that if anyone could survive this disease she could; she had to.

Being uncomfortable with the recommendation that she have an immediate mastectomy, and even though Elaine and George thought that we were being overly cautious, Don and I went home to do some research. Don spoke with a friend who is also a radiologist, and I combed the libraries of nearby medical centers, and the cancer center. I spoke with those doctors, some even in Europe, who had information relevant to Elaine's situation. My research concurred with the recommendations later made by the cancer center. I believe her surgeon, who recommended an immediate mastectomy, was more concerned with the cost consideration to his participating HMO than with her survival.

Don, her stepfather: A lot of responsibility was being placed on Joanne because Elaine was looking to her mother for guidance. Joanne was aggressive in digging up research, and demanding answers from doctors; consequently, she expected Elaine and George to follow through with what she found out. George, who does not like being told what to do, realized he could best help Elaine by taking a backseat. It was reassuring to both Joanne and me when my doctor friend agreed with the cancer center's recommendation by saying, "You're dealing with a vicious animal, so treat it viciously."

CHEMOTHERAPY AND COPING

Elaine: I found a local oncologist who was willing to work with the doctors at the cancer center. While telling myself to stay positive as I was being pounded with drugs that first cycle, my mind kept replaying the words, *Don't worry. It's not cancer.* I buried myself in the Downy-soaked blanket which I brought with me from that point on, and which was used to disguise the awful smells, and I learned to disconnect, to go into my own private world while the poison dripped into my body. Forty-five minutes later George would take me home. I'd throw up and then go to bed.

My hair was gorgeous, the kind people kill for. After telling myself, *I'm not going to lose it,* I was distraught when it began falling out in clumps shortly before my second cycle began. Several days later, after waking up and finding half of it on my pillow, I buzzed it off. Somehow it was then easier to deal with. Early one morning I heard Ashton screaming and rushed into his room. He took one look at me, stopped screaming, and sat down in his crib. In my hurry to get to him, I had forgotten to put on my wig. That was the first time he had seen me bald, and from then on began the game of Let's Pull Off Mom's Wig. George, who'd been telling me all along that I did not need to wear a wig, even though I couldn't bear not to, now would say things like, "Your head is beautiful."

George, her husband: Sitting on the floor, watching as Palmolive green and Indian summer red-colored drugs dripped into Elaine while she was curled up in her recliner, was the most helpless feeling in the world. As much as I wanted to, I could not help her. All I could do was to help keep the children's lives as normal as possible, and pitch in with the cooking and household chores.

Tara, her friend: I had flown in to visit because it was important to me that I just *be there* for her. My visit was over, and as Elaine and I were walking through the airport terminal to my gate, she turned to face me, and we both burst into tears. That was the moment I realized that my best friend, whom I've known since I was five, was sick.

MASTECTOMY SANDWICHED BETWEEN CHEMOTHERAPIES

Elaine: When my Reach for Recovery volunteer told me that she had removed a healthy breast I thought, *What's the matter with that woman? I'd never do that unless I had to!* However, as George and I became more educated it started to make a lot of sense. To find a doctor willing to do a prophylactic mastectomy was as challenging as it had been to find one willing to do a biopsy. It became evident to me during my search, that not only are older women discriminated against, but younger women are too.

After four sessions of chemotherapy my tumor had shrunk in half, and now measured "only" 3½ cm. It was time for the bilateral mastectomy; modified radical on one side, prophylactic on the other. I did not quite understand what I was being told about lymph nodes. I asked the general surgeon during our final meeting before surgery, "Why, if more than three lymph nodes were positive, would the plastic surgeon not do immediate reconstruction?" He screamed, "I don't understand why or how you expect to understand things that took me years of schooling and training to learn!" As the tears streamed down my face I wondered how he would feel if a doctor treated his two teenage daughters the way he was treating me.

On the night before surgery which was ten days before my thirtieth birthday, I took a bath and said good-bye to my breasts. They may not have been that great looking, but they were mine. By now I just wanted the surgery to be over. Reassuring myself that I would wake up with breasts was the only way I was able to keep a positive attitude. As I had learned to do during chemotherapy I disconnected myself from what was about to happen. When I awoke from surgery I felt as though a ton of bricks was on my chest. Even though three lymph nodes were positive, two microscopically, I was not denied the half saline/half silicone breasts I had so desperately wanted.

George, her husband: After losing her hair and breasts, Elaine lost her feminine identity for awhile. Neither was that big a deal to me, but I realized that she needed space and time, which I gave her, to deal with these issues. Emotionally, she needed to have reconstruction.

Joanne, her mother: Elaine can usually express her feelings, but when she becomes emotional she shuts down. Even when she didn't speak, I often knew what she was thinking, and would cry with her. When I told her one day, "I wish I could take your place," she responded, "I guess this is where I am supposed to be."

Tara, her friend: My grandmother had gone through chemotherapy, but I wasn't sure how to act with Elaine because no one my age had ever gone through it. We talked about that, and how she coped with losing her breasts. I told her how brave I thought she was and how wonderfully supportive George was.

CHEMOTHERAPY AGAIN

Elaine: Before even getting out of the car, I began vomiting. Just the thought of four more cycles was almost more than I could bear. Once I began taking Xanax, an antianxiety drug, I never threw up again, and my recovery time was quicker. I have continued taking it over the years whenever I am feeling stressed, or am having a panic attack. Fortunately I was never thrown into chemically induced menopause, but like many others I gained weight—twenty pounds.

Since I was estrogen receptor positive my oncologist put me on tamoxifen and strongly urged me not to have any more children. At first I felt as though another choice was being taken away. My gynecologist, on the other hand, was encouraging me to stop taking tamoxifen if I did want to have another child. Was I willing to risk a recurrence? The answer was no, and I am now at peace with my decision.

My oncologist and I did discuss whether I should stop taking tamoxifen after five years. Based on my particular situation, and the fact that the women in the trials were postmenopausal, we came to the conclusion that I should remain on tamoxifen for the rest of my life. Nine years have passed, and tamoxifen has not been the nightmare for me that it is for many women. I still get my period, and the hot flashes are manageable. Tamoxifen is my magic crystal, and the thought of not taking it petrifies me.

THE RECONSTRUCTION OF "BAYWATCH" AND "FRANKENSTEIN"

Elaine: Selectively hearing, "We'll see about radiation," I was under the impression that I did not need it. Only a month away from being completely reconstructed it was a blow to hear, "You absolutely have to have radiation now." Pleading for just a little more time was futile, and my oncologist insisted that there be no delays because of his concern that the cancer might be in my chest wall.

My plastic surgeon was inflexible, and refused to finish my reconstruction. "I will not get the result I want with an irradiated breast, the incision might not heal properly, and you could lose the implant." I never thought of getting a second opinion because I'd heard from other women how difficult working with an irradiated breast was. That was it—I'd have to live with my breasts as they were, and I was very unhappy with their appearance.

Five and a half weeks later, my breast and half my chest were fried a deep red, almost black color from the high-dose radiation I had been given. Although not painful, it was ugly; nevertheless, with time the color faded.

Tara, her friend: I never asked, and I'm not sure that I wanted to see Elaine's scars. But when she offered to show them to me right after her surgery, I was curious. They looked better than I thought they would. Actually, other than scars running through the middle of them, they looked just like breasts minus the nipples. Reconstruction is such a personal choice. You can say what you *think* you might do, but until you are in the position yourself, you just don't know what you *will* do.

Is There Ever a Victor
in a Lawsuit?

Elaine: Anger drove me in search of an attorney to see whether I had grounds for a lawsuit. I wanted *everyone* involved in my misdiagnosis to pay for my pain and suffering. Working from opposite coasts, my mother and I found a criminal attorney who agreed to take the case. A year later he resigned because of a conflict of interest; however, he did refer me to five attorneys which is how I found Janis Raynak *[see Part III].* Although it wasn't at the time, today her specialty is malpractice with an emphasis on failure to diagnose breast cancer.

After our initial meeting I got cold feet thinking, *What if we lose and I owe her a lot of money?* We discussed my fears the following day and she told me, "Forget the money. Just let me handle it." We sued two of my doctors. In my search for experts, I found one through a book my mother had read entitled, *Journey to Justice: A Woman's True Story of Breast Cancer and Medical Malpractice* by Diane Chechik, which is a woman's true story of breast cancer malpractice. Winning has a lot to do with how you play the game. Testifying during the hearing in front of the judge and ten men representing the defendants, I ripped open my dress showing my breasts. "*This* is what I have to live with because no one would do a biopsy."

In 1993, eighteen months after I'd hired her, we won. Janis had been correct when she had told me, "If you think the money is going to make you feel better, it won't." Those doctors had to be held accountable for what they did to me, and I deserve what we won. In truth what I felt was, "Big damn deal." What mattered was the fact that after the hearing was over, one of the doctors genuinely expressed his sorrow for the pain he had caused us. I would like to think that money had nothing to do with losing three friends, but it did. Janis again called it right when she said, "Some you think of as friends are only situational friends." By that she meant that some friendships are formed out of crisis. As the crisis disappears, so do those friends. And I know for sure that I lost one friend, whom I had thought of as my guardian angel, because she was jealous. Of what, and at what expense?

Having the right attorney is so important if you are considering filing a lawsuit. Find one who will fight really hard for you. How do you find an attorney? Ask around. Check with other attorneys or friends. See if there is an attorney referral line, and check out their specialty. Look for one who specializes in breast cancer malpractice. Make sure you get every single medical record available, and do it immediately. Then your attorney has to find and pay for the experts who will discredit the physician(s). That's the key to winning—the experts.

George, her husband: Right from the beginning Elaine's mother, whom we credit for starting the lawsuit, tried to get to the bottom of how this happened. It had never entered either my mind or Elaine's to sue. Other than being interviewed by Janis, my involvement was only during the negotiations at the settlement hearing. Elaine called the shots. Winning has not diminished my anger. What was done to Elaine was borderline criminal, and I will never forgive the doctor who did not apologize to us. We have to learn to stop putting doctors up on pedestals, and assuming that they, just by feeling a lump, know what it is. Do whatever is necessary to identify *what* the lump is, regardless of where it is on your body.

Joanne, her mother: It was a good thing that I insisted on getting Elaine's medical records immediately because, later on, they were altered. I also took pictures, documenting every phase of her treatment in case we needed them in the future. After winning I wondered, *In any lawsuit can anyone really affix a dollar amount for compensation to the person for his or her agony?*

Don, her stepfather: The final settlement infuriated me because it just did not resemble reality. It should have been an open-ended settlement, so that Elaine could get whatever medical care she needs for the rest of her life because of this misdiagnosis.

AM I HAVING A RECURRENCE?

Elaine: Two years after my diagnosis, and during the lawsuit, my plastic surgeon was at last going to remove the fill ports (that portion of the implant where saline solution is injected to fill the expander), and some of the fluid to help ease the discomfort I was experiencing from my very full, hard implants. Unexpectedly surgery was canceled. Apparently my surgeon developed "lawyer paranoia" after receiving a phone call from Janis wanting to know what type of implant I had, and its life expectancy. At his insistence we had a mandatory meeting during which he protected his own liability and surgery was rescheduled. It was only partially successful because he was unable to remove the fill port and tubing from my irradiated breast.

A year later the tubing seemed twisted and thicker, and was becoming uncomfortable. Once again, none of my doctors seemed concerned. It was not until 1996, when my new PCP insisted on doing blood work, that this problem turned into a crisis. After my CEA (marker for metastatic cancer) came back high he created panic by saying, "I think you're in trouble. This *lump* is a growth, not a reconstruction issue, and you need a biopsy." When I requested a prescription for Xanax he said, "You don't need Xanax. Go to church and pray." My oncologist was not on this HMO; consequently I couldn't use him. In desperation and still believing this truly was a reconstruction issue, I went to see my plastic surgeon; but he too insisted that I have a biopsy. George and I were beside ourselves, and, convinced by now that I was having a recurrence, cried for three weeks. To help me through this period, I began taking Zoloft, an antidepressant. Three days after surgery we got back the results. I did not have cancer; the lump was silicone gel. My implant was leaking.

George, her husband: We were so scared the nightmare was beginning again. Not wanting to expose my feelings as I had the first time, I told only a few close friends what was going on. My family didn't even know. Experience had taught me that their questions and concern put too much pressure on me, and threw me into an emotional tailspin. I would tell them later. Elaine's family, of course, knew. It got to the point where I wished people would not call. Just as I got one calmed down, another would call and then I'd have to repeat the whole process. The children might have had an inkling of how stressed we were, but we tried to hide our fears from them. In a confident manner I told them only that Mom needed to have a precautionary outpatient procedure.

THE CONTINUING SAGA

Elaine: Feeling no sense of urgency to have the implant removed, I began to research my options. Were there alternatives to the TRAM flap procedure (using abdominal muscle tunneled under the skin to form a breast) my plastic surgeon had told me was my only choice? A female surgeon I had found confidently said, "Of course I can do something." But my faith evaporated when I discovered that she had only worked on ten irradiated breasts. I investigated the free flap procedure, but decided against it as it is a very involved procedure. Continuing my search through a local breast cancer support group, I was matched with Betsy Roy *[see chapter 11]*. Her surgeon had reconstructed her irradiated breast using expanders and saline implants. After I met with him, he agreed to try the same thing with me.

When I awoke from surgery in excruciating pain, I discovered that he'd had to literally scrape the silicone from my chest and rib. He told me later on, "What a mess. I have never seen anything so horrendous." Both implants had been removed and replaced. "Baywatch," my non-irradiated breast is beautiful; "Frankenstein" is a nightmare—as my plastic surgeon continually reminds me. After being on antibiotics for three months while the incision healed, I was finally in the clear— or so I thought—when I went home for my sister, Julie Ann's, wedding. Two little blood blisters on the underneath section of Frankenstein where the skin was very thin, grew, opened up and began oozing a clear liquid. I was losing my implant.

The latissimus dorsi has been my plastic surgeon's most recent reconstructive endeavor (using the muscle and a flap of skin from the back to form a breast). To match Baywatch he put a saline implant behind the chest wall, and tried reconstructing another nipple which again flattened out. Even after two years I still have my fingers crossed that the incision won't open up. Am I satisfied with their appearance? Not really, but for now I am through with surgery. How could anyone who sees me in a bathing suit think that I intentionally did this to myself?

I did look into suing the breast implant manufacturer, but the settlement would have been worth only about seven hundred dollars because I had suffered no medical side effects. It wasn't worth it, and frankly, I was just grateful that I did not have cancer.

George, her husband: Breasts have been a very sensitive issue with Elaine, and I'm finally able to tease her a little about how much time she spends in front of the mirror. I'll admit though that I have put my foot in my mouth on more than one occasion.

Joanne, her mother: I have learned that I can't tell my daughter *not* to do something. After she lost her implant the second time I asked her, "Haven't you gone through enough? Why not just use a prosthesis?"

THE CHILDREN

Ashton: Dad and I talked about Mom being sick; about what happened, and could still happen. He tells me not to worry; that Mom's going to be fine. I don't say anything to Mom because I don't want to bring back bad memories.

Brandon: Even though my parents explained what cancer was, I wasn't scared because at the time, I didn't really understand what was going on. Two years later I realized that her cancer could come back. Ashton and I have pretty much kept what happened to Mom a secret. He has not told any of his friends, and I have only told a few. It's easier dealing with it that way. Dad asks if we want to talk to him about anything. I don't, but I get my answers from the questions Ashton asks like, "Is Mom going to be okay?" Dad always says, "Yes." I was really worried when Heather Farr, the golfer, died of breast cancer. I think about that sometimes, and hope that Mom won't die, but I also believe that she will be fine. *[Author's note: When Brandon was asked during the interview process if he might feel better talking to someone he said, "I don't want to talk about it. I don't like talking about it. I just keep to myself. I've made it my secret, and have put it in the back of my mind. It's kind of practice, in case anything else happens."]*

DEATH AND DYING

Elaine: I was skipping through life, starting my family, feeling like it was time for me to grow up, when I collided with reality. I could not see a future, and thought, *This is it; I'm going to die.* Crying, I walked

Brandon to his first day of kindergarten, while pushing Ashton in his stroller. I wondered, *Am I going to be here to take Ashton to his first day of kindergarten?* It dawned on me as I reached the playground and saw all the other mothers crying, that there are no guarantees for any of us. That is when I told myself, *Let go of the garbage, and move on. Stay positive, and just believe. Breast cancer is not a death sentence.* This is how I've lived my life *most* of these past nine years. There are moments of fear, anger, self-pity, and sometimes even panic attacks, but that is what being a survivor is all about. When I'm feeling low or have a pain, I think, *Oh my God!* If I share those fears with George we feed off one another. Like the time with my ruptured implant, or when I thought the cancer had spread to my lungs because I could not walk up the flight of stairs in my home without becoming breathless. Being a survivor means learning how to deal with those emotions. That is not an easy thing to do.

I know Brandon has had some fears about me dying because whenever there is anything on television about breast cancer he'll yell, "Mom, come here. There's this thing on breast cancer." That seems to be his way of dealing with it.

It was very helpful for George when my Reach for Recovery volunteer and her husband came to the house, to know that other men understood what he was going through. As a result of that encounter, he extends the same kind of help to those men whose significant other has been recently diagnosed.

My older brother, Michael and younger sister, Julie Ann, are still in denial. They are supportive, yet they act as though my cancer was no big deal. When I hear them say things like, "You're fine. It isn't coming back," I believe in one sense that it is easier being the one fighting the disease than being the one watching from the sidelines, feeling helpless and frustrated. My mother wants Julie Ann to take the genetic BRCA1/BRCA2 blood test, but I don't think she wants to know if she carries the gene. I want my sister to be vigilant, so that if something happens to her, she will have choices available to her that were denied to me. She is now the same age I was when I first found my lump.

George, her husband: Working out at the gym, with Ashton beside me in his playpen, was how I released my hostilities and aggressions.

Oddly enough, that was the best year I have ever had at work. It was also the only period in my life where I've wished time away.

It's strange, but while you are going through everything you don't look ahead, and that's a bad feeling. Finding out that the Reach for Recovery volunteer who'd come to our home had just finished reconstruction was reassuring in a sense because, to me, that represented "the end of the tunnel." If they could get through it, so could we. When Elaine finished radiation I was finally able to relax and let go of my emotions.

I am now on the lookout for odd behavior patterns. Elaine apparently reacted poorly to either the antianxiety medication or antidepressant she was on because, for about a month, her moods swung from being happy one moment, to snapping at me and the kids the next. I was glad to see her get off the drugs because I thought she was becoming too dependent on them.

Being actively involved in living makes it easy to sometimes forget that Elaine had cancer, until I am jolted back to reality. There was the time we thought she was having a recurrence, and I was so terrified I was literally scared dry of tears. When she becomes stressed a few days before her quarterly checkup, I try not to let it bother me until the actual day, and act like it is no big deal, but of course it is. I don't know if Elaine knows how scared I really am because I've never really told her how I felt, but I know we are both thinking, *Did they get it all?* I am still afraid that she could die, and I don't know what to do about those fears, other than try not to let them consume me. I just don't want her to die first, and leave me alone. Dying is not the worst thing that can happen; it's actually fear of the unknown. Her getting sick was a wake-up call for us, and we got our affairs—wills, estate planning, etc.—in order. How odd to plan your own demise; we were just entering our early thirties.

It still weighs heavily on me knowing that we could have caught her cancer earlier. I regret that I was not more in tune with her; that I was not more assertive; that I reached a point where I thought she was being a hypochondriac, and stopped listening to her screaming about her lump. I only hope that others who read this story will learn through my experience and not be complacent like I was.

Joanne, her mother: Elaine is the love of George's life. They have been together since she was sixteen and he was eighteen. I didn't know how he would react knowing that he might lose her and have to raise their children alone. How do you explain to them what is going on with their mother? They hear the word "cancer" and equate it with death. I wonder what my grandchildren think. What kind of worries do they have? I have been careful not to tell them that everything will be all right because I don't know that. George once asked me, "Is it possible for Elaine to give Ashton breast cancer through nursing?"

Parents never believe that something like this can happen to their own child. When it did, I felt as though I had lost a part of myself. Elaine once said to me, "Mother, until I had children I did not understand what you were going through and feeling." Parents think that when their children are grown, they no longer have to worry about them. That's not true; in fact, I will never take life for granted again. You can never let your guard down. I believe that God will take care of my daughter, and what will be, will be; but I also know how lucky we are to have Elaine with us today.

Don, her stepfather: Seeing what happened to Elaine was like watching a train coming at me, and being unable to do anything about it. It sucks the life right out of you. As a parent you almost have to operate on two levels. On the one hand, you have to be sensitive, reassuring and be able to lend emotional support; on the other, you need to remain objective. Keeping the two separate is not an easy thing to do because sometimes one overlaps the other, and we could not afford to let anything cloud our judgment.

Do I still have fear? Of course I do; every time I hear of someone I know who has died. I feel now as though I have come full circle. In the beginning I had faith that her lump was only a cyst; now I have faith that Elaine is a survivor.

Tara, her friend: It was important that Elaine knew that I supported whatever decision she made, regardless of how I felt. When she asked for an opinion I gave it. When she needed someone to listen, I listened. I was there for her during the good moments and the bad. Being in Washington, D.C., and participating in the Race for the Cure with Elaine was one of those good moments. Elaine was carrying a sign that said something about her misdiagnosis. Here she was, wearing short shorts, a little top, and cowboy boots trying to get on network television to get her point across. This is a woman who can teach and share her knowledge with others.

YOUNG WOMEN—BEWARE!

Elaine: When I was eighteen I asked my doctor to explain to me what a lump felt like, because I had them everywhere in my breasts. He said, "Know your breasts. If you examine them every month—at the same time, in the same way—you will notice a change."

I want young women to know that cancer knows no age. I want to get into the high schools and tell them, "Be responsible for your own breasts." A lump belongs in a bottle. If I had known then what I know now I would have insisted, after what happened with the needle aspiration, that they do a biopsy. My cancer certainly would have been caught earlier, and maybe choices that were denied to me would have been available. Too many of us are told, "You are too young to have cancer." Don't think, "It won't happen to me."

Postscript, February 2000

I am looking forward to my tenth anniversary of being cancer-free this coming July 6th. It does not seem possible that ten years have gone by. I am very encouraged by all the awareness and medical advances I have seen over the years. There are so many more choices available today than there were when I was first diagnosed. I continue to have my regular checkups and I am still on tamoxifen to keep my estrogen levels in check, but I am also very open-minded to a proven alternative.

It's funny, but I feel blessed by all the wonderful ways I have been touched because of my cancer experience. Inexplicably I believe it has brought more into my life in some ways than it took away. My oldest son, Brandon is six feet tall and is in high school! This past Monday he played on his father's softball team passing as an adult. I was quite angry at George for that, but how could I be when I could see Brandon's glee at playing next to his old man? My baby, Ashton will be eleven this coming April. He is big enough to steal his father's shirts to wear for school. He has his sights set on becoming a marine biologist. George and I will be celebrating our twenty-fourth wedding anniversary this coming year. If that is not enough I will be turning the BIG four-0 this July.

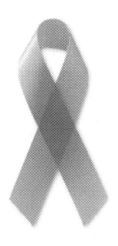

Nine

Marcia Storry

You Can Have Babies After Breast Cancer

Survivor Profile:

Age at diagnosis: twenty-eight (4/16/93)

Age at interview: thirty-one (6/15/96)

Type of breast cancer: infiltrating ductal

Size tumor: 2.2 cm; stage II

Three positive lymph nodes

Surgical procedure: mastectomy; prophylactic mastectomy one
year later on other breast

Treatment: chemotherapy

Reconstruction: bilateral immediately after prophylactic
mastectomy

Estrogen receptors: positive; Progesterone receptors: positive

Who's Who:

Eric Storry, her husband (Eric and Marcia began to date after
Marcia's cancer diagnosis and eventually married)

Sean Scott, her son (age seven at time of diagnosis)

Harry Gordon, her father

Maggie Gordon, her mother

Cheryl Rosser, her friend

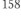

STUPID MYTHS

Marcia: One night, while taking off my bra, I accidentally hit myself in the breast and felt a definite lump. After my father, who's a family physician, checked it out I was comfortable with his suggestion to go through another menstrual cycle, and wait to see if there were any changes. There were none. I then had a mammogram and ultrasound which showed nothing because my breasts were so dense; consequently, I was referred to a surgeon who, like my father, thought I should go through one more cycle. When the lump remained unchanged both felt I should have a biopsy even though I was told, "Because of your age there's a 99.9 percent chance it won't be anything."

Still foggy when I woke up, I heard my surgeon say to me, "I have bad news. You have cancer." I kept thinking, *Wait, wait!* as my mind began racing, *cancer—death.* My mother, who had brought me to the hospital, came into the recovery room bawling. That first week I was in a daze thinking, *This can't be happening.*

My father pretty much handled the medical side of things; I was just there for the ride and did whatever I was told. The infiltrating ductal cancer in my breast was fast growing, so my father was pushing for me to have surgery as quickly as possible. Two weeks later, in April 1993, I had a modified radical mastectomy.

It was strange moving back into my parents' house with my seven-year-old son, Sean. I'd been independent since my divorce in 1988, and felt almost as though I were reliving my childhood in many respects; being bathed, having my mother change my bandages. When I looked at my scar I surprisingly wasn't shocked even though I don't like blood or gore. The flatness looked odd; in addition, I now had a peculiar numbness underneath my arm.

Maggie, her mother: It was apparent, just by the way her surgeon was walking towards me, that something was wrong. When she gave me the terrible news I asked if she would call Harry because I needed to see my daughter. She was sobbing, "Mom, I'm too young to die. I want more babies." All I could do was to tell her everything would be okay. That night Harry and I cried together. It was inconceivable that our twenty-eight-year-old daughter could have cancer. The next day the three of us met with her surgeon to find out what our next step was.

Harry, her father: Neither her mother nor I were concerned because Marcia has very fibrocystic breasts; in fact, I didn't think too much about it even when she went for her biopsy. When I received the phone call I was shocked.

Cheryl, her friend: Marcia was determined to show me her mastectomy scar. "You don't understand. I need to show you; I need for you to see what it looks like." I wasn't ready to see it, didn't want to see, and had no idea what to expect, but, was surprised at what it looked like. Her scars were still pretty raw and were much more evident than I thought they would be.

WHAT DOES A SINGLE MOM TELL HER SON?

Marcia: I've always been truthful with my son. Despite his young age I explained that cancer cells were mutated cells that grow into a tumor. Together we read a pamphlet I'd gotten from my oncologist's office that was written from a child's perspective. Chemotherapy was depicted in cartoon form with little Indians shooting arrows at the blood cells. As my son didn't display any emotion I'm not sure how he was coping, or even how much he understood. He's not a very open child.

My parents made an excellent suggestion that Sean spend the summer with my brother, sister-in-law, and their three children at their home in Alaska. As a result I was able to concentrate on me. We spoke frequently, and I sent him pictures of me bald.

Sean, her son: All I remember is my mom telling me that she had cancer, and then I went to Alaska for the summer. I wasn't scared because I didn't know you could die from breast cancer; in fact, I didn't know what having cancer was all about. It wasn't until maybe a year or two later that I was old enough to understand what my mother was saying. That's when I had a lot of questions, some she couldn't answer like, "How'd you get cancer in the first place?"

I didn't talk to my friends about my mother because, to me, it wasn't a big deal. Now I know better. If someone my age were to tell me their mom had breast cancer I'd tell them their mom has a good chance of beating it because mine did.

Eric, her husband: Marcia told Sean what she was doing in treatment, and also that she could die. He did ask some questions, but reacted like you'd expect a child his age to, such as, "That's grotesque" when she showed him her mastectomy scar followed by, "Okay. Let's go play now." I don't think it was denial on his part. It was more like, "Mom says she might die, but she probably won't, so okay." He'd say things to me like, "What are the other kids going to think when Mom picks me up at school, and she doesn't have any hair?"

DEALING WITH CHEMOTHERAPY

Marcia: In a total panic as I looked at all the old people sitting in the waiting room I wondered, *What am I doing here?* For three hours, as the Adriamycin and Cytoxan dripped through the IV, I could feel the movement of the drugs throughout my body, had an almost metallic taste in my mouth, and felt not a burning, but something like a cold wind rushing through my nasal passages.

Having been forewarned by my oncologist that I would lose my hair I'd already bought a wig. Two weeks later, it was evident my hair was about to fall out. It looked dead. Not wanting to stop up the shower drain in case it did fall out, I was washing my hair in the bathroom sink when suddenly clumps were in my hands. "Help me! Come in here!" I screamed and my fifteen-year-old brother Matt, who was the only one home, came running. First we looked at one another not knowing what to do; then, he helped me rinse out the soap, and I gathered what was left into a ponytail. Scooping what was in the sink into a Baggie, I dressed, and went over to my aunt's where I was expected. Calling out as I walked through the front door, "Sorry I'm late," I tossed the Baggie onto the table my family was sitting around, and added, "but I'm having a bad hair day." They all just cracked up.

Later that afternoon we all came back to my house to participate in a "Let's-shave-Marcia's-head party." My father had the honors. It's hysterical, even now, to watch the video as I kept repeating, "Oh my gosh" as my father shaved what remained of my shoulder-length hair. I was so afraid I would look stupid, or really bad; but my family and later my friends kept telling me, "You have the cutest little head," or "You look so good bald."

Chemotherapy wasn't something I'd want to repeat, yet it wasn't nearly as bad as I'd envisioned. After each treatment I felt drugged, almost as though I were in a daze. The Compazine I took as soon as I got home worked well because I only vomited twice although I was frequently nauseated. By the end of the summer I'd lost thirty pounds, but to me, that was a positive as I'd dance ecstatically through the house wearing my mother's size-four pants. What was disconcerting was the memory loss I experienced, which my oncologist attributed to stress, and not being able to sleep. Once chemotherapy was over sleeping was no longer a problem. Psychologically it was difficult to be told, "Sorry, you have to come back next week" when my white counts were too low, and treatment was postponed. I was mentally prepared only to have to go through the process all over again the following week.

My father became quite angry because I defied his wishes and went water-skiing when my brother, his family and my son came to visit for a week in July. Picture a bald woman with a scarf around her head, on skis, being pulled by a boat. That was me having the time of my life.

I used to think that anyone who went through chemotherapy was going to die. Now I know better. Chemotherapy became my net; once it was over I got scared, and found myself saying things to bolster my confidence like, "Okay. They got it all." A substitute that works well for me are the quarterly checkups I am still getting.

Eric, her husband: When I arrived to pick Marcia up for our date everyone was sitting on the back porch, and thought it hilarious that she had shaved her head. It didn't matter to me that she was bald. By her third and final treatment, which I took her to, we had become very good friends. It was interesting to see what chemotherapy was all about. Afterwards we went out for a little, but I brought her home before she began to feel ill.

Maggie, her mother: We might all have been laughing on the outside as Harry was shaving Marcia's head, but inside we were crying. Most of the time she had a really positive attitude, yet there were occasions she'd be down; furthermore, there were days she was so weak and tired she could barely get out of bed. We had some confrontations. Things surfaced that had been buried for years; however, much good came about as a result of them. Never could I have imagined how strong my daughter was, or that she would handle things emotionally as well as she did.

Harry, her father: After she developed a 104-degree temperature I put Marcia in the hospital. Infection is probably the most common reason people die during chemotherapy. Here she was in isolation, with a white count around her ankles, and I stood quietly in the doorway watching the nurses trying to figure out how someone so sick could be joking and laughing. That's how my daughter copes.

She was in a clinical trial, and her protocol was very aggressive; one that was being given to young women under the age of thirty. Her three doses were equivalent to the usual six. Marcia dreaded hearing me get up in the morning because that meant it was time for her shot of Neupogen, an experimental white cell growth factor, which I gave her in the thigh. Sometimes she got two in one day.

Marcia thought the reason I was angry with her that day she went water-skiing was because I didn't want her to get sunburned. With only 114 pounds on her five-foot-seven frame she looked sick, and I was concerned it would be too strenuous for her.

BEING STRONGER THAN YOU GIVE YOURSELF CREDIT FOR

Marcia: Between the time I found my lump and was diagnosed, I ended a three-year physically and emotionally abusive relationship with Dr. Jekyll/Mr. Hyde. Although he was supportive on the one hand he was also becoming more abusive, which I attribute to him feeling guilty for cheating on me. Despite having broken up I still needed and wanted his support. Stupid me; I kept trying to rein him in, he kept trying to pull away. For instance, he showed up at the hospital with flowers *after* surgery was over, or took me to my first two chemotherapies, but dropped me off so that he could go over to his girlfriend's. It wasn't until he said to me, "The only reason I'm talking to you is because you have cancer" that I realized not only how strong I had become, but that I no longer needed him in my life.

SOMETIMES YOU DON'T RECOGNIZE A GOOD THING

Marcia: Eric, who was my supervisor at work when I was diagnosed, came to the hospital with a tape of songs he'd made for me, and flowers. Throughout the summer we dated. I'll admit to having feelings for him, but I wasn't ready for a relationship with anyone. Besides, I wasn't all that attracted to him because he didn't have a lot of hair. Who was I to talk? I was bald! To think that I almost passed up a wonderful man because of my shallowness.

Eric, her husband: I was a little shocked when Marcia told me she had cancer. Her diagnosis didn't cause me to turn away from her; in fact, I suppose in the back of my mind I wanted to pursue our friendship. That summer we acted like two high school kids not wanting to admit to the other how we really felt. We were dating, but she was apprehensive about getting involved with me because she was dealing with issues of mortality resulting in an almost "What's the point?" kind of attitude. In addition, she still had feelings for her ex-boyfriend. It was probably good that her counts were slow to rebound because it forced us, or at least gave us an excuse, to move more slowly in the development of our relationship. Those at work who didn't know us well would say things to me like, "You're such a great guy for being there for her."

After what Marcia's been through I can understand a woman's apprehension, even fear, about getting involved in a relationship. At what point does a woman confess to having only one breast, or none, or that the breasts she does have are reconstructed? Marcia doesn't have nipples. When would she disclose that? Her breasts were no big deal; it was the whole package. You don't love someone because of a body part. If that were the case I'd say it's time to think about ending that relationship. Women need to know that all men aren't shallow. There are some good guys out there.

SUPPORT AND SUPPORT GROUPS

Marcia: Although support groups were helpful I found that they have a tendency to turn into bitch sessions. That's counterproductive, particularly for those who are attending for the first time. A support group for women my age, even one for single women of all ages, would have been really beneficial. Had I not gotten burnt out on cancer in general I might have started one for young women.

Eric, her husband: Between Marcia, my mother, some close friends, and my coworkers, even though the talk at work was mostly superficial, I never felt the need to go elsewhere. Marcia has pulled away from being a hotline volunteer as her time and energies are now focused on working full-time, being a mother and wife (we were married in March of 1996), and being pregnant with our first child.

Maggie, her mother: Marcia made a number of good friends her age whom she met through the support group. She has this kind of visionary complex where she's going to save the world. This gave her a real mission; in addition, it allowed her to deal with her own problems. She became absorbed in doing something for other people, and frankly it amazed me that my normally shy daughter was so outspoken. In fact, she did some public speaking for the organization she belonged to.

Cheryl, her friend: It's important to realize that it's okay if you don't understand what someone is going through. They don't expect you to; all they want is for you to be there for them whether that means going to a movie you really don't want to see, hanging out at the mall and having people stare because your friend is bald, or even going to support group meetings, which I did for a year. Be a friend; don't back away, but know when to give them space.

TIME TO GET ON WITH LIFE

Marcia: Sean was coming home, school was about to start, chemotherapy ended and I wanted to move out on my own again. My father thought that was the dumbest thing I could do. I've always looked up to my parents; in fact, I have felt guilty when I didn't listen to their advice, but for the first time in my life thought, *Why live like I'm going to die?* Their support was wonderful, but I needed to break away. Despite my parents being upset, Eric and I went apartment hunting, and I found the perfect apartment not too far from where he lived. Knowing how important it was that I get a fresh start and move on with my life, I nonetheless hoped that I was making the right decision.

HOW DID EVERYONE COPE?

Marcia: When you live with someone you don't notice changes that might be obvious to anyone else. When my brother came to visit he said, "Mom's aged so much," and even about my father, who's not one to show his emotions, "He's worried sick." My mother allowed me to see that she was visibly upset. For instance, she'd say things like, "I wish it could have been me instead of you." On the contrary, I knew that my father, despite his tough exterior, was crying inside.

Because my blood counts were so low, my oncologist recommended that I take a three-month medical leave of absence from work. Psychologically it helped knowing that my coworkers were concerned because they would call from time to time. When I did return to work any anxiety I felt over my appearance dissipated because they made me feel so welcome. Within two days I traded in my wig for the baseball cap I'd grown accustomed to wearing. I was very open about having had breast cancer, and would often wear my pink pin symbolizing that I am a survivor. It made me feel good being able to give advice when a coworker would say something like, "My mother found a lump. What should she do?" If someone asked why I was bald I would tell them the truth. I coped by constantly joking about my appearance, about the whole cancer experience which helped not only them, but me. If anyone wanted to see my mastectomy all they had to do was ask. Realizing how scary the unknown is I didn't want anyone to be shocked if they had to go through what I had.

In a strange way I grew to love having only one breast. To me it was like my war wound and I thought, *Wow, I can handle anything.* For the first time in my life I focused on me. It wasn't until everything was over that I felt a sense of accomplishment and realized, "I did this for me!" Maybe it's sick to say, but breast cancer came along at a time in my life when I needed something. It truly was a slap in the face kind of thing.

Eric, her husband: While at an outdoor concert Marcia and I ran into my brother and some of his friends. She was wearing a pair of shorts, a sleeveless top, her baseball cap and a little bandana. One of his friends asked me whether Marcia had AIDS. As we talked I realized that he was just someone looking in from the outside. Everyone responded to her in a very positive way because she was so open. Cancer didn't change her. No one made any negative comments to me such as, "Are you sure you know what you're getting into?"

Maggie, her mother: I'm in the church choir. One Sunday I was barely able to sing "God Will Make a Way" as the tears streamed down my face. It's so much harder on the parents.

Harry, her father: Even though it was expensive I kept up Marcia's apartment knowing how tough it is, once you've been on your own, to come back home. That way she'd have a place to escape to if she needed some quiet. I'm the type who quietly worries. It would have been easier if it had been me who had the cancer, and I've told that to my daughter. Thank God every time she calls me with an ache or a pain it turns out to be nothing. I never say to her, "I'm sure it's nothing bad."

Maggie and I relied heavily on our faith; in fact, our daughter's cancer only strengthened it. For awhile Marcia did, too, but she's reverted back to her old ways. Matt, our youngest who goes with the flow, didn't respond too much to Marcia's illness although they really bonded during that time. Our oldest was very worried about her.

As a result of my experience I have a new appreciation, a better understanding of what my patients are going through. You can't know what they're feeling unless you've been there. So, in one sense Marcia's having cancer has helped me to help my patients.

Cheryl, her friend: Throughout our twenty-year friendship I've been more the leader, and Marcia, who did everything to please others, the follower. Yet, when she became ill we all looked to her to help us cope. I could never have handled things as well as she did. She had her moments; however, it bothered me that she never cried because I thought she was keeping everything inside. Even she admits that she has difficulty crying, or letting go of her emotions. It definitely was not denial.

Until she met Eric she had always been in codependent relationships. That's the biggest change I've seen. Marcia now stands on her own two feet. Humor has helped her deal with her fears, and all the scary things happening to her. One night we were out, and had gone to the ladies room. Some girl who'd had too much to drink was complaining about life, and Marcia said something like, "I'm bald. I wouldn't complain." In disbelief the girl pulled Marcia's wig right off her head. Well, you can imagine her reaction. We walked out just rolling our eyes at one another.

She's been the focus of quite a bit of media attention: television, newspaper, even this book. Perhaps it's her young age. Regardless, she is a person for others to look up to. I've joked with Eric, "What's next? Movie of the Week?" What a strong person she's turned out to be. Of course she had it in her all along.

FAMILIAL BREAST CANCER

Marcia: My mother, who is fifty-six, is sandwiched between a mother and a daughter who have had breast cancer. I know she worries about that; in fact, when I called to tell her my good news about being pregnant she, too, shared hers. The lump she had found turned out to be nothing. She's told me my father still wonders whether the large mass removed from her breast, when she was in her twenties, was cancer.

Maggie, her mother: Oddly enough I don't believe their breast cancers are related. If you live long enough you're going to become that one in eight statistic. My mother, who is seventy-seven, is a four-year survivor. Harry was there when they aspirated my lump. I wasn't concerned; he was worried sick, and made no bones about how he felt. I'm not afraid. If I get breast cancer, I get it. If my daughter was strong enough to go through it, I can, too.

Harry, her father: One day Maggie shocked me by saying, "I think it's inevitable that I'm going to have breast cancer." When I asked why she said, "Nine women I know have it," and as she ticked off their names continued, "I think it's just a matter of time." There was no reason, at the time, to believe she was at high risk, but a month before Marcia's diagnosis her mother was out visiting and showed me an inflammatory red mass in her breast. It looked more like mastitis (an infection in the breast); nevertheless, I suggested she see a surgeon when she returned home. Nine out of thirteen lymph nodes were positive.

I FOUND ANOTHER LUMP!

Marcia: Exactly one year later I found a lump in my other breast, and was terrified. *Oh no. It's back. I've already had chemotherapy; my safety net's gone.* This time the mammogram and ultrasound showed something suspicious, and I was sure it was cancer. Both my father and the surgeon thought that, regardless of how the biopsy turned out, I should have a mastectomy followed by immediate reconstruction of both breasts. My mother was in recovery when I woke up. When she said, "It's benign" I was so relieved.

Eric, her husband: When Marcia had her first mastectomy we were friends growing closer. With the second, although still friends, our relationship had become somewhat strained. I was pushing too hard, but she needed some separation. I agreed with her decision; moreover, I feel strongly that it should be the woman's to make and no one else's. If having a prophylactic (preventive) mastectomy decreases the fear and makes a woman feel more comfortable, then I say, "Go for it."

Sean and I went to a ball game the day of Marcia's surgery. Afterwards I dropped him off at his father's, and went to visit Marcia. Finding her in a bad mood I stayed only briefly. Shortly thereafter, believing our relationship was going nowhere I decided to end it. However, a month or two later she expressed an interest in going out, and here we are today, married.

Harry, her father: The three of us had been talking about a prophylactic mastectomy, and then this mass just appeared. Alarms really went off. Based on what the frozen section evaluation revealed, she would have either a simple mastectomy if the lump were benign, a modified radical if malignant.

RECONSTRUCTION

Marcia: Doctors need to be more candid about the downside risks of reconstruction. My first mastectomy healed fine; however, the second one did not, I believe, because it wasn't given enough time to heal. At least two inches of the top section of the incision first turned blue, then black and then died. Although my surgeon kept trying to sew it back together I finally lost my implant. Six months later we tried again and it was successful; however, nipple reconstruction was not. The first two days my new nipples were beautiful; then, they both started to turn black, shriveling to raisins hanging on a vine, and died. We tried again. Same thing. Watching them die was the most difficult aspect of my entire cancer experience, and I've decided not to put myself through anymore emotional turmoil. It might sound silly, but all I wanted was little round nipples so that I'd look normal in a T-shirt.

Eric, her husband: Marcia asked my opinion: "What color should I make the nipples?" and after losing them the second time asked, "Should I try again?" I told her it didn't matter to me whether or not she had nipples, and it really didn't.

I'M PREGNANT

Marcia: Eric knew all along that I wanted another child. We discussed the fact that if I died Sean would go to his father's, but he would have to raise our child alone. Eric wanted to see some hard evidence that it was okay to become pregnant after a cancer diagnosis. So my friend Debbie, who'd also had breast cancer and was considering having another child, and I began researching the issue. We could find no information about pregnancy after cancer; only already being pregnant before a cancer diagnosis.

We combined our appointments with an oncologist at a well-known cancer center not too far from where we lived. Debbie is estrogen receptor positive, progesterone receptor negative. Because her estrogen levels were high (meaning her cancer was sensitive to estrogen) it was recommended that she not have any more children. If she chose to have children, then she needed to finish out her five years on tamoxifen, and wait six months to a year to make sure it was completely out of her system before trying to conceive. Even though both my estrogen and progesterone receptors are positive both are on the low side; estrogen seven, progesterone eighteen. Based on that, and the fact that I'm not taking tamoxifen, I was given the green light. We were told pregnancy does not cause cancer; it only causes a tumor to grow faster if cancer cells are already present.

Debbie had mixed feelings with her news while I, on the other hand, was ecstatic with a little bit of guilt mixed in. Had our roles been reversed, would I have gotten pregnant? Probably. You can't live your life like you're going to die.

Eric, her husband: Becoming pregnant was a very big decision for both of us even though we wanted children. Her father quite emphatically told her, "You can't have babies if you've had cancer. You shouldn't." That was the protective father and the doctor talking. Despite how both of her parents felt we decided to go for it when she was given the go-ahead. We hadn't been married very long before Marcia became pregnant, and frankly we are both excited and scared.

She sees her oncologist every six weeks which makes her feel more secure. I would feel guilty if something were to happen, but Marcia shouldn't. You've got to do what's right for you, and what we wanted far outweighed the risks, which we were willing to accept.

Marcia is not a hypochondriac, nor does she run to the doctor all the time; but whenever she gets an ache or pain she thinks the cancer's back. For instance if she's walking up a flight of stairs and becomes winded she'll panic, "Oh my God. It's in my lungs," and call her father who will say something like, "That's what happens when pregnant women walk up stairs; however, if it's persistent then look into it." She's more verbal and scared than she was before. Maybe I'm being naive, or still retain that high school mentality of being invincible, but I believe she's going to be fine, and tell her, "Don't get worked up. Let's get it checked out."

Maggie, her mother: Her being pregnant scares me. Besides, I'm not sure she was totally told "yes"; I think she wasn't told "no." She knows we're excited, and behind her, but we've also got our fingers crossed.

Harry, her father: Marcia was told there was no data one way or the other. Early on, before she became pregnant, I flat out told her she had to think about the possibility of a recurrence. Why bring a child into the world when you might not be around to raise it? I've only mentioned it once; however, I have thought it often since. I'm less concerned now because Eric's a super guy, and I know he'll raise the child, but still it's a pretty heavy thing for a child to lose its mother. We just have to pray that it works out.

Marcia's sense of humor was evident when she said to her plastic surgeon, "You've got a real problem as you're going to have to figure out how I can breast-feed this baby." Instead of dwelling on the negative she laughs about it.

Cheryl, her friend: Having also had cancer (melanoma) I can see the whole pregnancy issue from both sides. When you want a child so badly sometimes nothing else matters. Knowing how much she did I assumed they would have one, and I support their decision 100 percent.

FACING MY OWN MORTALITY

Marcia: Always having assumed I would die of old age I had to face my own mortality when I was diagnosed. It's not that I'm being morbid when I talk about cancer; on the contrary I'm being realistic. There's a 40 percent chance of recurrence, and it could kill me. After my diagnosis Eric's mother was diagnosed with cancer, type unknown, as the primary tumor was never determined. Unfortunately she lost her battle after only five months. It infuriates me that her doctors weren't honest with either her or the family, because they didn't know she was terminal until two weeks before her death. That's wrong. When Eric called to tell me she had died I went right over to his parents' house. That was scary for me because it was real.

I no longer dwell on cancer. If someone I haven't seen in awhile asks how I am, I wonder what's behind their question because the how is always a little more exaggerated. I don't think people realize they do that, and they should because that, and being labeled as I am by some of my coworkers, "that girl who had cancer," or maybe it's now "that pregnant girl who had cancer" not only bothers me, but makes me mad. I no longer think of myself like that, and don't want, or need anyone's pity.

Eric, her husband: Marcia had talked to me about her fear of dying, but until my mother's cancer diagnosis in August 1994 and subsequent death, it never entered my mind that Marcia's cancer could also be terminal. In retrospect I can now understand her fears, and even though I'm not frightened when she gets a pain or experiences a weird feeling, it does cause me to wonder, *Is it back? Is it terminal?*

In the three years I've known her, her attitude towards cancer and life have changed. She used to be paranoid about a recurrence; that she was going to die. Consequently, she was inclined to live for today, and not worry about tomorrow. I'm not sure when that changed, but she no longer sees death when she looks over her shoulder, or believes that cancer is an automatic death sentence. Now her outlook is more long-term; in fact, we're thinking about buying a house. My outlook is life needs to be lived and enjoyed.

Maggie, her mother: There isn't a day that goes by that I don't think about the fact that my daughter has had cancer; in fact, I probably will always think like that. Every night she's in my prayers. I've finally realized that you have to live for today, hope for tomorrow.

Harry, her father: Sometimes it takes something like this to make you realize you have only a finite amount of time to live. It took me many years before I was comfortable talking to my patients about dying. I guess that's because none of us wants to be reminded that one day we are going to die. It's easy to turn our back because someone's suffering makes us feel uneasy. You need to be realistic about an illness, whether it's terminal or not, and talk about it. Otherwise the patient isn't given an opportunity to vent their feelings. One of my terminal patients said to me once, "Nobody at work will talk to me. I feel as though I've been ostracized because of my illness." He had accepted dying, they hadn't. It's like Marcia said, "I didn't volunteer for this, but I've got to deal with it as well as I can." I understand when she calls to report on an ache or pain. It's scary for both of us, but it's normal to overreact to something that, in the past, you would have ignored. I pray every day that she doesn't have a recurrence. Your children aren't supposed to die before you do. I guess the passage of time, and seeing those patients who are twenty-, thirty-, even forty-year survivors, are what help me cope.

Cheryl, her friend: Even though Marcia's now a four-year survivor I don't believe she thinks she's in the clear. I understand her paranoia and you know what? It's not paranoia; it's just being realistic that her cancer could be back. Once she has her baby it's going to become even scarier because all of a sudden she's going to have this little person who's totally dependent on her, and maybe, just maybe she won't be around to raise him. I'm sure she's thought, "I could die, and he'll never know who I am."

Some people might think it's sick, but she's told me some of the things she'd want at her funeral. Furthermore, she has said, "Promise me that if something happens you'll make sure Sean's okay." I've repeatedly asked her not to talk like that because it scares me. When the movie *Beaches* came out a number of years ago we went to see it. I was Bette Midler, she was the actress who died of cancer. When she was diagnosed she wanted to watch that again with me. Of course it took on a whole new meaning.

Once she made a comment that she felt badly for what I was going through. I didn't understand because who cared what I was going through? Yet, when two people are as close as we are something like this is hard to deal with. I just can't imagine Marcia not being in my life.

Postscript, January 2000

Eric and I have three new additions to our family. Parker was born January 27, 1997 and the twins, Spencer and Blake, were born February 3, 1999. All of us are very healthy. Between working part-time, raising a teenage son and keeping up with three little ones, life is busy and exciting. My grandmother died two years ago from congestive heart failure.

Women need to follow their dreams because they really can come true. They should never, ever underestimate the power of their own strength and courage. I know that the dark cloud of recurrence is lurking over me at all times but now, besides my oldest son Sean, I have three more reasons to live. With that power I can conquer the storm if the rain falls.

Ten

Susan Scagnelli Tellier

Nursing Mothers, Beware!

Survivor Profile:

Age at diagnosis: thirty-five (4/11/91)

Age at interview: forty (7/3/96)

Type of breast cancer: infiltrating ductal and infiltrating lobular

Size tumor: 4.7 cm; stage II

No positive lymph nodes

Surgical procedure: mastectomy; prophylactic mastectomy

Treatment: chemotherapy, tamoxifen

Reconstruction: no

Estrogen receptors: borderline positive; Progesterone receptors: positive

Who's Who:

John Tellier, her husband

Dr. Burke Scagnelli, her father

Marjorie Scagnelli, her mother

Sarah, her daughter (fourteen months at diagnosis, age seven when interviewed)

Laura, her daughter (age nine at diagnosis, not interviewed)

THE STORY BEGINS

Susan: As a result of being diagnosed with fibrocystic breasts I had my first mammogram at the age of thirty. When I turned thirty-two I began seeing a breast specialist who recommended that I have another mammogram. Like the first, it, too, was negative.

Sarah, my second child, was born the following year. Because I was nursing, my annual checkup was postponed. Two things occurred during this time. Nursing hadn't been a problem with my oldest daughter, Laura, almost nine years earlier, but this time the milk wasn't flowing as easily. The milk felt engorged, as though it wouldn't release. Additionally I was feeling a new mass, at the nine o'clock position, in the same breast. When I saw the specialist after I'd finished nursing, he brushed aside my concerns with, "Your breasts are still too lumpy from nursing. You need to give them a chance to dry up, so come back in six months."

Thank God my father's a semi-retired family practitioner. That Christmas, almost a year after I'd first felt the new mass, I asked him to take a look. After feeling it, he urged me to return to the specialist and have a third mammogram because he was concerned. I did. This time there were calcifications in my breast. Once again I heard, "Come back in six months" which didn't sit well with my worrywart father. At his suggestion I saw my gynecologist for another opinion. Like my father, she, too, was worried. Even when the report came back that the fluid drawn from the needle aspiration was negative, she recommended that I have a tissue biopsy. My father wanted the entire lump removed.

John, her husband: What's so frustrating is that Susan did *everything* right. What infuriates me is their attitude, "Gee, you're too young to have breast cancer. Don't worry, it's nothing." Even though the mammograms came back negative, the doctor could feel a lump!

Burke, her father: When I felt Susan's lump I was really taken aback because even though it moved, it was hard and stony. I think I knew it was malignant, but then it never is until they tell you it is.

THE FIRST OF MANY DECISIONS

Susan: En route to the surgicenter, wrestling with whether to have just a tissue sample taken or the entire lump removed, I was sure that my father was just being overly cautious. My concern was that if they took out the whole lump (which they did), I'd have a pretty big indentation in my breast because the mass was about the size of a golf ball.

Surgery was over. Sitting alone in recovery, waiting for the results from the frozen section evaluation, I was unprepared when the surgeon knelt beside me and said, "It's malignant. Come to my office tomorrow and we can discuss your options." Shortly thereafter John returned from taking Laura to school, and my mother, who found me crying, came to take me home because John had to go to work.

John, her husband: The nine months prior to Susan's diagnosis had been hell. Both my parents and Susan's aunt were simultaneously going through health crises, and I'd been totally involved in litigating a civil trial. The impact on my family had taken its toll. When I'd get home late at night I would find notes from Laura, "Dad, don't you love us anymore?" Breathing a sigh of relief when the trial finally ended, I thought, *At last we can be a family again.* We never got that chance because within weeks Susan was diagnosed. I was dazed, in total shock because it had never entered my mind that something like this could happen.

WHAT NOW?

Susan: My parents, John, and I met with the surgeon the following day and were told, "Your cancer is a slow-growing, infiltrating lobular type. (Lobular typically mirrors in the other breast.) The lump is out. You can have radiation now, or you can have a mastectomy." At this point we were unaware that the 3.5-cm tumor he'd removed was not the entire lump. When my father saw the pathology report that weekend it stated that I had infiltrating ductal cancer—different from what we'd been told. Even though the pathologists have never agreed on my exact diagnosis, I believe I had both.

Electing to have a modified radical mastectomy turned out to be a wise decision because not only was there still 1.2 cm of tumor left, but the cancer was multi-focal—everywhere in the breast. I still wonder, *How could the surgeon tell us, after seeing the pathology report, that he'd taken out the entire lump?* Fortunately, my lymph nodes were negative.

My surgeon wasn't recommending chemotherapy, but the oncologist I saw for a second opinion was. He felt I was at high risk of recurrence because I was under the age of forty, and my tumor was large and had probably grown rapidly during my pregnancy the previous year. Additionally, other markers (indicators of recurrence) were poor. The cells were aneuploid and poorly differentiated, the cancer was grade 3, and even though my progesterone receptors were positive, my estrogen receptors were only borderline positive.

John, her husband: I was a mass of emotions: angry and upset because the doctors had been "watching" Susan for five years; frustrated and helpless because I couldn't fix her problem like I was able to with my clients; and scared because she was thirty-five and our youngest was only one. Even though Susan and I could talk, I was having problems coping. One day I realized, "We can't change anything. I'm too tired to spend anymore time feeling sorry for myself, so let's expend our energies doing something positive." That's when we started directing our energies toward learning as much about the disease as we could. We became experts by asking these kinds of questions: What do we do next? What are the treatment options? Who do we see? What is this that we're dealing with? After researching our options, we agreed that Susan's best course of action was to be as aggressive as possible.

Burke, her father: Lumpectomies weren't as common in 1991 as they are today; therefore, that was never an option I considered. Today's choices are so much more involved than they used to be. It disturbs me when I hear, "My surgeon was too radical. I didn't have to lose my breast."

CHEMOTHERAPY

Susan: My father was convinced that I should have chemotherapy, and that it be done at a teaching institution. It was a shock when chemotherapy was delayed because a chest X-ray showed a spot on my lung. Although never biopsied, all the tests indicated that it wasn't cancer, but rather old calcifications from a fairly common desert ailment, Valley Fever.

When I finally began chemotherapy a week later, I was given 5-FU and Adriamycin on days one and eight, followed by fourteen days of Cytoxan pills which, by the second month, was also being given to me intravenously. That helped to bring my blood counts up more rapidly as Neupogen (a white cell growth factor) wasn't yet available. Adriamycin was chosen because my oncologist believed, "You have one chance to cure it. What are you saving it for?" Like most, I developed complications although vomiting was never one of them. Instead I was plagued for a year with phlebitis (a painful inflammation of the inner membrane of a vein), and as a result was given the rest of my chemotherapy through a Groshong catheter in my chest. Antibiotics took care of an infection that developed in the tissues around the catheter. After the first month, my back, chest and face broke out horribly with acne. I didn't break out as badly after the second month, and even though my oncologist says that acne's not a side effect, I disagree. The same thing happened to a man I know in his early twenties also going through chemotherapy to treat his testicular cancer.

Because my oncologist was concerned about Adriamycin's potential to cause long-term damage to the heart, I was switched over to methotrexate starting with the third month. That thrilled me because I thought, *How wonderful. He thinks that I'm going to live to an old age!* His decision was also predicated on the belief that the four doses of Adriamycin I had been given should have killed 99 percent of any remaining cancer cells.

That summer, we spent three weeks vacationing in San Diego, California. I'd already gone through two months (four doses) of chemotherapy, and with doctor's orders in hand, went to a university hospital there for my next two treatments. Day one went fine, but imagine my disbelief when I was refused treatment on day eight because the doctors felt I was being treated too aggressively. Consequently, I immediately flew home. Had I not questioned my nurse who was about to put the Kool-Aid-colored drug into my catheter, I would have mistakenly been given an unnecessary and perhaps harmful dose of Adriamycin. Being the daughter of a doctor, I know that doctors and nurses are only human, and even they can make mistakes. You have to take responsibility for yourself. That's the reason I have difficulty understanding why so many women don't even know what drugs they're being given. Returning to California that evening, my energy levels were surprisingly good. When the suggestion was made to stay away from children because my blood counts were so low, which made me very susceptible to infections, I laughed. How was I supposed to do that? I resolved that issue by wearing a mask when I was around my kids, and taking my temperature frequently.

Maybe I should be more reserved and not tell the children everything, but there are no secrets in our home. I couldn't believe that a friend of mine, also going through the same thing, never told her children anything. Although I have no recollection of telling Laura that I had cancer, she knew; I'm guessing through an overheard conversation in the car. One day, while I was showering and she was sitting on the toilet seat, she asked me, "Mom, how do they know they got it all?" That's when I explained that was the reason I was doing chemotherapy. If there were any loose cancer cells, it would go after them and kill them. That seemed to satisfy her.

Of course I lost my hair. I'd held out hope that I wouldn't, but from days twenty to twenty-five every single strand fell out. Obsessively running my fingers through my hair, I'd think as the sink filled up with hundreds of strands, *I'm going to get today's allotment out.* It took John a year to finally confide that it was my baldness, not the mastectomy, that made him realize I was sick.

Laura, a typical nine-year-old, was okay with my walking around the house bald, but God forbid the doorbell should ring. Then I'd hear her scream, "Mom, put on your hat or wig." As the months passed, I grew more comfortable wearing a hat than a wig. A four-inch wide black headband, worn underneath the hat, helped to hide my baldness. I never completely lost my eyebrows or eyelashes, and in the fourth month, my hair began to regrow.

One day, to escape my illness for a bit, John and I decided to go to the movies. We went to an early showing of *The Doctor,* a movie that had been recommended as a good cry. With tissues in hand I was looking forward to purging my pent-up feelings, as I'd been on such an emotional roller coaster. Whispering quietly in John's ear as the movie began, I was shocked when the woman in front of me turned around, stared and yelled, "Shut up!" Now I was too infuriated to cry. When she whispered something to the man she was with, I hissed with a retaliating "Shhh." She whipped around in her seat screaming, "What's your problem?" I furiously responded, "My problem is that I've got cancer, and the lady on the screen doesn't. So don't treat me like . . ." Even with that, she still had to get in the last word. The movie ended, the lights came up and they remained seated. I handed John my wig, exposing my baldness to the world, leaned between the two of them and said, "Have a nice day." Hah! Not only did I feel vindicated, but I got in the last word!

I'd been prepared by my oncologist's office that it wasn't uncommon to suffer withdrawal-type symptoms when treatment was complete. I did. With the assistance of a psychologist I'd been seeing on and off for years to help with the ups and downs of married life I got through that.

John, her husband: It drove me crazy! Long, thick black hair was everywhere—in the sink, in the food, on the pillows. Have you ever seen pictures of really, *really*, old women who have little wisps of hair here and there? That's what Susan looked like. It wasn't until she lost it all that her baldness was easier to deal with. Laura sometimes showed off her mother, in front of friends, as though she were a dog performing a trick. When she'd say, "Mom, take off your wig and show them" the kids' mouths would drop open, and they'd get bug-eyed. Susan's seven- or eight-year-old nephew once asked, "Why'd you do it?" That's become a classic line around the house.

This was a very scary time for Laura who kept hearing horror stories from other kids about people who died from having cancer. Susan and I hoped that we weren't lying as we tried to reassure her that Mom was going to be okay.

There's an old saying about not killing the messenger. In my mind, her oncologist was the messenger, and he became the focus of much of my anger. Everything he said or did was wrong in my opinion. All the terrible things that were happening to my wife were his fault, including her wisps of hair! Plain and simple—he was the bad guy! Even though I've struggled with those feelings I still have displaced anger towards him, despite the fact that I like and respect him.

Burke, her father: It's not as simple as black and white, but I lean toward giving chemotherapy to anyone who's had an invasive cancer. In a sense it pleased me that the university hospital in California thought her treatment was too aggressive. I'm certainly not an oncologist, but I think that having radiation to kill any malignant cells around the area would be worthwhile. I don't know why, but I wish she'd done that.

THE TAMOXIFEN ISSUE

Susan: Despite the research in the early 1990s, which indicated that tamoxifen was more beneficial for postmenopausal women (today it's being given to more and more premenopausal women), and because my oncologist felt it would help prevent a recurrence, I decided to take it. By now I was using a male gynecologist who was in his mid fifties or early sixties, and who was flabbergasted with my decision to take tamoxifen, a drug with known anti-estrogen properties. This is what he had to say: "If you thought not having breasts was going to interfere with your sex life, just wait until you don't have any estrogen. You're five-foot-five now. If you take tamoxifen you'll shrink three inches and become all shriveled and dried up." Tears streamed down my face as I mentally reviewed my options. Live, but be old, ugly, dried up and not be able to have sex; or remain youthful, but die young because I didn't take it! When my oncologist heard that story, he sent him information.

Even after having gone through such aggressive chemotherapy I was still getting my period, although it was now much lighter and shorter than before. Chances were, according to my oncologist, I would continue to get my period while on tamoxifen (I did) because my body was still producing estrogen. This occurred in about 60 percent of his premenopausal patients who were still getting periods.

Within two months of going on tamoxifen I developed ovarian cysts. My doctor monitored them through pelvic examinations and ultrasounds. Surgery was never necessary. Supposedly there is no correlation between the two, but I find it strange that this also happened to a friend of mine who'd been on tamoxifen for six months.

Many women are plagued with hot flashes. I only have a couple a week. Doctors tell me that my waking up in the middle of the night and being unable to fall back asleep, is the result of a lack of estrogen. My biggest problem has been memory loss. It would scare me when the children would say, "Mom, you told me I could do that" and I had no memory of a prior conversation. It wasn't that the kids were trying to pull the wool over my eyes because this happened with other people, too. It seems as though there's somehow a short in my brain which I believe is estrogen related. Other women have commented to me, "I feel different," or "I don't feel as mentally alert," or "Do you feel scattered?" I find myself transposing numbers, something I've never done before, and words come out wrong even though, to me, they sound right. Like saying "sundee" instead of "Sunday." Then I get more scared because I think the cancer's gone to my brain. Weight gain hasn't been much of a problem, but it really annoyed me when a doctor, speaking at a support group meeting, had the gall to say, "Weight gain has nothing to do with tamoxifen. You're eating too much."

By October, 1996, I'd been on tamoxifen for five years. Research indicated there was no added benefit for staying on it longer than that; in fact, it was recommended not to stay on it. Going off tamoxifen has also caused problems. Every month since, a few days before I get my period, my face breaks out terribly with acne rosacea. I've also had some very severe bouts of depression and don't know why. Sometimes I think, *I wish I were dead,* and then immediately yell at myself, *How dare you say that! That could really happen.* I tried taking Zoloft, an antidepressant, but that caused so many insecure feelings to surface that I stopped taking it. The depression has lessened to a degree, but now I feel emotional surges—anxiety. There's all that estrogen floating around my body. Even though my crutch, tamoxifen, is gone I still keep it in the cupboard. Why? Maybe I feel that if the cancer returns I can gobble up those magic pills. John teases me by saying things like, "What are you going to stew about today?"

John, her husband: Tamoxifen's got its trade-offs, but it's sort of like the devil you know versus the devil you don't. I felt as though it wouldn't have hurt her to take it for another year. Because by taking it, at least you feel as though you're doing something to fight the disease. When you stop, you're left to wonder, "Am I giving this up too soon?"

Marjorie, her mother: Because I didn't want her thrown into menopause, I was against her taking tamoxifen. Since she's been off it, Susan seems a little more depressed at times. Whether that's tamoxifen related, or because of other changes in her life, I'm not sure.

MY OTHER BREAST: FRIEND OR FOE?

Susan: A bilateral mastectomy had never been an option discussed with me. It wasn't until I was finished with chemotherapy that I began giving serious thought to removing my other breast. I didn't want to, but I also didn't think that it would be true to me.

John and I met with a surgeon to discuss this. The tears I shed were because I was afraid he wouldn't recommend the surgery and that would have put the financial burden on us. Oh hooray, he recommended it. With mixed emotions I scheduled surgery, and knew I'd made the right decision when my breast was gone.

John, her husband: There was no question in either of our minds that Susan should have a prophylactic mastectomy. I married a person, not a pair of breasts. Even without them I find her very attractive. Will she still love me when I'm old, fat and bald?

AM I OKAY WITHOUT BREASTS?

Susan: I've never spent much time on makeup or nails; I'm not blue-eyed or blond; and I never had big breasts. I've never considered myself sexy, but then my image of a woman wasn't somebody with big breasts. I am who I've always been—just Susan. Sure I think about my breasts and wish I still had them. Not because they were sexual objects, but because now that body part is scarred. I think about all those strapless dresses I'll never be able to wear. How I never appreciated my body when I had the chance. My plan, when I finished nursing Sarah, was to get a great boob job. Hah! Little did I know!

It amazes me that some women don't know that reconstruction is a choice. I elected not to do it because I had a baby at home and I wanted to be able to hold her. Plus, I just didn't have the time not to be a mom. Besides, I'd heard too many women complain about how painful the whole process was. I won't say I'll never do it, but for now it's like, *mañana, mañana.* A women I know who'd held off having reconstruction for three years told me, "I never thought I missed my breasts until I got reconstructed ones, and I'm so glad I did."

John, her husband: The silicone breast-implant controversy was raging during the time of Susan's diagnosis and treatment. She looked good in a prosthesis and to be frank, we'd had our fill of surgeries. Besides, why put something in your body that might cause problems down the road? It doesn't bother me that she never had reconstruction. Maybe someday she will, but that's her choice. I love her just the way she is.

Marjorie, her mother: I was anxious for her to have breasts because I thought life might be easier for her if she did have them, and I didn't want her to worry that she didn't look right.

FINDING SUPPORT IN THE STRANGEST PLACES

Susan: My friendship with Donna, my "guardian angel," started the day of my mastectomy. She's a doctor at the hospital where I had my surgery and knows my father. When she called my parents' home that day my father's first thought was, *What bad news is she going to tell us?* Instead she said, "I was also diagnosed with breast cancer, and am currently going through chemotherapy. If your daughter wants anyone to talk to . . ." Without hesitation my father said, "Go see her now."

It's because of Donna that I've become an advocate. A few days before my prophylactic mastectomy we went to President Bush's Cancer Panel at M.D. Anderson Cancer Center in Houston, Texas. What an eye-opener that conference was for me. Nine months after my diagnosis I was asked to join the board of directors of the fledgling Y-ME of Arizona breast cancer support group. This was the beginning, for those of us with breast cancer, to be heard and taken seriously. All kinds of exciting

things were happening including the formation of the National Breast
Cancer Coalition.

As the years have passed, I think the time and effort I've put into
advocacy has taken a toll on my family. Laura's getting tired of hearing
about breast cancer and is constantly reminding me that I'm always
involved in *something* having to do with it.

John, her husband: Because everyone was so great, particularly
about looking after the children, my routine didn't change that much.
I'd call home three times a day just to see how Susan was doing, find out
what was going on. We tried to maintain a sense of normalcy around the
house because we felt that was important for the children. They needed
to know that life goes on.

Although I've always been supportive of Susan's involvement with Y-
ME, I also have mixed feelings about it. I understand this is how she's
giving back, and she's met some wonderful people, but at the same time
it's a double-edged sword. It takes so much out of her when a friend
dies. When that happens you think, *Oh God, that could be us.* But overall there's more of an upside than a downside.

I'm a pretty typical male—private about my feelings and fairly intro-
spective. It's difficult for men in general to talk about their feelings
because of how we were brought up. In the great scheme of things we
talk about nothing; usually business and sports. When I ask Susan what
the ladies talk about, she'll say something like, "Oh, we talk about our
emotions and feelings and . . ."

Sarah, her daughter: Moms need to make time for their kids. Kids
have a life, too. Sometimes it's like her support group is more important
than me. She went to a National Breast Cancer Coalition national conference in Washington, D.C., for five days. I was so proud of her, but I
missed her, and was scared even though she called home every night.
The only one who knew how I felt was my dog, Jazzie. When Mom
came home she went straight to a support group meeting.

Sometimes she's so busy she doesn't have time to tuck me into bed, or
kiss me goodnight until after I'm asleep. Dad does, but it's not the same.
I want Mom to do that when I'm awake. When I've asked, "Mom, could
you *please* spend time with me?" she'll say something like, "Maybe in a

little bit." She's too involved with the support group. I get mad at her for not taking care of herself. I'm afraid to tell her these things because she might not love me anymore. But I want to tell her how I feel. I want her to spend more time with me.

DEATH AND DYING—HOW DO WE COPE?

Susan: It always annoys me when, even three or four years after my diagnosis, people say dumb things to me like, "You look great," or "You're making it." Yet, I find myself doing the same thing to other women, and get so mad at myself for doing it. There's a group of women, all breast cancer survivors, who meet for lunch every couple of months. Some have metastatic disease, and it's with them that I don't always know the right thing to say. What do you say? "How are you?" What I do know is that just *being there,* regardless of what I might say, is important to both them and to me. I've learned that there are groups within groups. Those with metastatic disease are in a space we're not, and are going through things we don't understand. It's not like they want to exclude us, but they have their own sisterhood. Mary Lou, who has died, was a part of this group of women. One day, before a luncheon, she said to me, "I hope we're not just going to talk about breast cancer because I want to talk about vacations—about life." She was right. Life does go on regardless of where you are with your disease. But it's so hard when a friend dies.

Laura's a lot like me. She doesn't talk much about my having had cancer, so I don't know how she feels anymore. I do know that if something were really bothering her she'd talk to me. Sarah, who's now seven, is a different story. A teacher sent home a note one day along with a picture she'd drawn in class of a gravesite engraved RIP. She and I talked, and then had a good cry. To this day I'm plagued by fears that she nursed from a cancerous milk gland. Will she be okay? Although I've asked many doctors, no one has been able to answer that question. I guess only time will tell. Now, my dad didn't want to tell anyone that I had cancer. Those of his colleagues who knew would get only perfunctory, "She's fine, but let's not talk about it" kinds of responses to their questions. It was almost like my father was a failure because his child had cancer and he couldn't cure it. My mother, on the other hand, is an optimist, probably because she's been battling leukemia for years. She'd say, "You just have to make every day the best, and let's go on."

It's been five years for me, and I'm more afraid now than when I had one or two years under my belt. Too many women have had recurrences on or after this benchmark year. That's what's so scary about this disease— it can lay dormant for so long. It's like a sniper inside your body. I'm due for my five-year checkup, but I keep postponing it because I'm afraid my doctor will find something. I'm always feeling myself, and I always have scares. Even though my oncologist tried to reassure me by saying, "Sixty percent of all recurrences happen during the first two to three years," what about the other forty percent? When can you breathe easier? I don't think you're ever out of the woods. One of my friends said to me, "You know you're cured when you die of something else." But whenever I hear of someone who's had a recurrence I feel sick to my stomach— like someone has grabbed me by the throat. I want to grow old, and feel like, "Oh boy. I was loved. Aren't I lucky."

John, her husband: When Mary Lou died, I cried. Our families were friends. My fears surfaced and I thought, *Am I going to be facing this one day?* I just couldn't imagine trying to raise my children alone. You can't live your entire life dwelling on these fears, but there's this thing called CANCER that's moved into the house. It's always there; it becomes a part of your life. I deal with it by using humor, which I've been told is my defense mechanism. When things get too close, I make a joke.

Sarah only knows her mom with scars. While I was bathing her, when she was one and a half or two, she said, "I have boobies, sissy has boobies and you have boobies. Mom doesn't." When I responded, "That's right. Do you know why Mom doesn't have boobies?" she turned bright red as she answered, "I think I eat 'em off!" And I told her, "No. Mom had a disease, and the doctor had to do surgery and take them off because they were sick." That's become another joke in the family, but still—it's amazing what goes through the minds of children.

Susan has decided that she's not interested in taking the genetic BRCA1 and BRCA2 blood test. I agree with that decision. It's a great first step, but if you had the gene, this flaw, how would knowing affect your state of mind? How useful would it be to have this kind of information? It's okay that some people want to know, but I don't think I want my girls tested.

My dad used to say, "Life is hard. It's not going to be fair, you're not going to get everything you want, but you do the best you can." I think life's been damned unfair these past five to six years. Susan got cancer, both of my parents died, and now her mom is very sick. About once a month I'll yell and scream, even occasionally cry, for about five minutes while I'm in the car, and then I'm okay. I've gotten mad at God a lot because so much of what's happened in our lives just doesn't make sense. Sometimes I feel as though the school bully is after me. What did I do to get picked on? How much more am I going to have to deal with? I've gone through some pretty dark times. But a time comes when I have to stop feeling sorry for myself. I can't dwell on the thought, *Is the cancer back?*

Susan has repeatedly said over the years, "I just want to see my babies grown." Today Laura's in high school, and Sarah's in the first grade. What I want is for my children to have good memories of those they love. They will, no matter what happens to Susan, because our lives *have* gone on.

Burke, her father: When Susan was diagnosed I was knocked over; in fact, I still am. Cancer happens down the street; to someone else. I've handled it by not talking about it, other than to my wife. But even she has never seen my tears. Actually, none of us talks about it except on the rare occasion when Susan says, "Dad, will you feel this?" Then my stomach does a flip-flop. I may have put on my positive face when I was with Susan, but during those first few months I walked around with a funny feeling in my stomach because I was so worried. As the years have passed my fears have dwindled; nevertheless, we all know that a recurrence is a reality, and that there's nothing we can do to change that.

We've got five years behind us, but our biggest test might still lie ahead. Hearing her stories about other women just tears me apart. I suppose I'd be thrown into a tailspin if she were to have a recurrence. If that occurred, and I hope that day never happens, I don't know what I'd do, how I would react. That's my fear. To be honest, if it does, I hope I'm not around.

Marjorie, her mother: Because Susan, for the most part, has been so strong throughout this ordeal I rarely shed tears in front of her. I keep a lot of things to myself. Even though my friends were very sympathetic, I didn't have any one particular person to confide in other than my other daughter, Sarah. Lately it's been easier talking to my friends without getting weepy. I think the thing that bothered me the most was the fact that my daughter had cancer.

Susan would tell me when her Sarah was little, "She may never even know that she had a mother." Sarah still needs her mother, but I'm not as frightened now about Susan dying as I was before. That's one of the reasons I was so upset when I was diagnosed with leukemia. I thought, *I'm supposed to be around to take care of the kids if Susan's not.* Even though Susan doesn't say much, I know she's concerned about herself. I thought she was cured when she was five years out. But now, after seeing what's happened to some of her friends, I don't know.

Sarah, her daughter *[with tears in her eyes and a quiver in her voice]*: I try not to think about Mom getting sick again or about her dying, but sometimes I get scared. It's not as bad as when I was six, but I still get scared. Kids need to tell their moms when they're scared. Sometimes I wonder—what might it be like if Mom weren't here?

Postscript, January 2000

Over the last nine years there are moments when I want to tell God I have had my share of hard times. And then I wonder if he will respond, "When have you had your share of good times?"

Balance, gratitude and prayer are more of a focus now. I remind myself that the only guarantee in life is death. *When* is the unknown. Until . . . let me live to serve and enjoy life—my husband, daughters, family, friends and others. Amen.

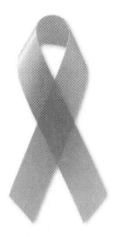

Eleven

Betsy Roy

All I Ever Wanted Was to Have Babies— Now They Tell Me I Can't!

Survivor Profile:

Age at diagnosis: twenty-six (9/92)

Age at interview: thirty (11/5/96)

Type of breast cancer: Infiltrating ductal

Size tumor: 3 cm; stage II

Five positive lymph nodes

Surgical procedure: mastectomy; prophylactic mastectomy

Treatment: chemotherapy and radiation

Reconstruction: both sides, not immediate

Estrogen receptors: negative; Progesterone receptors: unknown

   [Author's note: It was not until 1998 (six years after Betsy's diagnosis and two years after her interview) that she discovered her estrogen receptors were negative.]

Who's Who:*

Stanley Roy, her husband (not interviewed)

Nel Foster, her mother

Fictitious names by request (including survivor)

191

THE BEGINNING

Betsy: My husband, Stan, and I were in bed watching TV when I reached for the remote. My breast pressed against his arm, and that's when I felt it. I had been given a clean bill of health two weeks earlier when I went for my yearly gynecological exam, which included a breast examination. How did the doctor miss this lump? I figured one day I would get cancer because both my grandmothers and all my maternal grandmother's five sisters died from it—each before the age of fifty. But at twenty-six, I didn't think I had to worry. I made another appointment with my gynecologist.

My lump was almost under my arm and about the size of a quarter. When I saw the doctor, even knowing my family history, he said, "You're kidding, you're so young. It's probably just a fibrous mass." To ease my mind he sent me to a surgeon, but it took two weeks to get an appointment. I had my first mammogram, which was very painful, but showed nothing. Because the doctor got no fluid from my lump when he performed a needle biopsy, which would determine whether the lump was a cyst or a solid lump, we decided to do a biopsy. He took off my nipple even though the lump was under my arm. And I allowed it. What did I know then?

When I awoke from surgery, a nurse was patting my hand and telling someone, "Get a priest." I wanted to know why I needed a priest! The doctor came over to tell me I had cancer, and I started to cry. Stan came in. He wasn't crying. I told him, "I do not want a priest. I'm not going to die!" Because of the aggressiveness of my cancer, the surgeon asked Stan and me to come to his office for an immediate consultation. As soon as I was dressed, we went over and were told I had no choice of treatment options. It had to be a mastectomy because the doctor had not gotten clean margins (cancer still showed on the edges of the specimen), and he felt that radiation might miss some of the remaining cancer cells in my breast. My doctor told me I could get a second opinion, but when I checked with my HMO, a second opinion wasn't covered by my health plan. At that point, I decided that a second opinion didn't matter. I was scared and just wanted my breast off. Stan agreed.

Nel, her mother: I was with Betsy when she told me she had found a lump. Why, I could feel it just by brushing my hand against it. It was actually sticking out of her skin. Because of our family history, I think I knew what it was.

We found out that nothing showed on my daughter's mammogram because her breasts were so dense and firm. My son-in-law, Stan, and I were there for the biopsy. My husband had to work. It was Stan who told me she had cancer.

COPING WITH THE INITIAL DIAGNOSIS

Betsy: All I wanted to know when I heard I had cancer was, "Well, what do we do next?" That night I established the "no crying rule" and told my husband he had to enforce it. It makes things much worse knowing everyone feels sorry for you. People look at you with those big, sad eyes. I hated that and would tell them, "I'm not going to die from this. I'll be fine!" But I was not sure how to feel myself. I felt numb. It was a big blur. All I knew was that I was losing my breast!

Stan handled telling everyone. I didn't call anyone. I watched TV. I didn't want to think. If I didn't think about surgery, I could pretend it wasn't happening to me. And then . . . the flowers started arriving—lots of them. My house looked like a morgue because I was getting so many floral arrangements. I hated that. Someone gave me permission to throw them out. I did.

Nel, her mother: I "lost it" for the first time in my life when I found out my daughter had breast cancer. My entire body was shaking. I couldn't talk and couldn't remember my husband's work telephone number. When we did talk, we were both crying. We were all in a daze. My seventy-five-year-old dad took it very badly.

HOW COME THEY DON'T TELL YOU ABOUT LYMPH NODES?

Betsy: No one told me they were taking out my lymph nodes. No one had warned me it would feel as though a bomb had blown up underneath my armpit, that it would be numb, or that I was supposed to immediately start moving my arm! I was purposely keeping it still and using ice packs because it hurt. I thought only my chest would hurt from removing a breast. The following day my surgeon yanked my arm over my head. It hurt so badly I screamed. Now, would he have done that had I been older? They gave me arm exercises, but it took weeks for the pain to stop. Three years later, after one of my reconstructive surgeries, I started getting what felt like electric shocks up the back of my arm. Those sensations are gone now. No one told me about drains, either, these things that look like grenades that stick out from your side or about how painful it is when they are yanked from your body.

Nel, her mother: During Betsy's surgery, I was so nervous I went outside to get some fresh air. When I returned and stepped out of the elevator, an operating room nurse asked if I was Betsy's mother. When I said yes, she grabbed me, hugged me and left. That's when I realized how serious it was.

Five of my daughter's twenty lymph nodes were positive. The cancer was in her tissues, outside the breast area, which had been scraped. The surgery had been extensive, and the doctor felt he had gotten it all. She still has no feeling on that side. It was a year before I learned that the cancer had spread beyond her lymph nodes. It was quite a blow. I'm not sure if Betsy thought she had told me, so I never let on I didn't know. She tells me things little by little. I knew she had an aggressive cancer, but until I learned about her tissues being scraped, I hadn't realized quite how bad her situation really was.

Shortly after surgery she said, "Get your crying done because tears won't help me. I need you to be with me and I want your support. You don't have to agree with me. But no matter what my decision, support me." So, that's what I did—I got my crying done and gave her my support.

CHEMOTHERAPY AND COPING

Betsy: Before I started chemotherapy, a Y-ME hotline volunteer matched me with a woman who had gone through treatments similar to what I would be getting. I wanted to hear her story. I wanted to know

what kind of treatment she'd had. I wanted to know what would happen next. When I finally talked with her, it was so valuable because I
knew so little at that point. No one had explained things to me.

Because I had such an aggressive cancer—stage II, estrogen receptor
positive, with five positive lymph nodes—it was recommended I do
chemotherapy first, followed by radiation. My protocol was to get one
heavy dose of Adriamycin along with smaller doses of Cytoxan and
5-FU, followed by more Cytoxan and 5-FU a week later. Because
Adriamycin is so powerful and my veins are so tiny, a Groshong port was
inserted surgically underneath my breast for drawing blood and admin-
istering injections. Until scar tissue formed, it was tender. Only later did
I discover that the port is usually put on the side of the breast for con-
venience; I never understood why they chose this placement for mine.

My six cycles over six months stretched into nine months because my
white count was too low for me to be given more drugs, and that caused
delays. As a result, I was given CAF only once per cycle. Neupogen, a
white cell growth factor, was still experimental but was given to me
intramuscularly in my second or third cycle. I had an allergic reaction to
it and ended up in ICU. My heart was racing and I couldn't get enough
air. I am allergic to almost everything; morphine, Percocet, Percodan,
Vancomycin (the antibiotic of last resort) and, now I knew, to Neupogen.
With most of these things, I break out in hives. Demerol is the only
painkiller I can use.

Although I was scared of my oncologist at first, today we have a wonderful relationship. The nurses were great, never misled me and always
answered my questions. When I asked how chemotherapy would make
me feel, they said like a really bad, achy, chilly flu. They said I would probably vomit so I should eat lightly after treatment, but I didn't listen. After
my first treatment I ate barbecue and violently vomited the entire night.
I also threw up the antinausea drugs (Zofran and Compazine) I was given.
From then on I took them as soon as I got home before I could even get
sick. I couldn't eat foods with strong odors, so I ate lots of eggs, toast and
graham crackers. To offset constant heartburn, I took Tagamet and ate five
or six small meals a day. For fluids, I drank a lot of juice. I was slender
when I started on chemotherapy. It wasn't fair, I gained twenty pounds!

Although I've always eaten well, during chemotherapy I became Vitamin Woman. I ate lots of broccoli and Stan started juicing for me. He gave me apple juice at first which was okay, but when he added carrots, I drew the line! That juice just looked so gross!

Other than the week I had chemotherapy, I worked full time. My treatment was on Friday, and I didn't get out of bed until Monday except to go to the bathroom and brush my teeth. Mondays and Tuesdays I regained my strength and practiced having a normal life, and Wednesday, I went back to work. During those first few days at home while recuperating from chemotherapy, I felt so sick—I'd either be sweating or freezing. And I was so tired. I didn't watch TV or read. I couldn't concentrate on anything, I just slept. Fortunately, I was never hospitalized, but because of my many fevers and colds I took lots of antibiotics. Taking acidophilus helped restore the good bacteria the antibiotics were killing. Unfortunately, I developed a very painful condition called thrush—a white fuzzy fungus which grows in your mouth because of the lack of good bacteria. Taking lysine (in pill form) eliminated my mouth sores and their pain, and I never had another one.

I was told I would lose my hair fourteen to twenty-one days after my first treatment of Adriamycin. My hair was halfway down my back and I cut it to shoulder length. I put it back in a little ponytail and didn't wash it because I knew it was going to fall out. After four days it looked really dry. I told myself it wouldn't fall out, but I knew it would and I'd better get ready. When it did start to go, that second or third week after my first treatment, Stan and I combed and pulled out four wastebaskets full of hair. Other than a few wisps, I lost every single bit of my hair that day. It was the worst day of my life, and I cried and cried. Stan was wonderful. He kept saying, "You look beautiful without your hair. I love you anyway. You'll get better hair when it grows back." My head was so sensitive, it hurt. I hear people talk about having a bad hair day. I say, "A bad hair day is better than a no hair day!" When my hair grew back it was two shades darker and curlier than before. It took one and a half years before my hair returned to its normal texture. I also lost my pubic hair, but, oddly, not my eyebrows, eyelashes or body hair.

Stan was concerned that I not go into a protective cocoon, so he kept me busy. That was good to a certain extent, but I needed to rest. He didn't understand how exhausting it was just to walk the dog around the block. He kept pushing, wanting me to do more. On the hour-long drive home from work, I would cry and have my own personal pity party! That was my private time to feel sorry for myself. No one knew I did that. Only recently did Stan tell me that his private time was when he ran. That gave him the time he needed to deal with his own feelings.

For me, radiation treatment was much worse than chemotherapy, mostly because of how I was treated by the medical team. For two and a half hours, I had to lie perfectly still and with my arm over my head, the side I'd had the mastectomy on. They marked my chest like a road map with a Magic Marker so they would know where to irradiate. I wore a white T-shirt between my skin and my clothes, so the marker wouldn't stain them.

One to two weeks later, and without my being told, they permanently tattooed me! They just held me down and gave me these ugly blue dots! One right in the middle of my chest. Makeup does not cover these marks. I was so angry. On top of everything, I was bald, was wearing a wig, was already self-conscious, and then they give me ugly tattoos.

I found the treatment degrading because they only gave me a little towel to cover my chest until I lay down on the table, and I was very modest. I was petrified I would be given too much radiation even though the machine had been programmed specifically for me during that first long session. During treatment, only the machine and I were in the room. When the door closed, there was complete silence. It felt like I'd been locked in a vault. That ten to fifteen minute treatment took forever. I felt like a piece of meat in a microwave.

They warned me of the possibility of the radiation hitting a portion of my lung, which did occur. I haven't experienced any side effects from that, but I was told that if I had been a runner, I would have. Still I felt exhausted. Lotion took care of the minimal burning it caused. The skin of my irradiated breast is a little darker, harder and more leathery than the non-irradiated breast. During reconstructive surgery I insisted that my surgeon remove the tattoos. I didn't care if they were supposed to be permanent so that a doctor could see the location of where I'd already had radiation in the event of a recurrence. The scars would tell him that!

When the treatment finally ended five weeks later, I felt as though a weight had been lifted from me. Stan and I celebrated.

Nel, her mother: I was at her house almost every day. It was difficult seeing her without hair. My husband and I got a hospital bed for her room. One day she was halfway up the stairs on her way to bed when she said to me, "Here, I've got everything money can buy, I bought this gorgeous home with all these bedrooms so I could have a big family, and now I have neither children nor my health. I would give this lifestyle up for that." Her comments broke my heart because they had both worked so hard to get where they were. Betsy had everything except what she really wanted.

LOSING A BREAST

Betsy: Stan and I have been together ten years since our sophomore year in high school. He told me it was my decision, I should do whatever I needed to do. But he also said, "I won't miss your breast. Get it off. Your life is more important." Looking at the scar wasn't difficult for either of us. I felt like "good riddance," and he has never looked at me any differently. My mom didn't ask to see the scar but I knew she wanted to, so I showed her almost immediately. Her mouth said, "It doesn't look that bad. He did a good job." But her face said, "Oh my God!" Even though she was my mom, I felt embarrassed showing her, even a little awkward. Other than one friend, no one else has seen my scarred chest. Even though my friends have never asked, I've never offered. And I won't.

I felt unbalanced with only one breast. Finding bras and bathing suits was difficult because most mastectomy bathing suits are designed for older women. I hated the, "You're so young. What a terrible thing," look the salespeople gave me. I resolved the bra problem by putting the prosthesis into a sports bra or an old bra and using self-sticking tape on it so that the prosthesis would adhere to my skin. Foam prostheses are the most natural because they don't have nipples that stick out all the time, like you're cold or aroused.

THE SECOND TIME AROUND

Betsy: A bilateral surgery had never been suggested. Even if it had, I don't think I would have done it because there just wasn't enough time to process all the information I was given. I didn't think it would be so bad having only one breast. I was optimistic. I thought, *You can just go out and get another one, Betsy!*

Almost from the beginning I wanted my other breast off. When I finished radiation, I obsessed about it. It wasn't just the clothing issue or having only one breast, but I hated it! All I could think of was, *You're not my friend, and you're going to get it, too!* As always, Stan said it was my decision, he didn't care either way. I told my surgeon I would lose my mind if he didn't take my second breast off. For my mental well-being, he did. And fortunately that surgery was covered by insurance. I gave a huge sigh of relief when it was gone!

DO I RECONSTRUCT OR NOT?

Betsy: Because I had gone through hell, was tired and still getting my energy back, I wasn't rushing into reconstruction. Eventually, I interviewed three surgeons who all felt I should have a latissimus dorsi (using the muscle and a flap of skin from the back to form a breast) or a TRAM flap (using abdominal muscle tunneled under the skin to form a breast) procedure. But I chickened out because I was too scared and couldn't deal with any more pain. Three years later, because of my company merging with another company and because I was worried that the new insurance wouldn't pay for the reconstructive surgeries, I decided to proceed. Although my surgeon recommended the latissimus dorsi or TRAM flap procedure, he felt I was a good candidate for expanders (empty silicone implants that are inserted behind the chest wall muscle, and filled weekly or biweekly with saline solution, stretching the skin while creating a breast mound), even though irradiated skin is less elastic and more difficult to work with. Many surgeons hesitate to use the expander procedure when a woman has had radiation therapy because of the possibility of not getting a good cosmetic result.

When I awakened from surgery, I was bound so tightly I couldn't breathe. Sleeping was difficult. I couldn't lie on my sides because of the drains or on my stomach because my chest hurt from the expanders being placed behind my chest muscle. And my back hurt. On my personal pain scale, the reconstructive surgery was a 10 (the highest), the fills only a four or five. After my weekly fill I would go home, take two Demerol and go to sleep. I'd have to take off the next day because of muscle spasms and pain.

Even though I had no feeling in my new breasts, I was in heaven. They were expanding beautifully. Thinking bigger was better, I went from a B to a D. Nipple reconstruction went fine and the ports (that part of the implant the saline solution is injected into during the fills) were removed. I thought my nipples looked huge, like eraser heads. I was almost healed when I noticed some white, goopy stuff by my nipple incision one Saturday. I panicked! When I called my doctor he scheduled me to come in that Tuesday. Over the weekend I thought I had the flu because I was throwing up and running a fever. The white goo was an infection. By the time Tuesday came, the infection was the size of a quarter and you could see a black spot through the incision—which was my implant. I lost that implant on Thursday. To eliminate my infection I was given strong antibiotics, and then I developed thrush for a second time. I was really peeved about losing my implant. I wanted it back!

Four months later we started reconstruction, again, and from scratch. This time, my doctor used less saline with each injection as he was being more cautious, and I was filled every other week instead of weekly, like before. As a result, the fill didn't hurt as much. Fortunately, the doctor was able to save my reconstructed nipple, which had flattened out, and which I much preferred to "eraser heads." If I had it to do over again, I wouldn't have reconstructed nipples. I'm still undecided about getting tattooed areolas.

I solved the problem of having different size breasts during the first two fills by wearing my prosthesis in a sports bra (a prosthesis works better for you when you are not reconstructed). After the first few fills, I got a more natural look by substituting shoulder pads as stuffers. I started with ten, stacking them back to back. Because of the Velcro, they stick to one another and the top one sticks to your bra. Each time I got filled, I peeled one off. You can be any size you want, and no one can watch you change. When I'm finished I'm never wearing a bra again—unless I want to be sexy, and then, I'll wear black! It's taken five surgeries for these breasts and I love them. I was really scared to have this reconstructive surgery, but it's the best thing I did for myself.

Nel, her mother: It wasn't the scars that bothered me, it was that they belonged to my daughter. When I looked at her scars, I saw somebody who had a better chance of survival. Her breast wasn't important; her life was. She asked my opinion about reconstruction, and I told her, I wouldn't do it. But I'm fifty and she's twenty-six. Although it was risky and I wasn't wild about her doing it, I told her it didn't matter if I approved. It's her body and her choice.

I felt badly when she lost the first implant. The irradiated breast has more of a melted look and the skin is a little smoother and thinner than the other breast. But they are nice and perky and look pretty darn good! I didn't realize they would look so real.

SUPPORT AND SUPPORT GROUPS

Betsy: I tried support group meetings, but I didn't care for them because I found some of the topics like recurrence of the disease too depressing. For some people, breast cancer is their sole existence. For me, it is only a part. I would reconsider a support group if it were just for young women.

All my friends wanted to talk about breast cancer because no one our age had ever had it. Getting so many cards made me feel special, but also sick. It also made me realize that people with cancer are categorized. Suddenly everyone knows how you feel because they've had an uncle with cancer or know someone who's been sick. My mom said, "It should have been me who got it," but I told her that was a stupid thing to say. She and I went wig shopping before I started chemotherapy. That's the best time to shop because you still have your own hair to compare to. I got the hair she always wanted me to have—"Buffy" hair, cheerleader hair! My husband and I detested it, so I bought another wig, one that looked like my real hair. Because I wanted the world to think I was fine, I never left home without it or my makeup on.

The first day I wore the wig was awful. My head felt like it was crawling with bugs. I was driving to work bawling my eyes out, and the man in the next lane kept staring. Finally I just whipped it off. You should have seen the look on his face! I never made it to work that day. Mom made me a head covering out of T-shirt material to go under the stocking that went under the wig. Although it was still hot and itchy, it felt better. During the winter my head was cold at night. My mom made me a sleeping cap but it was too uncomfortable, so I didn't wear it. I would never walk around the house bald even though Stan said he liked me that way. Instead I wore scarves. My friends only got to "peek."

My parents came over every night for awhile until their comfort level returned. My friends were great, but I was hurt by my younger brother's silence. I'm his only sibling. Even though he lives close by, I didn't see him or speak to him. He was in total denial and relied on my mom for information. It was his way of coping. I finally saw him, and we spoke just a little. His three-year-old son was curious when he saw me bald. He wanted to talk about my wig, so we did.

My dog was wonderful. She slept with me the entire time. She knew something was going on because everyone else was acting differently. It was nice having her there to talk to when I was feeling sad.

I ended a friendship during chemotherapy because this girlfriend kept telling me horror stories about another woman with cancer. I wanted her support or, at least, to lend an ear when I needed to talk. But she was unwilling or unable to simply listen. I just couldn't take her anymore. Her talk made me feel ill. A friend says, "You look good today," or, "That wig looks really good on you," even when you're looking your worst—something positive and supportive. Friends put you at ease, so if you want to talk about it you can.

DEATH, DYING AND COPING

Betsy: Cancer was my first thought every morning when I awakened. I was having a difficult time dealing with it. I was scared and felt it was unfair to be so young and have to deal with this disease. At night, my mind wouldn't stop working, so I took sleeping pills. I found I really needed validation that what I was feeling was normal and okay, so I saw a counselor three times. She'd had breast cancer and she understood what I was feeling. She gave me a wonderful piece of advice, "For every single bad thought you have, think two good ones." It was a program that worked! She said it was okay to be selfish. I used to be a house-cleaning fanatic, but I hated to do it. Now, I have a housekeeper. I never liked cooking, so Stan has taken over. If he's not in the mood, we eat cereal or vegetables! I'll never cook if I don't want to again.

I think it stinks that this happened to me, but it could have been worse. I could have AIDS or some other disease. I believe you will live if you think you will and, on the other hand, die if you think you will die. Attitude has a lot to do with it. I always thought deep down I'd survive. It's taken me two years to reinvest in my 401K. You know, I used to make sick jokes about my mortality, but no one other than Stan was allowed to joke along with me.

I don't think Stan likes to think about negative things. But out of this has come something positive. He now realizes the value of life, that you can't take it for granted, and that it's no longer a given. I think my having breast cancer made him face my mortality. He cried only once that I'm aware of, right before my first mastectomy. I caught him in the bathroom, gave him a hug and told him to stop crying because I wasn't going to die. I just reminded him of the "no crying" rule!

What I really do enjoy is being a hotline volunteer—talking to other women and helping them. Being a hotline volunteer forced me to think about all those things I try not to think about. It makes me realize that maybe I haven't dealt with everything as well as I thought I had, or maybe I haven't dealt with it at all and I chose not to think about it. I tell women that living with cancer gets easier and easier. I don't have a magic solution for getting to the stage where I'm not thinking about it all the time, but one day I woke up and I just didn't think about it anymore.

I don't like hearing people say "Breast cancer is a blessing" because that's certainly not completely true. Some positive things have come about because of it, but I certainly don't think it was a blessing for me or anyone else. It really does make you look at your life and reevaluate your priorities. You certainly do learn a lot from it. So what? You have to live day by day. Maybe you just don't plan ten years in the future.

Nel, her mother: I was angry that she got sick when other people who abuse their bodies have good health. She said to me, "Everything happens for a reason." But I told her, "When you figure out the reason, you tell me. I sure can't come up with anything."

My husband is a "Mr. Fix-It" type of man. He felt helpless because he couldn't fix her. He doesn't think her cancer will ever come back because she had the other breast removed so there's no other breast to get it in. We've talked about the fact that it could. And he should know this already because he saw it come back and kill his own mother. I don't believe he's in denial. But he still thinks that if the cancer were to come back, she could fight it off because of her youth and also because she's healthy and strong. He honestly feels that way.

My son, Brian, who was twenty-two at the time, thought surgery would take care of everything and she would be cured. He didn't cope well. I had to tell him there were no guarantees. It's taken him four years to realize maybe her situation was more serious than he thought. He did say to me though, "It should have been me that got the cancer. I was always the one who was raising hell. She was always the good one."

As for me, I'm with her whenever she wants. She calls and I drop everything. If she wants to talk, we talk. If she wants to go out, we go out. But I let her initiate it. I don't think I've told her "no" in four years.

Betsy and Stan are wonderful together. He says he copes just by living their lives and taking it one step at a time. I think he copes by not dealing with it or thinking about it because it bothers him too much. He can't talk to anyone about it except Betsy because the whole thing's just too close to him, too personal. Nothing in his life ever scared or stopped him until this. I think he now realizes that life doesn't always go as you planned.

I REALLY WANT A BABY

Betsy: My periods, regular during chemotherapy, became very sporadic when I completed this part of my treatment. The doctors suspected a pituitary tumor, but when that was ruled out I was sent to a fertility specialist. Although I was given no remedies, after three years my periods are almost regular again. They told me being regular wasn't a big deal. But it is, if you want babies. I won't go on tamoxifen because that would throw me into menopause.

I want children more than anything in the world, and I'm being told not to because I'm estrogen-receptor positive. Pregnancy dramatically increases the estrogen in a woman's body and my cancer feeds on estrogen. Stan keeps saying, "no." He knows having a baby could be dangerous to my health. We've talked about all kinds of alternatives including having my egg and his sperm artificially inseminated into another woman. That's problematic because I have no female family members to ask, and we feel that asking a friend to do this is crossing the friendship boundaries. My maternal need would be satisfied by adoption, but he would have to accept not being the biological father. Could he, and would he, still love the baby? This whole baby thing is a tough issue for him and although I've tried to get him to see a therapist, he won't. He just doesn't want to think about it, so at this point we handle it by not talking about it. If I have our biological child and live through it, what happens if I do have a defective gene for cancer and pass it on? It would be worse if our child were a girl.

I'm coming up on the fifth anniversary of my diagnosis. My mom and I are going to get tested for the BRCA1/BRCA2 gene. In general, the requirements for being tested are: more than two generations are affected, e.g., mother and grandmother, and at a young age. However, the breast cancer gene can also be passed down on the father's side, so it might be his sister and mother. I won't have a baby if I carry the gene. You know, if I don't carry the gene, then why did I get breast cancer? What did I do to have this kind of life?

Nel, her mother: I believe the gene was passed down and feel that it's my fault Betsy got breast cancer. Had I known so many women in our family would get breast cancer, I might have considered not having children; however I can't picture my life without them. I wouldn't have married a man who didn't want children. Maybe I would have adopted instead.

Betsy wants me to take the genetic test for breast cancer and thinks that if I do carry the gene, I should have a prophylactic (preventive) bilateral mastectomy, just to protect myself. I can see her point, but I don't know if I could remove healthy breasts even if my insurance would cover it. Well, I have to take the test to see if I do carry the gene before I make any decision on that.

It makes me sad that I won't see my daughter as a mother and also that I won't be a grandmother to her children. The doctors recommended a hysterectomy, which she refuses to have. She says, "Maybe, if I go a few years and it doesn't come back . . . ." Accidents happen and she told me she would never abort, and that scares me. Adoption? I doubt it.

DOCTORS DON'T LISTEN WHEN YOU'RE YOUNG!

Betsy: With few exceptions I don't think you're listened to or treated as a thinking, feeling person when you're young. I felt pushed around and treated like a "case." That's why Stan came to all my appointments. I liked my oncologist; however, I detested my radiation oncologist who spoke only to Stan, never to me. It was as though I wasn't even in the room. His attitude infuriated me.

The nurses think I'm a bitch because I won't let them give me IVs anymore. I'm very polite but tell them I'll only allow the anesthesiologist to do it. Even he has difficulty getting the IV into a vein on the first try because my veins are so tiny. Even though working out with weights is supposed to bring them back, mine still collapse.

It's taken me four years, but I now demand respect from others. I've learned that you need to speak up for yourself. I'm no longer intimidated by anyone. If you don't want them to do something, tell them. If you have to, stand on the biggest chair you can find and scream at the top of your lungs. Make them hear you. You need to make sure they don't hold you down to tattoo you. Don't let them do anything to you unless they tell you first what they're planning on doing and you've given them your permission to do it. I didn't do that then, but I do it every time now because I've changed; I'm no longer treated as a kid or just another case.

Nel, her mother: In the beginning, Betsy was poked so many times both of her hands were black and blue. That made me angry, and I told her she didn't have to let them do that to her. Now she's assertive and questions everything. The nurses refer to her as "the woman from hell." They forget how to be sensitive.

DOES IT EVER END?

Betsy: I get aches and pains all the time, but I'm not constantly on the phone with my doctor. My big downfall is in not telling the doctor when something's bothering or hurting me. It's been difficult walking the past two weeks because of a deep pain in my leg. We don't know if it's muscular or in the bone. The doctor suggested keeping a medical journal for the next two weeks to see if the pain lessens or goes away. If not, I'll need to get a bone scan.

Postscript, December 1999

I didn't think it comical at the time, but . . . While scuba diving on vacation my saline implant deflated caused by either the pressure from the deep dive, or from carrying heavy gear. I never had the inflater tube removed, and that was the part responsible for the deflation. As a result I now have silicone implants which are more natural-looking and feeling. Now I can continue to go on deep dives. Giving up diving was *not* an option.

My health is great, and I have never felt better or stronger. I am married to the same wonderful man. To this day he has never missed a doctor's appointment. There are no children in our lives. My heart continues to yearn for a child. Adoption is the only choice as my doctor feels it is too risky for me to bear a child. I feel it would be worth the risk; my husband does not. Adoption is a huge decision for us.

Twelve

Melba Adamson

Nobody Told Me
Life Without Estrogen
Was Going to Be Hell!

Survivor Profile:

Age at diagnosis: thirty-seven (8/90)

Age at interview: forty-three (11/22/96)

Type of breast cancer: intraductal (DCIS), multi-focal with microscopic invasive tissue

Size tumor: .8 cm; stage I

No positive lymph nodes

Surgical procedure: lumpectomy; mastectomy

Treatment: chemotherapy

Reconstruction: no

Estrogen receptors: negative; Progesterone receptors: negative

Who's Who:

Barry Adamson, her husband

Bernice Fagerstrom, her sister

Donna Grant, her friend* (see chapter 14)

Lolly Champion, her friend (see chapter 16)

Rachel, her daughter (six at time of diagnosis, not interviewed)

Lauren, her daughter (four at time of diagnosis, not interviewed)

All names other than Donna Grant's last name are real

DISCOVERY

Melba: At the urging of a close friend who was dying of breast cancer, I finally went in for a baseline mammogram. By the time I got home there was a message on my answering machine informing me of calcifications that warranted a biopsy.

Because of my medical background as an occupational therapist, I thought that having a biopsy would be "no big deal." It did not prepare me for the trauma of the procedure which involved laying absolutely still while the radiologist did the wire needle biopsy. Even with my breast numbed it was painful. I did not expect that the biopsy would be positive. Neither did the doctor. After all, I was only thirty-seven.

I clearly recall my doctor's late-night phone call. I was alone in my bedroom. He said, "I'm really sorry, but it's malignant. You have invasive breast cancer and need surgery." I could hear the shock in his voice, "because I'm so young." When I hung up the phone I was numb.

Bernice, her sister: I'm almost six years older than my sister and I'd been on her case to get a gynecological examination and mammogram because I had been diagnosed with precancerous cells in my cervix. One night she calls me hysterically sobbing, "I have breast cancer." Then she called back and said, "I don't have it." Then she called a third time to say, "I do, but it's microscopic." My thoughts were: *My God, she has breast cancer!* . . . *Phew, she doesn't* . . . *Oh, she does!* There was such confusion over her diagnosis. What a harrowing experience!

WHAT DO I DO NOW?

Melba: During my meeting with the doctor the following day, he told me and my husband that he had given me the wrong diagnosis over the telephone. He had not been reading from his notes and instead of my having invasive breast cancer (a much more serious diagnosis), I had intraductal cancer (also called DCIS). I knew that wasn't as serious because I had talked to some nurses I knew the day of my biopsy, and they had given me general information about breast cancer.

A lumpectomy was scheduled for the following week. Because I had

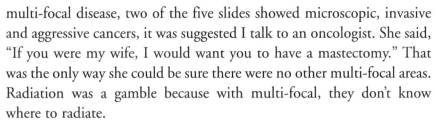

multi-focal disease, two of the five slides showed microscopic, invasive and aggressive cancers, it was suggested I talk to an oncologist. She said, "If you were my wife, I would want you to have a mastectomy." That was the only way she could be sure there were no other multi-focal areas. Radiation was a gamble because with multi-focal, they don't know where to radiate.

Two people helped in my decision-making process. One was my pastor who said, "Make decisions you can rest with, in your heart. It's not your parents', your husband's or your doctor's decision. It's yours." The other person was a woman who had recently undergone a mastectomy. She shared with me the reasons for her decision, which were very beneficial and helped me realize how important support is during the time of diagnosis. So many women are unaware that they can get a second opinion, or that they usually have time to get one.

Barry, her husband: Melba and I debated whether or not she should have a lumpectomy after being told by the doctor that he had not gotten all the cancer. She had the lumpectomy and then I turned my attention to getting as much advice and information as I could. Then I had to decipher it. As an attorney, I'm used to that approach. It became apparent and frustrating that neither the surgeon nor the oncologist really knew what to recommend. All we kept hearing were statistics. Then, when I asked the oncologist for her recommendation, she said she couldn't say. I told her that was ridiculous. She later called to apologize and, at that point, recommended a mastectomy. Melba and I were undecided. The decision to have a mastectomy was a joint decision. However, it was reached from different perspectives. Mine was based on the information we had; hers was more emotional.

CHEMOTHERAPY AND COPING

Melba: My surgeon had gotten clean margins (no cancer on the edges), and my lymph nodes were clear. He wanted me to see an oncologist. I was told that in cases like mine, there were no strong protocols. Statistically, chemotherapy would not greatly improve my odds; however, I had an aggressive cancer. After the mastectomy I thought I was finished having to make choices. Yet I was faced with another one. I elected chemotherapy because I wanted to do everything I felt I could. My protocol consisted of getting injections of 5-FU and methotrexate (which took about twenty minutes to administer), and Cytoxan pills. This is referred to as CMF. For the first two months I felt great, like I wasn't even on anything. Around the third month, my hair started to thin. I was losing hundreds of hairs a day. It stopped falling out in the fourth month. I have heard that if you still have hair around the fourth month, you'll keep what you have. I only lost about one-third of mine, but what was left looked lifeless. I was also fortunate not to lose my eyebrows or lashes, and I never needed that wig I ordered. Then the fatigue started. By the fifth or sixth month, I was wiped out by mid-afternoon. Neupogen (white cell growth factor) wasn't yet on the market and my white count was low. Even three months after the completion of my treatment, my count was only half of normal. I couldn't eat rich foods, but I was gaining weight anyway, which the doctor said was normal.

I went to a licensed acupuncturist during chemotherapy to help boost my immune system. The Chinese herbs I was given helped diminish my hot flashes and did not aggravate the psoriasis I'd had for years. My oncologist was aware I was using these herbs and had no objection, as long as I was not given estrogen.

During this time I started a support group with three other ladies who were older than I and had been through chemotherapy-induced menopause. As my friends and I were too young to have experienced menopause I thought I was going crazy when I started to experience things like hot flashes and a dry vagina—it felt like sandpaper. These ladies explained to me that being thrown into menopause and the lack of estrogen is what causes the vaginal tissues to become thin and dry, and that I wasn't crazy. There were creams like Replens that would help. As we talked and laughed I experienced moral support, or maybe you'd say some kind of swapping of human understanding I couldn't have gotten from my husband or friends.

Breast cancer is like a ripple effect. What I refer to as "battle fatigue" others refer to as post-traumatic stress disorder or stress. I used this analogy with some of the women in my support group:

Picture that you are going through a tornado. When it hits (read this as diagnosis and shock), you go down to the basement where many of us store our boxes. While waiting for the tornado to pass, and since you can't yet go back upstairs, you start rummaging through those boxes (just like you're going through treatment). You hope the tornado misses, but if it does hit you hope that all you'll need to do is put a few things back in place and move on. It passes; there's been some damage, but you've survived (your treatment is complete). Now you know you're going to live, but you also now need to clean up the mess. And you know what? You realize some boxes can be brought upstairs, but some of the "stuff" in the boxes is broken and needs to be thrown out. It just won't work anymore. And when everything is cleaned up, you'll never see things in boxes or outside the house quite the way you did before.

I tell other women that it's not just a matter of having surgery and then, boom, it's over. There was a treatment plan and lots of doctors' appointments; there was structure. When it ends, some women feel stranded. You know it's time to get on with your life, but something's changed. Maybe it's your partnership relationship or the fact that you're not good at nurturing yourself, or perhaps you're having to face how you look at yourself. With me, it's not like I planned on looking in my boxes, but I did. That's why I can't arrange my life the way it was before. Because when I went into "my basement," I discovered that I am a different person now. I think many of us go to the basement and look into our boxes. Those who go into deep depression and can't snap out of it have to understand that life can't be seen in the "as usual" mode when treatment is complete. Look at what has changed for you. Many people have never done that. For me, I went into therapy. Perhaps, just perhaps, cancer was my trigger.

THE TRUTH ABOUT CHEMOTHERAPY-INDUCED MENOPAUSE

Melba: One little ripple you're told very little about before starting chemotherapy is menopause. Fifty percent of women my age (thirty-seven) go into it. All the doctors say is that they'll give you things for it. It was not suggested that I see my gynecologist to discuss what it means to live without estrogen. No one told me that my risk, or any woman's risk, of heart disease increases or that bone density often decreases when we stop producing estrogen. When I was tested three years later for bone density, it showed I had the density of a seventy-year-old. I don't know if bone loss is chemotherapy-related, but my doctor suspected I'd had low bone density years before I started chemotherapy because mine was so low. I wish I'd had the test done before I started chemotherapy because that way I'd have known for sure. Three and a half months into chemotherapy my periods stopped, I was plagued with hot flashes and was fatigued. My vaginal tissues were starting to thin and become dry. Everything seemed dry. Even my eyes were so dry that I couldn't wear contacts. I was not a candidate for tamoxifen, which is given to women with positive estrogen receptors. Mine were negative. I was having a mental and emotional coping problem.

Six months out from chemotherapy, my period returned for two months, then stopped again, this time permanently. There is no doubt in my mind I am a different person without estrogen. My gynecologist wanted me on estrogen because he felt my risk of dying from heart disease was far greater than a cancer recurrence. But I disagreed and didn't take it.

I decided to work with a naturopathic physician. He put me on Ostaderm, a cream with phytoestrogens (plant compounds with estrogen-like activity) in it. I rub one teaspoon onto my skin twice a day. I've been on this for three years and have noticed that the thinning of my vaginal tissues has pretty much reversed.

Bernice, her sister: There are lots of tears when Melba talks about the hot flashes, the vaginal dryness and not being able to sleep at night. She thinks menopause and its side effects are worse than the mastectomy. It's been hard relating to menopause because I'm not in it. My doctor feels I'm not at any increased risk of cancer even with my family history. He also says that I am a candidate for hormone replacement therapy. I don't know what I will do because Melba goes on and on about how miserable she is, and you know what I think? I don't want to live like that.

THE CHILDREN

Melba: My husband and I told our four- and six-year-old girls that Mommy had breast cancer. We explained a little about what Mommy was going to go through, but kept it simple. We wanted to keep their lives as steady as possible. However, children are intuitive and pick up on a lot through overheard conversations, seeing tears, etc. They didn't have very many visual signs. Had I *looked* sick it might have been different, but the drains came out in the hospital so they didn't have to see them. I never vomited during chemotherapy and my hair only thinned. I was tired, but I looked fine and was doing everything.

Six weeks after my diagnosis, my oldest child broke out in shingles. She internalizes a lot, so I think this was a reaction to stress. The four-year-old? There's only so much a child that age can process. I did show them my scars and explained I had only one breast. My six-year-old asked, "Will I be like that when I grow up? Will I get cancer, too?" I truthfully explained there are no guarantees, but chances are that she wouldn't since her grandma didn't have breast cancer. I told her that simply because I didn't want her to live her life wondering about it. I told her that when she was older, we would talk about it more. In retrospect, I wish we had talked more about it then and had gotten an outside opinion on what was happening within our home, so we could give the girls an outlet. It might have helped had someone said, "Draw me a picture of Mommy's illness." Women have their own perceptions of their children and what they're feeling. Someone outside the family might have had a different perception of how the children were coping. We need that—different perceptions.

Barry, her husband: My children are fairly typical. Who knows what's bothering them? They don't mention cancer. They just know something's not right around here.

Donna, her friend: Melba thought that because of her fatigue during chemotherapy that she had abandoned her girls and hadn't spent enough time with them. It seems to me, she has put this huge burden on herself to make up for the last five years. Now, she feels she has to be there for them all the time, so she's babied them way too much. Her kids are spoiled rotten. She lets them whine and get away with things, and they don't help around the house. It was difficult at first to be around the children, but I realized I couldn't let her mothering skills (and my disapproval) destroy our friendship. Her children are affected by something, either the cancer or the relationship between their parents, I don't know which. The children have never talked to me about her situation.

Melba was pretty open about letting her children see her torso without a prosthesis. They have only one bathroom. My girls are the same age as hers. I didn't intentionally hide myself from my girls, but I also didn't go out of the way to show them what it looks like to have a mastectomy. I don't think such awareness of things like that are necessary in a child's life. It's one thing when they become teenagers if they want to ask about it or know about it.

Visual things have a tremendous impact on children. When I was younger, my family went camping. My mother was modest. However, my aunt was not, and she took off her clothes in front of us to shower. Now this woman was healthy and whole, but I still vividly remember her breasts and that black bush. It's an image that has stayed with me all my life! So I wouldn't just say to my kids, "Look, this is what it looks like."

Bernice, her sister: My sister wasn't very strong after surgery. She was having difficulty sleeping, was nauseated and just didn't feel well, all as a result of the chemotherapy. Her daughters didn't seem to understand what was going on and were very demanding of her. At that time, their mother just didn't like attending to their needs. They are now eleven and thirteen, and I think Rachel and Lauren are getting mixed messages. The children think everything that their mother tells them to do is negotiable because Melba negotiates everything with them. She needs to say what she means and mean what she says. Those children run her every way but loose. They are demanding because they're allowed to be demanding.

Lauren, the youngest, was too young to have fears about her mom dying. All she probably knew was that her mom was sick. I'm sure Rachel had some of those thoughts and feelings. I think all children equate cancer with dying, to some degree. But with time, those feelings have probably faded. Children always know when there's tension between two people, when things aren't right, when their parents are angry, even without a lot of fighting. This has caused a lot of problems for the girls. I believe the reason one of the girls is overweight is because of the household tension and her feelings about that and herself.

THE LOSS OF A BREAST

Melba: At first I was thrilled to be alive. Who cares about losing that sagging fatty tissue! Still, I was self-conscious and felt as though everyone was staring at my chest. The first few weeks after surgery when friends came to visit, I wore a borrowed prosthesis. About three months after surgery, I started sobbing in the shower. You can fake it most of the time but not in the shower where you can't hide from it. I missed my breast, and I revealed that to my husband one night. He hadn't said a whole lot about this thing, but instead of saying, "Oh, I don't care," he said, "I miss it, too." I knew he had been sad for me, but I hadn't realized, until that moment, that I had needed him to acknowledge that he did miss it. I was tired of hearing that it didn't matter. I wanted it to matter at least a little!

It has now been six years, and some days I want to throw the prosthesis in the toilet. It's hot, heavy and is an inconvenience. I'm small-shouldered, large-hipped and wear a C/D cup. It's obvious when I don't wear it. I have two daughters who are both starting to develop breasts, and they get embarrassed about anything having to do with breasts, so they have fits if I leave my prosthesis in the bathroom.

Barry, her husband: It really didn't bother me that Melba had only one breast. What bothered me was her scar. When I was a child I had a very serious accident which caused me to have many surgeries. I am fine today, but to this day I get physically weak and dizzy at the thought of surgery and looking at scars. Even though I've tried to reassure Melba that I'm okay with her scar, I'm sure that she thinks that I'm lying.

NOT EVERYONE IS A GOOD CANDIDATE FOR RECONSTRUCTION

Melba: Initially I didn't want to think about reconstruction, but five years later I did. Unfortunately, I am not a good candidate. I have very thin skin around my ribs and back, and when they removed my breast, there was barely enough skin to close me. You can see my heart pumping, my ribs are right there. Because I'm not flat across the chest and I cave into my armpits, I would be cock-eyed. I'm not sure I have enough skin on my back for a latissimus dorsi. I could have a TRAM flap, but I'm chicken. Besides, that's a six- to seven-hour procedure followed by seven days in the hospital. All that for just a breast? I would still need to wear a prosthesis or have a breast reduction on the other side for my breasts to match. Obtaining symmetry is difficult. I have felt deformed at times. Why couldn't I be as good a candidate as others?

Barry, her husband: It's a shame she wasn't a candidate for reconstructive surgery because I think having that breast gone has affected her attitude.

Bernice, her sister: Melba hates her prosthesis because it's so heavy. Even I was blown away by its weight. She has problems finding tops to wear. When I asked her why she hadn't had the surgery (her insurance wouldn't pay 100 percent), she hemmed and hawed. I've wondered, *Is it that she isn't a candidate or is it the money issue?*

STARTING A SUPPORT GROUP

Melba: Three weeks after my mastectomy, the local newspaper interviewed me. It was October, Breast Cancer Awareness month. As a result of that article, I received a call from the local hospital asking me to start a support group, which I did three months later. I ran that support group for almost two years until I left to work on some personal issues. During this time I also started a business in which I educated women about their options, before having surgery. We talked about their concerns, and I helped provide insight and solutions. We talked about things like sleeping on the opposite side of the bed if you're having difficulty physically getting out of bed because of the surgery, and that it's easier getting into a blouse that buttons down the front after surgery, and how to pin a little something into your blouse which will give you a little shape so that you're not completely flat. Just simple things.

This networking brought home to me the many blessings that get missed. I can't believe how many women I've been able to laugh with! We all need that, but can't do it except with others who have been through the same thing.

Barry, her husband: I think it's a terrible thing to have to face alone, so I feel that support groups are worthwhile. She met some great people and I think that overall, the good probably outweighs the "pity party" effect. But the negative side is that you can get too self-involved and angry and consequently, forget everything else as a result of continually being around and talking about cancer.

Donna, her friend: I went to Melba's support group and felt she offered a lot of "survivor" insight. There were a lot of young women in the group. Melba always tried to match us with someone who had a similar medical history, same tumor size, number of positive lymph nodes, etc. That's really comforting when you're going through it. A support group helps you to know you're not the only one it's happened to, and that you have someone to talk to and find out what happens next.

COPING WITH LIFE AND DEATH

Melba: My six-year-old brother died of leukemia when I was thirteen. I never got to say good-bye. My two older siblings were away at school. No one in my family dealt with his death. We just kind of put our lives back together and never talked about him much. So it was especially hard having to call my parents, who lived out of state, to tell them I had cancer, too. My dad started crying and moaning, "Oh no, oh no." Even today my mom does this telephone thing. I know what she means when she says, "Well, how *are* you?"

It wasn't until after I went into therapy that I learned to write in a journal. Many hidden issues surfaced. One was the realization that because my parents didn't have a pattern set up to talk to me as a child, I didn't have the skills to talk to my own children. Another was that I equated cancer with death. I found I was more petrified of death than I ever realized. Old feelings surfaced, and I felt furious with God for letting my brother die! As a result, I lost my faith. I've had to fight to get God back into my life. I'm still working on it. What I eventually came to realize is that I can be angry with God and can still have a relationship with him. I've learned how to have a voice and that it's okay to make mistakes.

My husband is tender but hides a lot of his feelings. I found support in having him there to hold me. But even early on in our marriage, I had a problem expressing to him what I really wanted and needed. When I was diagnosed, he went on autopilot and his role was more, "I've got to take care of this home and the children." So even though I did get some support from him, I got more from my relationship with God and other women in terms of really working through the process and the different stages.

It's been hard losing friends to this disease. We take all kinds of preparation classes; marriage, birthing, etc. But what about death preparation classes? None of us has a clue how to do that. Once you can admit to that or admit to having feelings of loss, you can move on. Through therapy I've acquired a wonderful healing tool, laughter. Even in tragedy you have to find something to laugh about sometimes. You can laugh through your tears, and that doesn't mean you are in denial.

Barry, her husband: Our marriage was fair to good before her diagnosis, but since then it has gotten worse. I think there were deeper things going on, and cancer was the "trigger." Melba became very self-absorbed in the cancer thing and involved with cancer-related projects.

Breast cancer was a turning point for her. I believe it made her realize she was angry about a lot of things, family things, childhood things. She was also angry about being thrown into menopause. At one point, life turned into a self-pitying party, and I am so sick and tired of hearing about breast cancer that there are times that I just want to tell her, "Move on with your life!" It has been almost seven years, and she can't let it go! After working fourteen years with the same law firm, I quit my job because I didn't feel my career was going anywhere. I took a year off to try to figure out what I wanted to do, and as a result of that Melba started working full time. Right around the time I started my own practice, she was diagnosed with breast cancer. She blames me for her cancer saying that because I took a year off, she got sick. That's irrational. Worse, Melba constantly reminds me of all she went through and that I wasn't there for her. Yes, she did go through a lot, but no one else could do the chemotherapy treatments except her. I couldn't help that she was nauseated, but we *were* there for her and didn't let her go through all that by herself, even though that's not her perception of what happened.

I needed to confirm with some of our friends that I wasn't just imagining the changes in Melba. They noticed changes, too, and wanted to know what was going on with her behavior. Finally I realized part of the blame was mine. I was codependent and needed to change that. I finally made it clear that there was a problem, that she needed help. There needs to be a resolution of all that because I can no longer be accommodating.

Donna, her friend: When I met Melba in 1991 she was physically healed but still angry about things that had happened to her during chemotherapy, like being thrown into menopause. She was sad, not clinically depressed. We became friends and I was the "up" person in her life. It's important for friends to listen or to talk about the cancer. Friends shouldn't be afraid to ask how the person with cancer is dealing with this or that and whether they feel like talking about it. By asking, you are giving the other person the opportunity to say "no" without probing. My friends know what's going on with me, but it doesn't consume our relationships.

With Melba, cancer is still utmost in her mind. It dawned on me recently that as long as I've known Melba she's been involved with cancer in some fashion—support groups, doctor groups, etc. She's stuck in the cancer rut, and her entire life revolves around it. Someone needs to shake her and tell her "There's life after cancer!" I say, "Try to do fun things, go out to lunch, have a glass of white wine, people watch, see a funny movie. Don't talk about cancer all the time!" But she persists because that's who she is.

Lolly, her friend: We all have our own personal battle plan. Hers is being won by giving service to others. That helps Melba deal with her own pain. She is very effective at it. I've known her five or six years, and I think she is still having trouble facing her particular private issues. My feeling is she hasn't come to terms with having breast cancer, but I don't believe any us ever do. I think you have to take time to take care of yourself because no one is going to be more responsible for you than you.

Maybe she'll deal with it, maybe she won't. It would be nice though to see her more at peace with her own situation.

Bernice, her sister: When I stayed with Melba after her mastectomy, I cleaned her house—a lot! That's how I cope when things are out of my control. I had already lost a little brother to cancer, and I was afraid she was going to die. Those first couple of years I kept waiting for that phone call telling me she had a recurrence. As the years have gone by, I've become more comfortable.

Barry and I have very different viewpoints on the role of women and "their place." We don't get along, and I felt awkward staying in their home. They've been together seventeen to eighteen years, and there's a lot of tension between them. I think there are serious marital problems going on that I don't believe are specifically related to breast cancer and her mastectomy. Because he's always been undemonstrative towards her, I wasn't shocked at his behavior after her surgery. Yet I was awestruck at his coldness, his lack of empathy and how he was handling it. I couldn't believe a man wouldn't be more tender after what his wife had just gone through.

His behavior upset me, so I asked my husband, with whom I have a wonderful relationship, "Does the loss of a breast impact men that much that he should be so cold?" I needed to know if Barry's attitude was the norm. I had seen her scar, and it was bigger than I thought it would be. Did men have such a hard time handling the loss of a breast that they couldn't touch or hold you? My husband said, "It doesn't have a damn thing to do with that. You could have no breasts tomorrow, and it wouldn't change one thing between us." I had to know that if I were ever in that position, my husband would be there for me, helping me cope.

I feel extra sorry for Melba because she doesn't have that. I've never actually heard Melba tell Barry she blames him for her breast cancer. She has, however, told him she feels he is constantly judging her and that she comes up short in his eyes. Breast cancer has exacerbated their problems. I don't think the real problem is money. My feeling is that neither of them has been willing to sit down and face the real issue—which is how they feel towards one another and where they're going.

Both Melba and I were raised to be caregivers and to give little atten-tion to our own wants and needs. Breast cancer was her wake-up call, the beginning of taking an inventory of her needs. I've learned that regardless of my love for my sister, I have to let go. I have my life and she has hers. Whatever problems she has, she has to face them herself.

Postscript, January 2000

Wish list:

Wish I had gotten a second opinion.

Wish I had looked into reconstruction and the possibilities available to me before surgery. It is now not possible.

Wish I had kept a journal and that I'd had my children write down their thoughts or draw a picture—something to remember.

Wish more doctors would consider hiring therapists for both before and after surgery.

Wish I had paid more attention to stress.

Wish I would celebrate more often.

Additional Postscript

Dear friends:

I use the word "friends" because I have come to deeply value even those of you I haven't met. Maybe I'm learning a great lesson to value everyone not just those I am particularly drawn to. One who comes alongside is a friend. Each of you in reading this book has in some way come alongside me and others to listen, possibly learn and grow in your own understanding. I believe that is how we help one another. Many of you will face this diagnosis or some other life crisis. I suppose we're all in training to walk whatever our journey is without fear or intimida-tion, and to not be overwhelmed by life but to live it. Interesting but I now think I may have been living in more fear than I realized a few years ago. The kind of fear that comes from inside. The kind that is there yet hidden. I believe we must do more to know and care for each other whether that involves helping someone cope with cancer, adoles-cence, aging parents or single parenthood. Hopefully my vision of com-munity is much broader than before cancer.

I continue to live in the same community with my two wonderful teenage daughters. I'm divorced and work part-time as an occupational therapist with children. I believe women still need more information and someone to come alongside them in the beginning when they hear a breast cancer diagnosis. I did have the opportunity to work with a group of surgeons who spoke with women both pre- and post-operatively. There are lots of little things that don't necessarily get discussed with doctors that can be discussed and shared in order to avoid unnecessary worries and hassles whether a woman is thirty-seven or seventy. I hate to see the concerns of older women minimized because of their age.

I have low bone density so I walk a few times a week. I used to lift weights, but have stopped for now. And yes, in many ways I take better care of myself. Life is definitely different without estrogen. I still use natural remedies. Occasionally I receive a phone call from a woman just diagnosed, and we simply talk. Somehow reassurance becomes more real with a person, not just books or pamphlets. I wish everyone could get that kind of personal involvement.

Unfortunately my dear friend Donna Grant died in 1997. This past summer my sister had a lump the doctors were almost sure was malignant. It was not. We need to wait, take more deep breaths and develop our spirits and life's work. I am now celebrating ten years cancer free. May God richly bless all you who continue to fight and hope.

Thirteen

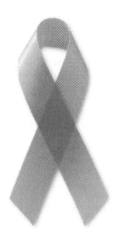

Tania Katan

The Creation of *Stages,*
an Autobiographical Play

Survivor Profile:

Age at diagnosis: twenty-one (11/92)

Age at interview: twenty-five (11/20/96)

Type of breast cancer: infiltrating ductal

Size tumor: 4 cm; stage II

No positive lymph nodes

Surgical procedure: mastectomy

Treatment: chemotherapy

Reconstruction: no

Estrogen receptors: negative; Progesterone receptors: negative

Who's Who:

Joelle Katan, her mother

Fran Troy, her significant other

How It All Started

Tania: I was twenty-one and in college. While doing a breast self-examination, I felt a lump so I went to Planned Parenthood. They said I probably had fibrocystic breasts and that I should limit my caffeine intake and come back in one month. A month later the lump had grown and was very painful. I went to my primary care physician who suggested I take vitamin E, stop caffeine altogether and watch my condition for another month.

After a two-month delay, I had an ultrasound which showed a mass. The surgeon couldn't get any fluid from it. As a precaution, he suggested doing a biopsy even though he didn't think it was anything.

Joelle, her mother: We all thought it was just a cyst! She was told by everyone she had fibrocystic breasts and needed to stop drinking coffee. Tania kept telling them it was getting bigger and more painful but was told that if it's painful, it's nothing to worry about! I finally insisted on accompanying her on an appointment. It was Tania who insisted on a biopsy. Was the surgeon's hesitancy because of her age?

I fell asleep in the waiting room during the biopsy and was awakened by a nurse who said the doctor wanted to see me. He said "I have some really bad news. I know for sure this is cancer."

I was having a hard time coping. Eleven days earlier my twelve-year-old stepdaughter, Megan, died from an inoperable brain tumor. My husband and I had gone through nine months of hell—experimental chemotherapy and radiation. I was exhausted, drained and depressed. And now, I was being told *my* child has cancer and the doctor thought a very aggressive one! I thought, *No way! We just had cancer in the family.*

After the biopsy, the doctor left it up to me to tell her she had cancer. I felt that was wrong. He should have told her. Was it because she was still sedated or because of her age? Before I told her at home I went into my bargain with God thing. *Why did you give this to my daughter? Aren't I good enough for you?* When she awakened, I had on that fake "Everything is okay" mask, but she saw through it. I was so uncomfortable. How would I tell her? What would I say? It was such an incredible weight. I didn't tell her the doctor suspected it was the worst kind of breast cancer because we didn't yet know for sure. So I just told her it was aggressive and that we were still waiting for the pathology report. I wanted to tell her my fears, but instead just held her and cried. Half smiling she said, "Mom, it's okay. I'll be okay."

Subconsciously, I was thinking it can't be true. *What if they made an error?* I was angry thinking about the lack of money spent on breast cancer research. Part of me felt that my daughter was the sacrificial lamb. She was only twenty-one!

NOW WHAT?

Tania: The next day the doctor told me that I had a 4 cm, grade 3, quickly spreading, aggressive, infiltrating ductal carcinoma. My options were to have either a lumpectomy or mastectomy, and I needed to make a decision quickly because my cancer had grown from the size of a small jellybean to the size of a golfball in one month. The doctor explained everything, but I was hit with so much information at one time that I was unable to process it all, not only because it was a blow that I had cancer, but also because I really didn't have a good grasp of what he was telling me. Aesthetically I understood what it meant to have a breast removed but I wasn't sure which procedure was better for me or the benefits of doing one over the other. I opted for a modified radical mastectomy with chemotherapy because to me, the less tissue left, the less likely it was to return. Because my surgeon seemed competent I did not get a second opinion.

Today I think, *Are you guys idiots? How could you not know? How could you just pass me around? A lump that grows from one size to another quickly and is painful? A mass that's solid?* I was classic. The only way I wasn't classic was being twenty-one . . . that's just ridiculous!

Joelle, her mother: When I found out she did not have the worst kind of breast cancer, I felt as though we had won the lottery. Tania told me she wanted to be the primary person asking the doctor questions. I understood this was her experience and the decisions were hers, not mine. I allowed her to be the adult she was. I respect Tania's space because she is so assertive, and sometimes that bites me in the nose. But I did ask questions.

THE HOSPITAL EXPERIENCE

Tania: In the hospital I had a self-dosing morphine machine, because I'm pain sensitive and painkillers make me vomit. I hated the IVs, everything was so painful. But because I was in a daze, I just accepted it. I was visited by a social worker who gave me pamphlets on what to do and support groups. I was overwhelmed and blown away by the entire experience. I felt as though I were in a maze and had to choose A or B. So, I dealt with it by not dealing with it for awhile.

Within two weeks I was playing tennis and was able to start school when semester break was over. I healed quickly.

CHEMOTHERAPY AND COPING

Tania: At the beginning of spring semester at Arizona State University I started chemotherapy. It had been about a month since my mastectomy. Although I told some of my teachers what was going on, I didn't think it would be a big deal. I was in total denial!

My regimen was to take Cytoxan pills and get injections of methotrexate and 5-FU in my hand which only took about one minute. I hated the injections and feeling the chemicals in my body and tasting them in my mouth. I imagined it was how bleach and cleaning agents would taste. For five minutes I felt sick and wanted to vomit, but I couldn't move. Then I would drink some water and be all right. I discovered that running my hands under hot water and opening and closing them right before the injection helped my veins to stop rolling.

When I started chemotherapy, one of my theater major classes was playwriting, which was a perfect outlet for me and I decided to write "my story." *Stages* was my therapy. It took me two years to write, modify and produce. It has been performed throughout the United States. I won a National Playwright Award in 1996, and I was interviewed by the *New York Times,* as well as being on radio. The play has gone over well.

Not just because breast cancer is a hot issue, but because I was twenty-one and it was autobiographical. *Stages* uses a lot of humor, because that is how I dealt with it. There was no resolution for my main character, Lisa, because in my life, there was none. Lisa says that maybe it could come back and maybe it won't. It isn't optimistic or pessimistic, just realistic. Once you have cancer you're not the same. The truth is . . . it could come back. I didn't set out to be an advocate, it just happened. I needed to write my story and purge. I'm so happy people can relate to it.

Fran, her significant other: Tania and I had started dating around the time she started chemotherapy. The hardest thing for her during this time was not being in control of her body or her life. She's a doer and a goer, and she couldn't work out or do the things that she normally did. Here's a woman who's master of her universe and this was something she couldn't master and couldn't control. She cried once. That was out of frustration with her body and not being in control. Despite her young age she got respect from her doctors as well as sorrow and disbelief . . . because of her age! And that pissed her off! Tania has a commanding presence but is also funny and knows how to work a room and situation to her advantage.

WHY I CHOSE NOT TO BE RECONSTRUCTED

Tania: Initially, I didn't think about the aesthetics when I lost my breast. I thought, *In order for me to live, it has to go!* Wearing a prosthesis or having reconstruction didn't occur to me until I was recovering and was visited by a Reach for Recovery volunteer. She brought me this silly little stocking thing with stuffing in it. I became angry, because it was as though everyone would be much happier if I "had a booby." It wasn't my fault I had lost my breast, and I didn't feel there should be any shame involved. At that point I became adamantly against reconstruction.

I didn't wear a prosthesis for three years because I wanted to become comfortable with who I was, having only one breast. I'm a lesbian and for me, having only one breast was like "coming out" all over again. When is it a good time to tell someone? Do I have to tell them? Is it an

issue or a non-issue? Maybe if every woman opted not to have reconstruction, everyone would grow more comfortable with it. I know it's
difficult to function in society without breasts, but if we all said it's not
our fault and we were comfortable with it, people would have no choice.
A classmate who didn't know me well one day asked if I stuffed my bra.
When I told her I had lost a breast to cancer, she felt terrible. In a way
I was glad she was honest.

Most days I feel comfortable not wearing a prosthesis but it is easier
having two breasts, because then it's a non-issue. I wore my prosthesis
to a job interview. Why? Because I didn't want to go through potential
discrimination. If I don't wear my prosthesis to work I wear baggy shirts,
simply because I don't want to deal with it. I like having the option.
Sometimes though I do think about reconstruction, particularly when
my clothes don't hang right. But those days are far and few between. I'm
glad I made the decision I did. In *Stages* Lisa's therapist asks her whether
she will wear a prosthesis when school starts. She replies, "No. No prosthesis and no bra. And I'm going to wear something tight." I did that
sometimes just to see the kinds of reactions I would get from people.

I was fired as a camp counselor because I only had one breast. When
the director found out, he asked what would I tell the girls when we
were showering together? I told him I would answer their questions and
educate them. Shortly thereafter I was fired with full severance. Was the
bottom line what would the children think? What impact would that
have on their parents? Or was it because I'm gay? I was discriminated
against, but I've chosen not to think about it in those terms.

Fran, her significant other: Tania and I talked a lot about reconstruction. I felt she should do what she wanted. What I really thought was,
*Don't go back to surgery, something could go wrong! You need a breast for what
reason?* My opinion was and still is, why not just have a prosthesis? Have
a breast when you feel you need one, for clothes or body image or when
you just don't want people looking at you differently. This way there's no
danger. I knew it wasn't true when Tania told me she didn't care what
others thought, because I'd see her putting in her prosthesis. I was saddened because I knew what that was all about. But, she has to deal with it.

Joelle, her mother: I accepted Tania's decision not to have reconstruction. Because she set the tone, I had a less difficult time handling that decision. On a physical level it was just a scar. Maybe the fact that Tania is gay had a lot to do with my accepting everything better. I live in a heterosexual world and understand the male perspective about what a woman's breast represents. Although I know little of the lesbian lifestyle, I suspect that women as a whole are more accepting of other women.

SUPPORT GROUPS

Tania: I went to a Y-ME support group meeting during chemotherapy specifically to talk to other women who had lost one or both breasts. I'd hoped that sharing their experiences would help me become more comfortable with having only one breast. At the meeting, my mom and I were taken to the bathroom so all these ladies could show us their reconstructed and altered breasts! I felt they were "covering up" their cancer, not dealing with it! We had obviously gone through the same thing but was my response different because of my age? I wanted to deal with deeper issues, not surface ones like reconstructed breasts and where to buy a wig!

Months later I tried a different support group. I was now angry about having breast cancer, the thought of reconstruction, everything! That women who had something go wrong with their bodies were trying to cover it up! I just wanted someone to say, "I can understand where you're coming from, but this was my choice and here's why I chose it." That would have given me some insight into why someone did what they did. No one could understand my reasons for not altering my breast. I could not find anyone to relate to. Instead of sharing, they became defensive. It's not fair to ask someone to accept you when you don't accept yourself. I didn't know how to respond to them because I had no shame, and I felt they did. For me, these types of support groups were counterproductive. What did appeal to me was a breast cancer art group. As an artist, I met others who had learned to express their experience through their art.

Joelle, her mother: When all those women whipped off their tops to show us their reconstructed breasts, it was almost like men showing off: "Look, this is what I got in the war!"

LIFE AND DEATH

Tania: I equate cancer with death. So, when they told me I had breast cancer, I really thought I was going to die until the doctor told me I wasn't. Then he explained I had invasive cancer. What does that mean? That I could die!

I coped by writing my play. Sometimes, I'd be on my way to class and would inexplicably find myself crying. When that occurred, instead of going to class, I'd go to a coffee house and sit there crying and writing for hours, writing about what I had experienced. I am more afraid of dying today than when I was diagnosed five years ago. My mortality has been questioned. In *Stages* Lisa says, "Oh God, my head hurts. I have a headache. Is it cancer in my brain?" And that's the reality of this disease. Statistically I can die.

My friends and family coped by using good-natured humor, and it was beneficial to me knowing others could joke about cancer. I think some people are uncomfortable and don't know what to say (myself included) when they're around other people with cancer. If the one with the cancer feels comfortable with it, their attitude puts others at ease. My male twin and younger sister didn't talk about it. Maybe they thought they were treading on thin ice. Or perhaps, they were in denial. Seeing the play allowed them to see what I was feeling. My sister, Tessa, told me she wasn't sure how to approach certain things with me like how I felt about it. We had to feel each other out with what was okay to talk about. They both wanted to see my scar but were afraid to ask. So I had to initiate that and let them know it was okay. They did care. Tessa now freaks out about everything. She checks her breasts all the time and goes in for regular gynecological examinations.

I went to a therapist a few times, but it wasn't my gig. Ironically, I ended up dating one, Fran, who became my significant other and major supporter. It's important to know you're a good person, that you're not losing a part of yourself that is essential to your being . . . that defines you. If you feel this loss, then go into therapy!

My parents are divorced, and I have a good relationship with both. Cancer has brought my dad and me closer. His sister died of breast cancer, and he has never really dealt with her death. He just holds me a lot which is his way of caring. Mom told me, "I wish I were going through this instead of you." They're so cute. If I tell one I'm not feeling well, I get a phone call ten minutes later from the other asking if I'm okay. I like them being so supportive.

I'm Jewish but don't go to temple. I believe in, let's just call it, a big energy. Sometimes I thank God for being alive, but that may mean something entirely different to me than to someone else. Whether it's coming from me or from some other place, I'm thankful for it. Essentially, I'm the same as I was before. I wouldn't want to repeat the experience, but I'm thankful for the insight it has given me. I'm more appreciative of life itself, I don't take certain things for granted and I don't want to be sucked dry in relationships. I've become more selective about choosing friends. I've learned to demand and expect respect and support from those around me. If they can't do this, I choose not to have them in my life.

Fran, her significant other: I'm the type to take care of everybody and everything. Only a few years ago did I learn to express my own feelings. After Tania's mastectomy, I wanted to talk through my anxieties about death and mortality. I was crying about her cancer, and she was detached from it. She said, "What's the point in feeling bad? It's a done deal, it's out of me. My lymph nodes are clear, and I don't want a pity party." Was the disparity in attitude caused by our fourteen-year age difference?

I needed to talk openly and honestly, but it was difficult not knowing when I might say or do the wrong thing. Just because we joked about it one day didn't mean it was okay to joke about it the next. I needed to be aware of that and let her be there for me, too. She didn't always want to be the one being taken care of. It's okay to say the cancer word because saying it makes it real. It's like when you see a person in a wheelchair and you try to pretend they're not in the wheelchair so you kind of talk around it. You don't want to make them invisible. Validate the experience.

Sometimes Tania would exhibit crazy behavior like eating fatty foods, drinking, smoking cigarettes or going on shopping sprees we couldn't afford. She knew I'd be irked about the shopping, but that's how she'd cope. One part of me said, "It's okay, it's the cancer thing." The other felt frustrated and shut out because I knew this was how Tania dealt with her feelings. Instead of talking to me she'd spend money. I think I shocked her once when I said, "I'll kill you if you die and leave me with all this stuff you bought because you didn't deal with your cancer!"

As she was writing, I watched her evolve as she learned to express her feelings through her play. I sat back and watched her scream about being out of control through Lisa. It was her way of giving life to those feelings.

Joelle, her mother: My stepdaughter Megan's death was a tremendous blow. I was exhausted from lack of sleep and having to be my husband, Steve's, support. On top of that, I was dealing with Tania's health situation. Because of exhaustion, I'm not even sure I consciously thought she might have cancer. When she was diagnosed I was overwhelmed, incredulous and angry. I understand the importance of not being afraid or too proud to reach out for help. Yet I couldn't talk to Steve, who was wrapped up in his own grief. Tania had always been my confidant, but I felt she had enough to deal with. And I didn't want to burden my friends. That's when I realized, prejudicial or not, that women feel things at a higher, more complex level than men do. I was drained. I couldn't say a sentence without wanting to cry. And for nine months I was near suicidal. As a result I saw a therapist, on and off.

Being a social worker I'm well-versed in death and dying. It has been a fascination, as well as a fear, of mine. I thought a lot about Tania dying and my frustration was knowing I would want to die with her since I didn't know if I could survive the pain. Even though I have two other children, that's how I felt. One day I told Steve to just shoot me and put me out of my misery. You've heard people say they want to die because of such and such. Having gone through the experience, what I believe is really being said is, "I have this incredible need for somebody to make me feel better, and I don't think anybody is capable of giving me that." What comes out instead is, "I'm suffering and I want to die" or "I want to die."

My marriage to Steve has been lived in what I call "crisis management." He copes by burying himself in work and sports. I coped by overeating and not exercising, which I must do to maintain my own health. I finally made a choice and decided to save my own life. We have separated, and I am moving out of state.

Stages was my daughter's catalyst to say something really important about what happened to her and how she reacted. If only one person is affected, what a gift she has given. She showed you can laugh through your tears. Tania is like many children who risk things when they're young, because they are fearless and they think they're indestructible. I taught her that she could do no wrong, that nothing could happen to her. It only proves, even with all the right components, something can.

Is It Ever Over?

Tania: I went in for a routine Pap smear two and a half years after my breast cancer diagnosis. During the examination the doctor said, "Oh my God!" You don't say that to a woman who's had cancer! I immediately panicked. Because experience had taught me how valuable it is to bring a tape recorder and a list of prepared questions to doctor's appointments, I was prepared for the consultation. I had by then learned that I was the customer and had the right to ask lots of questions and not be afraid to ask. Instead of the vacation Fran and I were supposed to take, I had surgery. We didn't know if I had cancer again or just a large mass. I didn't think it was cancer, but I didn't want to jinx it by thinking about it. So many scenarios were going through my mind: hysterectomy, colostomy, cancer!

My mom and Fran were screaming, "It's not! It's not!" when I came out of recovery. What a feeling to know you have this large mass that is just a large mass and not cancer!

Fran, her significant other: The routine gynecological examination where the doctor found "something" in Tania's uterus was the hardest time for me because I wasn't with her when the breast cancer was discovered. I missed the waiting, the fear of the unknown and my fear of her dying. I'm usually positive but thought, *She's had cancer before. Who's to say it's not cancer again?* I'd picture the doctor opening her up and then immediately closing her because it was too late. We would have periods of high anxiety, and then we'd crash. It was really hard being the significant other because I had to deal with the possibility that the person I loved could die. Nights were the most difficult for me. I would look at this young woman sleeping next to me and become fearful and angry that bad things happen to good people. I talked to both Tania and my friends about my feelings. Was that fair? I think so, because she has to be there for me, too.

The day of surgery arrived and Tania's mom was driving both of us crazy with inane remarks like, "I hope it's going to be okay." She wanted to express her feelings but didn't know if she should or could. Even though each of us had our own support team there, we all supported one another. Through this experience my awareness of giving support to others was heightened. It was a happy ending. Tania had a non-cancerous fibroid. I cried nonstop for three hours from relief. Then I was angry because we had been so focused on breast cancer that Tania skipped her annual gynecological exam. It could have been discovered a lot sooner. She'd had symptoms. Her periods had been getting worse, and she was urinating frequently.

Tania and I are no longer together. When we broke up I felt some relief. We both needed to grow. Tania needed to experience taking care of herself, and I needed to stop caregiving. But when I learned that she'd had a routine Pap smear and had gotten back a funny result a part of me said, *Now what do I do? Do I go back and resume a relationship because she's sick?* I realized I didn't want to be in a relationship because of illness. Even though I still love her I can't go back. And I felt a sense of peace because I knew I didn't want to be there because of that. I had a profound thought. It wasn't about Tania, it was about me and illness. Would we be together today if she hadn't had cancer? I don't think so.

Postscript, January 2000

I had breast cancer, I survived and I'm thankful for the insight it provided me. However, I would prefer never to repeat it again! I am happy, healthy, surly and sassy and have moved to San Francisco where I am a professional playwright with a day job.

A word on one-breast visibility. Since my mastectomy I have appeared half-clad in numerous publications including: *The Advocate, Mamm* magazine, *Girlfriends* and others. I recommend taking off your shirt for national publications or just for your neighbors—it increases visibility and is JUST PLAIN FUN!

Fourteen

Donna Grant

It Just Kept Coming Back

Survivor Profile:

Age at diagnosis: thirty-four (5/91)

Age at interview: thirty-nine (8/6/96)

Type of breast cancer: infiltrating ductal; breast cancer other breast (11/93): infiltrating lobular

Size tumor: 6 cm; stage III; three positive lymph nodes

Surgical procedure: single modified radical mastectomy; breast cancer other breast (11/93): mastectomy

Treatment: chemotherapy and radiation; recurrence 4/93: radiation; recurrence 4/95: tamoxifen, Taxol, radiation, bone marrow transplant using stem cells, Arimidex

Estrogen receptors: positive; Progesterone receptors: positive

Who's Who:*

Tony Grant, her husband

Jessica Grant, her daughter (age six at diagnosis)

Emily Grant, her daughter (age three at diagnosis)

Emma Pazos, her mother

Anthony Pazos, her father

Melba Adamson, her friend [see chapter 12]

*Fictitious last name of survivor, husband and children by request. All other names are real.

IT BEGINS

Donna: I had a small lump removed in October of 1990, and it was benign. The baseline mammogram that was done in December showed nothing, but a month later I noticed another lump in the same place. Assuming it, too, was benign I did nothing; however, by April it had grown considerably. My doctor wanted me to have a biopsy. I was thirty-three.

When I woke up from surgery, Tony and my surgeon were standing beside me. When my surgeon said to me, "I hate to tell you, but it was cancer," my first reaction was, "You're kidding, right?" I was absolutely floored. Tony looked very shaken and was too speechless to talk.

At the meeting the next day, my surgeon told Tony and me that the lump he had taken out was a 6-cm (about the size of a large plum) infiltrating ductal cancer. Because of its size, and the fact that I was small-breasted, my only option was to have a mastectomy. I was infuriated when I was informed that I had already been scheduled for surgery three days later. My surgeon had taken the first available operating room. After brooding about it for a day, I realized I really had no other choice.

Tony, her husband: I called the surgeon's office to see if Donna was out of surgery and was told, "You had better come to our office," so I did. When her doctor told me that Donna had cancer my first question was, "Can it be treated?" and he said, "Yes." I did not care that Donna was going to lose a breast when we were told a mastectomy was her *only* option. My only thought was, *God, just don't let her die.*

Emma, her mother: My husband, Anthony, and I were really shook up when Tony called to tell us the news about Donna. I immediately booked a flight to Portland, Oregon, where they lived at the time, so I could be with them. It's a good thing I went because Tony practically collapsed in my arms when he picked me up at the airport. That night the three of us talked about what to tell the girls. I thought they should be told the truth; Tony did not; and Donna wanted to protect them and do whatever Tony wanted to do. Since we were at an impasse, I invited myself to pray for the two of them, and we joined in a three-way prayer. It seemed afterwards as if we were all calmer and more able to cope.

Anthony, her father: I felt as though my world had collapsed. The more I thought about it, the more I cried. *How can this be? There is no cancer in our family, on either side!* Then I kept trying to reassure myself, *It's going to be all right.*

THE DAY ARRIVES

Donna: That Friday I had a single modified radical mastectomy. Terrified of developing lymphedema, I began to exercise my arm in the middle of the night. The girls came to visit on Sunday since it was Mother's Day.

Even though my doctor had left both silicone implants from the breast augmentation I'd had done the year before, I was scared to look at myself when the bandages were removed. If he had taken out the implant I think I would have been a wreck. When I did finally look, I thought to myself, *That's not so bad!* There was no nipple, but at least I still had some shape. Once I was home the girls assumed that things were back to normal. Emily wanted to give me hugs and be picked up, but I could not do that. I told her, "Mommy is sore and has a big boo-boo." She understood as much as any three-year-old could.

Tony, her husband: Donna took losing her breast pretty hard. We did not have an unveiling. She showed me her breast when she was ready.

Those first couple of weeks were a blur. I felt as though my adrenaline was pumped up, and that I had to "do" something. I was constantly on the phone telling family and friends about Donna. We told the children their mother was going to be okay.

CHEMOTHERAPY— ## ITS BARK IS WORSE THAN ITS BITE

Donna: Three of the twenty-three lymph nodes I had removed were positive, so I needed to have chemotherapy. Tony did not want to tell the children how serious my situation was; I did. I had heard from a breast cancer survivor, who later became a good friend, that we should tell them the truth, because children are very perceptive and know when something is wrong. We kept things basic and told them, "Mommy has cancer. Cancer is a disease that can kill me if I don't treat it. Medicine will kill the cancer, so Mommy needs to have medicine." Jessica understood it could be serious, but Emily was too young to absorb what we were saying.

That summer I began four cycles every three weeks of Cytoxan, Adriamycin and 5-FU (CAF). Having been forewarned I would lose my hair fourteen days after my first treatment, I had already bought a wig, which I wore only to work. I bartend, and the night it did begin to fall out, I had plastered my hair with hair spray. Fortunately, my hair did not fall into any of my customers' drinks! The next day Tony bought a bottle of vodka, we had a drink and then he shaved my head. He must have prepared the girls because shortly thereafter, when we were all sitting in the hot tub on the deck outside our house, the girls just stared at me. Then they were okay. My only request was that they tell me when someone was coming over to the house so that I could put on a scarf. None of them, including Tony, were very good about that!

About my whole chemotherapy experience a friend said to me, "One day you are going to break down because you just bulldozed your way through it." I told her, "No I'm not. I'm strong!" Truthfully, chemotherapy was not bad. I did vomit the night of a treatment, and I had some problems with smells, but even though my energy levels were somewhat diminished, I continued to run three miles every other day. When I was finished with treatment I felt terrific. *It's over!* Or so I thought.

Through a mutual friend I received a phone call from a woman named Melba Adamson who invited me to a breast cancer support group she had started. I was not too enthusiastic about going because Tony and I had attended a support group meeting, and it had not been a good experience. The women were much older than I, and all they did was complain. I told Melba, "I might come, and I might not," but I did end up going. Melba met me at the door, and made me feel very comfortable. This was a positive experience, because I met other women I could not only relate to, but who helped me to not feel so alone. Some of them, including Melba and Lolly Champion *[see chapter 16]* became close friends. After about a year, I stopped going because I wanted to move away from the whole cancer scene, and concentrate on being healthy.

HEARTBREAK—A RECURRENCE

Donna: It was January 1993 and I had almost reached my two-year anniversary when I felt a tiny lump on my mastectomy scar, so small I could not see it. Neither my doctor, nor the breast surgeon he sent me to, thought it was anything to be concerned about, so I wasn't. Tony wanted me to have the lump taken out, but I did not want another scar. Three months later when it became evident the lump had gotten considerably larger, I returned to the surgeon and said to him, "Humor me. Take it out." He did. The next day, a Friday, I received a phone call. "Doctor wants to see you in his office Monday." I knew something was wrong. Tony was infuriated they would tell us nothing. He called my oncologist, explained the situation to him, and asked if he could find out what the results were. When I got home later that day, Tony told me the bad news. The lump was tiny, only 2 mm (about the size of a small BB), but it was cancer. I have often wondered, *Was that first lump* really *benign?*

I began six weeks of radiation therapy and was given the maximum dosage a person can be given. I am still angry that my doctor led me to believe I would walk away perfectly normal. My entire chest was irradiated and became discolored, brown and burned; and my implant got hard. As scar tissue formed, it compressed the implant so that my breasts were very uneven—one considerably higher than the other. My energy levels were quite depleted; however, I had made a commitment to participate in an eighteen-mile race, run over a twenty-four hour period. I did run, but it was very embarrassing to shower in a public facility with all those women. They tried to look away when I undressed because they could see my discomfort. I thought to myself, *I am every woman's worst nightmare. I could be their future.*

OH MY GOD! *AGAIN?*

Donna: I have always found my lumps. This time was no exception. I had gone with Tony on one of his business trips. While lying in bed I was doing a breast self-examination as I frequently did, and felt a tiny lump. I told Tony, whose immediate response was, "Have it checked out as soon as you get home." I think I cried the rest of the night. The next week I met with the breast surgeon who had refused to give me my results over the phone six months earlier. He apologized to me and said, "You have taught me a lot. I have learned not to make my patients wait." Again, he thought the lump was nothing, but he agreed to biopsy it the next day. Tony was with me. It was bad news. But this time I had lobular cancer—a totally different cancer.

Some women remove both breasts because they do not want to deal with the threat of getting breast cancer in their other breast. Breasts were too important to me, and I wanted to keep mine for as long as I could. However, my surgeon recommended that I once again have a modified radical mastectomy, so on January 1, 1994, I did. This time my lymph nodes were negative. The lump had been tiny—only 3 mm. Both implants were removed and replaced with tissue expanders which would eventually be replaced with saline implants. To be honest, I had immediate reconstruction because I was chicken to wake up with no breasts.

I went into a terrible depression for about two months. I was constantly crying, was lethargic and did not exercise. All I wanted to do was to run away from home. When I finally told Tony how I felt, he suggested that I visit my sister in California with whom I am very close. We had so much fun. We laughed and cried, and told one another how scared we were. I was afraid I was going to die. She was so terrified of getting breast cancer that she could not bring herself to have a mammogram. With her I felt comfortable swimming in her pool topless. She told me, "Your breasts just do not look right without nipples, but they're not so bad." It meant a lot to me that she was so honest. Another friend was the total opposite. She made such a point of giving me privacy that she made me feel very uncomfortable.

RECONSTRUCTION

Donna: Every week I had my tissue expanders filled. My irradiated breast always hurt. It felt as if an ace bandage was wrapped too tightly around my chest. Six months later the tissue expanders were taken out, and replaced with my permanent implants. Less than six months later I developed an infection in my irradiated breast. Once again scar tissue formed which compressed the implant. In January of 1995 my surgeon removed the scar tissue around the implant; however, I developed another infection, the incision opened up and began to ooze a clear fluid, and a month later I lost the implant. Why was I not told that there is a 50 percent chance of implant failure with women who have had radiation to their breast? I was heartbroken. For the first time I was flat-chested.

ANOTHER RECURRENCE

Donna: It was April, 1995 and my lower back had been bothering me for the past six months. My oncologist had never found anything wrong, but now I asked him to order a bone scan. When the technician began to take extra pictures I knew I was in trouble. Again it was Tony who told me the bad news. "Your doctor called. Something is wrong with your bone scan." I thought to myself, *Oh no! Now what? What else can go wrong?* While I was having the MRI my doctor had ordered, I was thinking, *This* can't *be happening!* The MRI revealed that the cancer had spread to my vertebrae. I never associated my stiff neck with cancer. I was having symptoms, but I did not recognize them for what they were! The tumor marker blood test he had also ordered came back abnormal. Somewhere in my body a tumor was growing and shedding cells.

For the past five years Tony had been traveling three weeks out of every four, and was home only on weekends. He now realized he needed to be home with the girls and me, but good jobs in high management positions are hard to find. He was offered an excellent position in Arizona, which he accepted. None of us wanted to move.

At the time of my diagnosis my oncologist had mentioned, "Perhaps you should think about having your bone marrow's stem cells collected just in case." I had not given it much thought then, now I was. There was an excellent cancer center only a two-hour drive from where we were going to be moving, so I called and made an appointment. Life, however, threw us a curve ball. Shortly after my second recurrence, Tony's brother died after battling a long-term illness. Within days of my third recurrence, his mother died—we believe from a broken heart.

Funeral arrangements were left up to Tony. We had a whirlwind trip. First we flew to the memorial service in California, then to Arizona so I could see the house Tony had bought, and then to the cancer center to meet with the doctor to see whether I was a candidate for a bone marrow transplant. I was. To be honest, I can see *why* Tony shut down.

It took five months for my insurance carrier to approve the procedure. In the interim I began four cycles of Taxol which was given to me intravenously. Again I lost my hair, but by now the girls were used to me bald. Jessica would say to me, "Mommy you're beautiful." I had no nausea, but I felt like a little old lady because I had so much bone pain, and I was very weak when I walked. Halfway through the treatment we moved, and I had to find all new doctors. That was very stressful. I finished my Taxol treatments in Arizona, and then had radiation.

UH OH—NOW WHAT?

Donna: In August 1995 I went to the cancer center for two weeks of tests, and to have a Hickman catheter put into me, which is how I would be given my drugs. In addition, they collected my stem cells over a four-day period, three hours each day. That was painless. My mother had been with me the first week, and one of my sisters had come for the second. I sent my sister home that morning to spend some time with Tony and the girls because my only remaining test was a bone scan. I felt I could handle this test on my own. As I was getting ready to go home, the radiologist came to see me: "Tell me your history." When I asked why, he said to me, "We found five new hot spots." A hot spot is a site of activity which could be arthritis, a mended broken bone or cancer. In my case, after comparing bone scans, it was cancer that had now spread to my ribs, my skull, both arms and my left femur. I was in such shock I was incapable of driving home. My brother, who lived near the cancer center, came to pick me up and I spent the night at his house. Tony, who was absolutely devastated, flew down, and we met with the oncologist the next day to see whether I was still a candidate for the procedure. My prognosis was now not nearly as favorable, but the transplant was still a go.

LET'S DO IT

Donna: It was August 28, 1995, our wedding anniversary. The children left for school knowing I could be gone for as long as six to eight weeks because today I was checking into the hospital for my transplant. Shortly after they left, the phone rang. Emily was at school in tears, and wanted to come home. Tony picked her up, and the three of us drove to the cancer center. When it was time for them to leave, Emily and I sobbed. Both of the girls had given me their stuffed bunny rabbits to keep me company. I gave Emily's back to her. I thought she needed it more than I did.

My brother and sister-in-law rescued me later that afternoon, since treatment would not begin until the next morning. We went for a picnic, ate junk food and drove into the mountains so I could watch the sunset. The next day it began. I vomited a lot. After a week I was unable to eat, and had to be given nourishment intravenously. I had no pain, but I began to hallucinate, and I could no longer determine what was real and what was not. When I woke up I was not sure where I was, or what I was doing. When I spiked a 105-degree fever the doctors finally traced the source of the infection to my catheter, and had to remove and replace it while I was awake. The pain from that was excruciating. It was my worst day. Tony, who could only visit on weekends, came that day. He thought I was going to die. It was written all over his face. He kept staring at me, and taking my temperature. Finally I yelled at him, "Stop staring! I know I look like hell!" Two weeks after it had begun, I was given back my stem cells.

Emma, her mother: I used my son's house as a home base during the four weeks Donna was in the hospital. We were then going to stay in an apartment near the hospital because she still needed to be monitored. The day before she was released from the hospital she was given a three-hour pass. All Donna wanted to do was to breathe some fresh mountain air. So I drove twenty miles, in an unfamiliar car, up a *very* steep mountain and was a nervous wreck the entire time. When we reached the top, Donna got out of the car, took a couple of deep breaths and said, "Okay. We can go back now!"

Her counts bounced back so quickly that four days after we moved into the apartment she was released. We called to tell Tony and the girls the good news. We planned on going home the next day, but we were so anxious to leave I packed up the car and we drove home that night. We probably should have waited. They were still in the midst of cleaning the entire house when we arrived, and it was turned upside down. Donna just sat down in a chair and watched.

Jessica, her daughter: My parents explained to Emily and me that Mom's cancer was back, that she needed to have a BMT, and what was involved. I was worried because even though the percentage was small, she could die from it. After she began her treatment, one of my teachers asked me to explain to my classmates what Mom was going through. Most of them are my friends, so they already had an idea what was going on. They were old enough to understand what cancer is. My teachers also had them write letters to my mom, which I think she appreciated getting. Emily and I only saw her twice, but we talked almost every day. It was almost better to talk to her than to see her because she looked so sick. Seeing her would have made me feel worse than I already did.

Emily, her daughter: I did not really understand what my parents told me about the BMT. When we went to see her we had to wear masks. Mom looked normal except for her eyes, and her voice was really hoarse. I did not like it when my teacher talked about my mother in class one day. I had to leave the room because I knew if I stayed I would cry. Plus, I did not want to hear what she had to say. The only adult in school I felt comfortable talking to was my counselor because she understood my feelings were private, and that I did not want my feelings to be shared with anyone. I did not want the kids in my class to write letters to my mom. Why should they? The only reason they wrote to her was because my teacher made it an assignment!

LIFE AFTER A BONE MARROW TRANSPLANT

Donna: That first month home I was so paranoid about germs I wore a mask. Tony kissed me on the cheek, but we did not follow *all* the rules.

My jaw felt off skew, and food tasted like cardboard. It took almost three months before my taste buds came back. It was so overwhelming to be home that I cried constantly. I wanted to "do" and "be a mommy," but I could not, because I had no strength. When I came down with shingles —*herpes zoster*—the cancer center was not surprised since it is often caused by stress. Antibiotics cleared it up. My mother stayed an additional four weeks. She was the one who encouraged me to walk every day. Less than a month after getting home from the hospital, my mother and I were participants in my new hometown's Race for the Cure. We walked the entire 5K—3.2 miles!

Emma, her mother: Portland held their Race for the Cure the day Donna was being given back her stem cells. One of her friends sent us a video. The DJ, who was emcee that day, shouted into the microphone, "Right now one of our runners is in the hospital in Arizona fighting for her life. I want everyone to give a cheer for Donna Grant. We hope to see her next year!" As the camera panned the crowds, thousands of people were clapping and cheering for Donna, wishing her well. Every time I watch that video I cry.

LET'S TALK TURKEY!

Donna: I had spent five years developing my own interests and friends, and building a network, because Tony was never home. We moved at *the* most crucial time in my life when I needed my friends. Living in Arizona has been a strain on our relationship. I do not know how much of the strain is cancer related, or just the fact that we have been married sixteen years. Tony was more supportive by the time I had my BMT, but as far as I am concerned he has handled nothing pertaining to my cancer experience well, and I think he would agree. We seldom talk about the fact that I have cancer because Tony does not want to face the truth—I can die from it. I think he feels if we do not talk about it, then everything is okay. He keeps all his fears inside, and I cannot reach him. I do not think Tony wants me to see his fear. Even his friends are unable to get him to open up. When they try, he says things like, "Leave me alone. I do not want to talk about it!" When we do talk it is only about *me,* how *I* am coping.

Tony wants to fix everything and he cannot. I think he feels weighted down by the responsibility of taking care of his family, and as a result he retreats behind work and his computer, which he is constantly on. But I know he is thinking about the cancer because he always asks when I have a test coming up, "How do you think it will turn out?"

Many books I have read say that when a person gets cancer they value every day, every minute because of a newfound appreciation for life. I have become more dissatisfied with my life as I have gotten through each recurrence because it is not the way I want it. I am not happy *just* to be alive. I want more. I want it to be better.

I STILL HAVE CANCER, BUT . . .

Donna: Six months and two bone scans later, everything was stable. I was tired of dealing with a prosthesis. I wanted two breasts! My family was behind my decision to have more reconstruction. The plastic surgeon I met with felt we would get good results with a latissimus dorsi. He took muscle from my back and tunneled it underneath my skin to form a breast, and also put in another tissue expander, which would be replaced later with a saline implant so that eventually both breasts would be the same size. This was a very easy surgery for me, and so far there have been no complications! Neither girl has seen my breasts. It's not that I am ashamed of them, but I have never shown them my breasts—even before this happened! If, in the future, Jessica wants to see what I look like, I will gladly show her.

HOW DID MY FAMILY COPE?

Donna: My family is huge. Right before my transplant we had our first family reunion. I postponed radiation because, as I told my doctor, "I might never get a chance to see everyone together again." My parents and siblings, three sisters and two brothers have been great. They have "been there" for me—strong. They allow me to cry when I need to cry, even though they do not cry in front of me. I try not to cry in front of my mother because I feel as though I have to be strong for her. Besides,

I am so afraid she will say to me, even though she never has, "Buck up. Turn off the waterworks. You are going to be fine!" My father is definitely the most nervous person in my family, although my older brother is a terrible worrywart. My father called the cancer center five times a day when I was having the BMT just to check to make sure I was okay! When my family tells me I am going to be fine, I feel as though they are in denial, not facing the reality of the situation. No one, including my doctors can tell me that. Maybe saying it makes them feel better, but I still feel that my cancer is going to kill me one day.

Tony, her husband: Donna's family are wonderful, God-fearing people who do not have a fault to them. Both Emma and Anthony rely on God, but they are not holier than thou. They remind me of Ozzie and Harriet, and have raised six kids who are all doing well. I know they care about me, and they would probably be a great source of strength for me if I allowed myself to talk to them, but I do not want to add to their burden. They are having a rough time. I saw what happened to my mother when she lost a son.

Emma, her mother: Each time Donna has a recurrence Anthony and I are devastated for a few days, and then we just gear up again and get ready to fight.

Anthony, her father: Emma and I always stressed to the children that when someone in the family is in trouble all of us are there to help. Now we are living what we preached. We all know it is a possibility that Donna can die, but none of us talk about it. Tony is very pessimistic about Donna in front of me, but at least when he is around her he is very up.

HOW HAVE THE CHILDREN COPED?

Donna: Tony now realizes we did the right thing by telling the girls the truth about me. I think we have struck a pretty good balance in giving them just enough information, but not too much, and I feel they have handled things fairly well. When I tell them I have had a recurrence and have to go back into the hospital, they ask me things such as, "How long will you be in?" and "Is this going to cure you?" Jessica is very stoic and tells me, "Mommy, you are going to be fine." She is very mature and has accepted responsibility when she has had to. Recently she was in

Portland visiting friends. She remembered I was having a bone scan, and called home. I had not gotten back yet, and she said to Tony, "Make sure Mommy calls me when she gets home from the cancer center." Emily, on the other hand, is more emotional and is always worried about me. She wants to know when I am going to the doctor, and what my test results are. She cannot grasp the concept that the reconstruction I am now having is just to give me a breast because every time I go for a fill she says, "Is this going to help you so that you don't get cancer anymore?" I feel badly because they both worry about me. They have lived with cancer for so much of their lives.

Tony, her husband: I would never offer advice to other parents because they are not me, and their kids aren't my kids. I have tried to be honest with mine. They know they can ask us anything, and we will not shade the truth. When they ask me if their mother can die I tell them, "Yes." There is a three-year difference in their ages, but I tell them both the same thing. Obviously Jessica can grasp what I tell her more than Emily can, simply because she is older.

Jessica, her daughter: I do not remember my parents telling me that Mom had cancer, but I do remember that she went through chemotherapy. Until her transplant, my memories are vague. Dad does not have anyone to talk to here, although he did when we lived in Portland. Maybe being in Arizona, and mom having cancer, is too much for him to deal with, because I think he hides behind his computer and going to work. His computer seems to have taken the place of a friend. It's as if he's running away so that he does not have to deal with Mom having cancer.

Emily and I talk more to our friends in Portland about Mom than we do with our friends in Arizona, but that is just because we have known them longer. To be honest, none of our friends really understands what we are going through, just like we can't understand quite what our mom is going through because we are not her. Her support group was good because she was able to talk to people who really understood what it was she was going through. Now she gets more sympathy than empathy.

Emily, her daughter: It is frustrating talking to my friends about my mom because I have to explain the same thing five times before they sort of understand what I am telling them. I wish I could be in a family that did not have anything wrong. I wish my mom did not have cancer.

Melba, her friend: I think Jessica handles things a lot like Tony. In my opinion they are exactly alike—she handles her mother's cancer with intellect. I am sure she has her moments, but I wonder, *Does she share her feelings with anyone?* Even though it seems as though she handles things on the surface like, "Okay, we'll get through this," deep down I think she is probably quaking in her boots. Now I think Emily is a petrified little girl who has a lot of grief inside, and is screaming for help and no one is noticing.

IT NEVER ENDS— AN INTERVIEW FROM 12/12/96

Donna: I just had nipple reconstruction, and I pointed out some bumps on my abdomen to my doctor. He biopsied four different places, and three were lobular cancer. When I called my oncologist to tell him the news, he immediately took me off Arimidex which had replaced the tamoxifen I had been taking since my second recurrence. I am seeing him next week because I have hundreds of little bumps on my abdomen. The cancer has metastasized (spread) to my liver. A verse from the Bible has helped get me through some *very* scary times since this all began: "God has given me the spirit not of cowardice, but of strength and love." I repeat over and over, "I am strong. I am not a coward."

I have read several books that have affected me in different ways. *The Cancer Conqueror* by Greg Anderson is about having a healthy, positive outlook, in addition to being nonjudgmental and loving people for the way they are. As a result of reading this book, I pray throughout the day and ask God, "What am I supposed to be learning from this?" I feel as though I keep having recurrences, because I am just not getting whatever message I am supposed to be getting, although I do not feel that I caused my cancer. Another book that has helped me enormously is *The Cancer Battle Plan* by Anne Frahm. I have decided to fight my battle with alternative methods, and this book outlines a detoxifying and cleansing program I am now following. Recently I finished a ten-day juice fast. I have also seen a naturopathic physician who specializes in nutrition, and I am now eating tofu, grains, vegetables, fruits and fish. This is a low-fat, not a no-fat diet. In addition I am drinking Essiac tea, a very powerful herbal blood cleanser and intense detoxifier that has anti-tumor properties. It feels good to be so proactive, but I wonder, *Am I doing all this for nothing?*

HOW *ARE* WE DOING?

Donna: When the cancer metastasized to my liver, I realized we could not move. I decided that it was time I made a life for myself in Arizona, and I have. I now refer to Arizona as home. Most of the people here do not know that I am sick, and that is good because I want to be treated like a "well" person. Cancer does not have to be the focus of my life with my new friends. The last time I was in Portland was horrible. By the fifth day I was in tears. Lolly had just come over and I said to her, "I can't stand it anymore. Everyone is depressing me. They all think I am dying! It's pouring rain, it's freezing cold, I feel lousy and I want to go home!" It started the day I got there. One of my friends said to me, "So. What are you doing to prepare? Are you making a videotape for your girls? Are you writing them letters?" I told him, "Until I am sick, I do not want to think about it or talk about it, so let's change the subject." Even Melba asked me things like, "What scares you the most about the future? What are the things you are going to miss?" They all think I am losing weight because of the cancer. I am very thin, but it is because of the diet I am on!

Tony cried for the first time when I told him the lumps on my abdomen were cancer. Things finally began to surface with him, and we cried *together*. Obviously that makes me sad, yet it was good for me to be able to see that he is affected by this, and that he can be emotional, because I have been so worried that if I die he will shut down, and the girls will have no one to turn to. The girls react to how Tony and I are acting, so we try to be as positive as we can. Jessica tried to hide it, but she cried a little bit when we told her. And Emily was very upset. I don't think they think about it that much now, because they never talk about it, so we just go on about our daily lives.

It has been extremely helpful that Tony and I have seen a psychologist. He has helped to steer Tony toward being more a part of the family. Tony is trying to take more time off from work, and he has stopped spending so much time on the computer. The psychologist has helped me to understand that Tony cannot automatically turn off being a manager the moment he gets home from work. He has also shown me that Tony will be able to cope if anything does happen to me.

Jessica, her daughter: Cancer is a part of my life. I always worry about it, and I am afraid my mother will take a turn for the worse, or die, even though she tells Emily and me that she intends to live long enough to see us married and have children of our own. I try not to think about it, but when I do, I talk to my parents. I want to know what's going on. My parents have always been honest with me. There have been times when they have asked me not to tell some news to Emily because she might not understand, or it might upset her.

Emily, her daughter: I do not feel comfortable talking to my mom about her cancer, because she is the one who has it. When we do have long talks, she cries. That makes me cry, which I don't like to do because then I think about it all the time. When that happens, I want to talk about what I am feeling, but I do not really want to talk to her! I found out the cancer had spread to my mother's spine because everyone in the house was acting so weird. Finally I asked my mom, "What's going on?" I could *feel* that something was wrong. Sometimes I know something is wrong because my dad gets grumpy. He also becomes more easily frustrated now. And my mom is a little more sensitive than she used to be.

Emma, her mother: I could not function when I found out this latest news. Anthony called all the children. I was incapable of getting on the phone. We both came home early from work that day, and consoled one another. Ever since then I feel as though God is carrying me. I feel like a poem I read that goes something like this: A person was walking along the beach. When they turned around there were two sets of footprints in the sand. After awhile there was only one set of footprints, then two, then one. The person asked God, "Why in my hardest times is there only one set of footprints? You weren't with me." God replied, "That's when I was carrying you."

Donna's positive attitude has helped me to have a positive attitude. She is fighting this, and both Anthony and I believe she will beat it. She almost fell apart five years ago, but since then she has taken every blow, and she bounces right back. Donna has told me she is not afraid to die, but she would like five more years so that she can raise her girls.

Anthony, her father: I have lost a lot of sleep over these last five years. One night, shortly after the cancer had spread to her liver, Donna called me. She was crying and said to me, "Dad, I'm scared." We talked for a long time which helped both of us to calm down. I was trying so hard not to cry, because I knew she needed my strength. I told her, "You've got to take one day at a time. There's still hope." That's when she told me about the diet she is on, and that she was not going to have any more chemotherapy. I feel more positive with this than I did when she had her BMT.

Melba, her friend: I do not think Tony has strong coping mechanisms. I can remember one time he was standing in his kitchen in Portland, and he said to me after Donna's second recurrence, "It is going to kill her. It is just a matter of time." Then he walked away. It is almost as if he goes on automatic pilot so that he does not have to deal with it. I am sure he is thinking that he might have to raise those two girls himself. It was huge step when Donna told me that she and Tony grieved together.

TONY SPEAKS

Tony, her husband: Shortly after Donna was diagnosed, I read a book called *What to Do When a Loved One Dies* by Eva Shaw. I still feel guilty thinking she can die, but there has been a side to me, even from the beginning, that thought, *What will I do if she dies? How will I handle raising my small children?* And because I was traveling so much at the time, *What will I do with them?*

Donna's doctor told us that the transplant did not work, and that barring a miracle her cancer is terminal. The funny thing is, her doctor never used that word. He took a piece of paper and drew a line with an arrow pointing one way and wrote the word "treatment." Then he drew another line with the arrow pointing in the opposite direction and wrote the words "quality of life." Then he said, "You know Donna, we found the cancer on your liver by accident, not through symptoms you were having. Some people in your situation might say to me, 'I'll come see you when I start to have symptoms,' and I might not see them until then. Others feel the need to do 'something.' You need to ask yourself, 'Do I want to go through chemotherapy again, lose my hair again and feel sick?' or 'Do I want to feel good for as long as I can?'" I thought his delivery was very sensitive. That is where we stand right now.

I read somewhere that what I am going through now has four stages, just like grief: disbelief, denial, negotiation and finally acceptance. Each recurrence is like a grieving process, and with each I am a little better prepared, and I am able to reach the acceptance stage more quickly. It is an American myth that the male ego is supposed to be strong and can handle anything. I was completely twisted sideways for a couple of months the first time. My head was not screwed on, and I could not think or sleep. This time I was only like that for a few days. I do not want to be thought of as cold or insensitive, but it is how I cope. Donna having cancer is something I cannot control. I have to ask myself, "Do I let it eat me up alive, or do I go about my life the best way that I can?"

The pressure I am now feeling is from things like, "Am I doing the right thing, and how do I do the right thing? What do I say to Donna? What do I say to my kids, and how do I handle them?" Right now Donna is feeling good, but I know I am going to need some kind of support in place when she goes into hospice. That is why I talked to my pastor this morning and told him I wanted to get some professional counseling for myself and the children—someone not attached to the church. I do not want to wait until the last minute to do these kinds of things. The network needs to be in place now. That will take some of the burden off of me because I know that I am taking care of my family, and that what I am doing will help them. This isn't about me. It's about taking care of my family. I am more worried about my children, and I want to make sure they do not develop phobias or hang-ups because of this. If there is anything left of Tony when this is all over, I will deal with me then. Right now I do not have the time.

I am very happy that Donna is finally beginning to meet people, because I still feel guilty for moving my family to Arizona. They have been so unhappy. When I mentioned that to Donna this morning she told me, "Let it go!" We could have a big support network in Arizona like we do in Portland, but we have to make the commitment to develop that network. I think Donna is now ready to do that.

That "benign" lump she had taken out in 1990 was *not* benign. I do not know if we were given a copy of the pathology report and at the time did not understand it, or if I got a copy of it at a later time, and by then understood what I was reading. It clearly states that Donna's lump was "precancerous." I thought seriously about suing the doctor who took the lump out, but I did not want to put my family through that. Had we known, we could have attacked this thing when the cancer was really small, before it had a chance to get into her bloodstream. Maybe if we had known, she would not have cancer right now, and we would not be going through what we are.

Donna and I have not talked about death, and probably will not until it is staring us in the face. We are both aware of it, but talk about it only in a humorous way. She will say things such as, "If something does happen to me, you have to get remarried, because the girls will need a mother." And I will say to her, "I am never remarrying, and that is that!" We have not yet reached the point where we need to say, "We need to look at how much time we have," and "What do we need to do to get done between now and then?" Donna having cancer has made me stronger, has made our marriage stronger, and has certainly helped me to get my priorities straight as far as raising the children. I have cut down on the amount of time I spend on the computer, because I need to make sure that when I am home, I spend it with my family. I go on the Internet after everyone has gone to bed. That is when I get some "me" time.

FROM ONE KID TO ANOTHER

Jessica, her daughter: Find out as much as you can. Do not hold your feelings inside the way I do because when you do, you feel worse. Talk to whoever you need to. I do not think a counselor would help me, because even though they are supposed to be "experts," they do not know what is happening in our family. They have not taken a course on kids whose parents have cancer, so they cannot talk about it from personal experience. I think I can deal with this myself. I would tell someone my age that breast cancer is a disease they have not yet found a cure for, but they are working on it.

Emily, her daughter: It is hard to talk to any adult about what is happening, because how can they understand what I am going through if they haven't been through it themselves? I would tell a kid my age, "Don't think about the future, because you do not know what is going to happen. If something bad happens, then worry about it."

THE FINAL INTERVIEW—6/10/97

Donna: It has been really good that my parents are visiting. They are in a quandary right now. They do not want to leave, but they know they cannot stay indefinitely. I need some time alone with my family, and I also want to spend time alone with my friends who are now starting to come out to say good-bye. I need to tell that to my mom. All my brothers and sisters have been out to visit. No one can say good-bye out loud.

I am in the process of writing cards to the girls that Tony will give to them on special occasions. I am also deciding who gets what pieces of my jewelry and certain "things" in the house. I get depressed because there are so many things I want to do, but I do not have the strength to do them. The girls and I have talked, and they have cried just from the sheer magnitude of it all. Every day Emily asks me, "Mom, how are you feeling?" She thinks if I start to feel better, then I am getting better.

Tony took me to Northern California, to all our special places, so I could see them one last time before I die. We were supposed to go to Europe, but I was too ill. Instead we went to Portland. We are talking, but not about the things I am prepared to talk about now. He wants to plan for the future: how he is going to lease the house; who will do the property management; how much income he will make from the house. I cannot think that far in advance. It is going to happen when it happens. It is pointless to dwell on it or worry about it, because Tony and the girls are not going to move until it is all said and done. It just seems that our time would be better spent trying to enjoy what there is of each day, rather than getting all wrapped up in the future. I am taking it moment by moment. Tony is becoming depressed. At first he did not want to move back to Portland. When I asked him why, he said to me, "I won't be able to handle the rain because you won't be with me." He has since changed his mind. I think we both feel better about his decision.

Postscript written by Jessica Grant, Donna's daughter, 3/4/2000

It was June 30th, 1997. I had spent the night at my best friend's house because the doctors had told us that my mom had at least a few more weeks. I got a phone call, "Come home." When I got home they took me into the next room and said, "Donna died about twenty minutes ago." It almost seemed as if they were waiting for some kind of reaction from me. They did not get it. I did not cry; I did not speak; I just nodded and accepted what they told me, because I knew that was what I had to do. By trying to keep some semblance of normal life during such a hard time, I missed the chance to say good-bye to my mother.

Three days later I celebrated my thirteenth birthday, and received a card from my mother. In the card she told me how proud she was of how I had grown up, and how much she loved me. I think remembering how much she cared about me and my family is what kept me strong through the whole ordeal. After my grandparents and everyone left, and the hospital bed was gone, my dad told me that Mom wanted us to move back to Portland where my sister and I had grown up. I was devastated. Although I had spent my childhood there, I grew up in Arizona. I had changed so much during the two years we lived in Arizona, that it felt as though I had lived there my entire life. Nonetheless, at the end of August we were on our way back to Oregon.

At first I think it was difficult for all of us to be back in Oregon because it was so full of memories, but after a while we all learned that it was not the past we were living in, it was a future we were making for ourselves. My dad began to remodel our home shortly after we moved in. I am sure it was a way for him to escape from the tragedy that had just shaken his life. Emily was able to move on fairly quickly. She was back with her friends, and she was happy. After two and half years we have all found that it is entirely possible, and even normal for life to move on. Recently my dad became engaged to a good family friend. The remodeling slowed to a halt about six months ago because I think he finally accepted what had happened, and he no longer needed the added distraction. Emily is now in the seventh grade, and is becoming a wonderful, strong, young lady because of all she has been through. I honestly believe that my mother's battle with cancer has also made me a much stronger person.

Until now I thought it was strange that it was so easy for me to get over losing my mother. I thought I was wrong to feel that way, and that I should always miss her. But now that I see my family is also moving on with their lives, I know that it is only natural to live your own life after the death of a person you love.

[AUTHOR'S NOTE: *I requested a postscript from Tony Grant, Donna's husband. It was just too difficult for Tony to write even though Donna died almost three years ago.*]

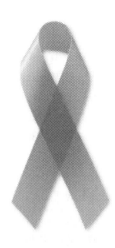

Fifteen

Ben Bunch

What Do You Mean
Men Get Breast Cancer?

Survivor Profile:

Age at diagnosis: fifty-five (4/15/91)

Age at interview: sixty (11/12/96)

Type of breast cancer: infiltrating ductal

Size tumor: 1 cm; stage II

Two positive lymph nodes

Surgical procedure: mastectomy

Treatment: chemotherapy

Estrogen receptors: positive; Progesterone receptors: positive

Who's Who:

Sue Bunch, his wife

Ed Bunch, his son (age thirty-four at diagnosis)

Bob Ferguson, his friend

DISCOVERY

Ben: One of my nipples had been itching for about a month. I had been using cortisone cream which seemed to help. My nipple was kind of looking downwards. Like most guys I didn't think much about it. One night I forgot to use the cream and was awakened in the middle of the night because it itched so badly. While scratching, I felt a lump near my nipple.

The next day I was playing golf with a doctor friend and mentioned the lump. He said it was rare that men got breast cancer but I should have it checked. When I got home I told my wife, Sue, about the lump and made a doctor's appointment. After being examined, I was told it was probably an infected cyst and that I should soak it in hot salt water for a week. That helped the itching, but the lump remained. It was then recommended that I see a surgeon.

Sue, his wife: When Ben discovered the lump we didn't really think much about it because like most people we just naturally assumed that men do not get breast cancer. Silly us!

THE NEXT STEP

Ben: The surgeon was a friend. Both he and his associate said, "It doesn't look like there is any big concern, but we really should take it out." They weren't worried, so Sue and I weren't. Three weeks later, on a Friday, I had a biopsy. My surgeon told me later that as soon as he cut into it he knew by the color that it was cancer.

Sue, his wife: The surgeon told me that men rarely get breast cancer. We never thought it would be cancer. It couldn't happen to us or to anyone we love. I was shocked when he said, "I'm sorry Sue, he has breast cancer." I probably would have been more prepared if the diagnosis had been mine. I think I was in denial when I called the children to tell them.

Ed, his son: We're a family business. Dad walked into my office one day looking concerned and said, "I found a lump. What do you think about it?" He opened his shirt, and I felt this hard lump by his nipple. I suggested he get it checked out, but I knew it wasn't breast cancer because men do not get breast cancer. He was worried, but the family downplayed it a bit.

I wasn't at the biopsy because I had something really important to do. My wife and I had made the difficult decision to put one of our dogs to sleep, and the house vet was coming over to pick him up. I loved my dog and needed to say good-bye.

ARE MEN GIVEN CHOICES?

Ben: I was already scheduled for a single modified radical mastectomy by the time I came out of anesthesia from the biopsy. I was not given a choice.

Because everything happened so quickly, I never had time to worry. My only concern was whether I would need chemotherapy or radiation. The day after my mastectomy, on the way home from the hospital, I had Sue take me to the plant, drains and all. They couldn't keep me down. For six months after surgery, fluid would build up in my breast area. The doctor had to keep aspirating the fluid with a needle to drain it. Because it was numb it didn't hurt, although it was uncomfortable.

I have talked with a number of women in their thirties and forties who have had breast cancer. Many have had lumpectomies and some have had recurrences. I can understand their reasons for doing a lumpectomy, but I think if you get breast cancer you should let them take your breast.

Sue, his wife: Immediately after the biopsy our surgeon asked, "What do you think?" I said, "I think we should schedule him for surgery as soon as possible. I don't know how he is going to handle this. He's a man who has never been in a hospital or under anesthesia of any sort. It's unfortunate we can't do this today, but let's do it as soon as possible." A lumpectomy was never recommended. I don't know whether they do anything other than mastectomies for men.

The weekend before his surgery Ben and I operated on automatic pilot. Our attention was focused on the fact that he was having surgery. Not what the surgery was for.

Ed, his son: My wife and I were sitting at our kitchen table very upset over having put our dog to sleep. We assumed it was the veterinarian when the telephone rang. It was my mom saying, "It's a bad day." I said, "Yeah, it really is a bad day. The vet just took our dog." Her words weren't registering even though I knew my dad had gone in for a biopsy. Then she said, "Your dad has cancer." It never dawned on me that my dad, the biggest, strongest person I had ever known, who was impervious to everything, could possibly have breast cancer. Men do not get breast cancer! Within a few seconds our lives and priorities changed. I did not think about my dog for another week. I love animals and I love dogs, but I would trade one thousand dogs for my father.

When I talked to my dad on the telephone I cried. It's not something I do all the time, but I realize it's healthy and I certainly felt better after having done it. That weekend, before surgery, all of us kids went over to our parents'. It was kind of uncomfortable because no one really knew what we could do to help. It's as if you are there for them, but you don't know exactly what it is that they need. I was feeling a little funny about how to help. I just kept saying, "Everything is going to be okay, don't worry."

POSSIBLE CULPRITS

Ben: Eight years prior to being diagnosed I was driving to work in my convertible when an overhead electrical transformer shattered and showered me with PCPs, a coolant now discontinued in most transformers across the country. When I called the electric company to report what had occurred, they immediately sent a team down to clean up the residue. They washed my car, and suggested I immediately take a shower, all the while assuring me I had nothing to worry about. But the next day, men in white protective gear were picking up the earth around the blown transformer. It wasn't until later that I learned there is a link between PCPs and breast cancer.

My tumor was 1 cm. It takes about eight years to grow a tumor that size. Coincidence? Five years prior to that, I was two hundred miles from Chernobyl when the nuclear plant blew. I think the PCPs are a much more likely reason I got breast cancer.

THE IMPORTANCE OF A SUPPORT NETWORK

Sue, his wife: It helped talking to friends of ours who have had cancer because they have been through the process. Their spouses also understood and called me specifically to see how I was doing. I don't think you can give the same kind of support unless you've personally experienced it. Our family also was very supportive. I say that if you don't have a good support network, get help from a psychiatrist or psychologist. Because you cannot do it alone.

Although Ben has always been supportive, since his cancer he has become emotionally supportive. Before he got sick his support was more the good-ol'-buddy type of thing. Now he is so loving and caring, and you know he's making a difference. He will call people with cancer and talk with them. He will say things like, "I've been there. I've had this worry. I know where you're coming from." Our relationship today is so much richer because of his attitude change.

Ed, his son: I was glad I worked with Dad because it gave me the opportunity to see him every day. Being a close family, we had a great support network. Only my close friends asked how I was doing. That was okay because, at the time, I felt it more important for my dad to be nurtured than me.

Bob, his friend: Sue took really good care of Ben. She sheltered, encouraged and prodded him. Being close family friends, they had my support as well as my wife's.

When someone has a serious illness the best thing you can do is to lend your support without too many strings. Don't expect anything and give them room. I get angry when an employer treats a sick person like a sick person. If a person can only work thirty minutes a day, let them work thirty minutes a day. Those thirty minutes are important to them because it means they haven't given up. The person who is sick should be able to say, "Let me tell you when I'm sick or when I'm not able to work." Ben knew what he was capable of doing.

CHEMOTHERAPY

Ben: I did chemotherapy because two of the fifteen lymph nodes they removed were positive. I interviewed oncologists, and one really caught my attention when he said if I were to have a recurrence, castration was a consideration. That supposedly would help stop hormone production. I had a monthly injection of Adriamycin and 5-FU, followed by two weeks of Cytoxan pills. Even today, five years after my diagnosis, there is no difference in treatment between men and women as far as I know.

Sue was with me for all my treatments. I was fine after my first injection, but went a little crazy after my second. On the drive home I felt as though I were jumping out of my skin. I could not stand being confined and had to restrain myself from jumping out of the car and running . . . while we were going sixty miles per hour. What a funny feeling. I guess the doctor put a tranquilizer in my IV after that because I never experienced that feeling again.

I worked the entire time. But I was tired and lacked energy, so I put an air mattress in my office and napped when I had to. I lost all my strength, almost as if my muscles had deteriorated. I was so weak I had difficulty taking tops off containers. Many times my car would stay at work because I did not have the energy to drive it home. I also did not have the energy for golf the first two weeks after treatment, and I am an avid golfer. Even though memory loss was a problem, this period was very productive for me and my company. I'm an inventor of business machines, and we got six to eight new patents during this time. My memory returned within a year of finishing chemotherapy.

I could not bring myself to shave the fringe of remaining hair. Other than the fringe, all my body hair fell out and I only had to shave every two to three weeks. I gained about twenty-five pounds because I was constantly eating to get rid of that funny taste and dryness in my mouth. It wasn't until my last treatment that the oncology staff told me that lemon sourballs help remove that awful taste. I did not drink alcohol because even one beer gave me a three-day hangover.

Finishing chemotherapy is what I imagine it must be like to be released from jail. I couldn't wait, and it felt like the world was taken off my shoulders. I thought twice about taking that last Cytoxan pill. I was going to save it . . . but I did take it. No one suggested tamoxifen.

Sue, his wife: Watching the people in the reception room at an oncologist's office is scary. They looked old and as if they were dying. It worried me and I thought, *Is this it? Is this what it's like?* We interviewed oncologists and rejected one because of the clutter in his office. If his office was cluttered I wondered what happened to the blood samples they took. What our minds can do to us! We also changed oncologists after the first treatment because we wanted someone local, not someone two hours away.

Out of a whole month, Ben had one week, at the end of the month, when he felt even halfway normal. That was a tough week because you knew Monday, when he would start the cycle all over again, was right around the corner. I tried so hard to let him do things for himself because chemotherapy is so imprisoning. It's "the ruler, king of the hill" and calls the shots. It hurt to see such a vibrant, strong person down. And you couldn't do anything to help. His concentration was totally destroyed. He could not pull up information like before, and he was so tired. Because his reflexes and coordination were off and he was lurchy, it was very scary when he drove. He would have had difficulty touching a finger to his nose had a cop pulled him over. When he drove, he had this sheepish, little boy look on his face like, "I know I shouldn't have driven but . . ." Even his eyesight changed. You live in a crisis mode but you focus on the fact that it will end.

Ed, his son: Even though I put on an optimistic front I was worried sick about my dad. He looked like hell, and I was afraid he would die. My sister would tiptoe down the hall at the office so she would not disturb Dad while he was napping. Dad always kept a small container of cranberry juice in his office to help rid him of the metallic taste in his mouth. Either an employee or family member would always check, unasked, to make sure it was full. You did the little things, just to show you cared. It becomes a part of normal life.

Bob, his friend: Ben had good days and bad days. He slept on the bad days. But he kept up his sense of humor. Like the time his doctor told him he wasn't sure whether or not Ben's hair would grow back curly. Ben was laughing when he said, "I can tell you it's not. I have been getting it permed for years." His doctor cracked up.

What's It Like for a Man to Lose a Breast?

Ben: I have a male friend who is four to five years younger than me who was also diagnosed with breast cancer. When he heard about me, he came to my plant and pulled up his shirt to show me his scar. We were a perfect pair. Like me, he is fine today.

I intentionally bring up the fact that I have had a mastectomy when I meet new people. I do it to get across to guys in particular that they can get breast cancer and that they need to check themselves. When a TV station asked to interview me about having breast cancer, I agreed. I felt it was important that men know their risk. It felt really good being an advocate.

I believe if a woman wants to be reconstructed, she should. It was suggested I have a nipple tattooed. But after giving it some thought I decided, "Enough is enough. Let's leave it as it is." Had I known at the time of my surgery what I know today, I would have had both breasts removed. But no one suggested it. And I do not want another surgery.

I believe that because breast cancer is still viewed as a "woman's disease," men have not given enough money for breast cancer research. Funds have been short for years. Yet men will spend a lot of money on other things, like prostate cancer research. They're going crazy on AIDS research, yet breast cancer kills more people than AIDS. They should be spending more money on breast cancer than on AIDS. Maybe we will get more funding.

Sue, his wife: I do not think psychologically that breasts are as important to men as they are to women. Ben said to me after his treatment was complete, "I will probably never run around shirtless again." This was a man who would, before surgery, walk around nude with the windows wide open. A man who would be completely comfortable at a nudist colony. Ben is vain to a certain extent, and I wondered if he was feeling the loss of a breast or the fact that he had a 10-inch disfiguring scar on his chest. His turning point occurred six months later when he exposed himself . . . to another man, our gardener. Ben told me later, "It was really strange. I watched him looking at me. His eyes wandered down, the eyes came back up. I knew he was thinking, 'That can't be what I think it is.' " From that moment on Ben accepted his mastectomy. It was like he had never lost anything and he can now kid about it. Except when the media neglects to mention the fact that men can get breast cancer.

Ben is great with our female friends. They want to see what a mastectomy looks like because it's a reality for them. We want to know what it looks like in the event it ever happens to us. Women are much more hesitant to show other women, other than maybe a best friend. But Ben has no hesitation and just whips off his shirt. I think it's wonderful that he does that. His scar isn't bad. I think the anticipation of what it looks like is worse than it is.

A friend of mine lost her mother and sister to breast cancer when they were both in their mid forties. Even though my friend did not have breast cancer she elected to have a prophylactic bilateral mastectomy (preventive removal of both breasts) because as she told me, "I don't think I want that to happen to me and all indications are that it could. I'm going to take charge of the situation before it ruins my life." She decided not to wait until she was forced to make a decision, when she is at the crossroads. Ben and I have discussed what would happen if I were diagnosed with breast cancer. He's all for my having a mastectomy. It's a personal choice, and I truly believe that today I agree with him. But the reality is, you never know how you'll react until it's you.

Ed, his son: Dad's got a strong self-image, and I don't think he's concerned with having only one breast. I've seen his scar. Who hasn't? If a perfect stranger asks how he is he'll say, "Not bad for a guy with only one boob." Sometimes they'll bite and ask what he means. He wants the world to know that men can get breast cancer.

About a year after Dad's diagnosis, Joe Garagiola hosted *The Today Show.* They were doing a week-long series on breast cancer. A guest started to talk about the fact that men get breast cancer and Joe cut him off to go to commercial break. Dad reacted like a tornado and got him on the telephone. On the show the next day Joe said, "I had some interesting calls yesterday, especially from one of my old friends in Arizona. I've got to tell you . . . men get breast cancer, too." I am really proud of my dad. Does he know Joe? Maybe. They both live in the same city and he also plays a lot of golf.

Bob, his friend: Ben's scar isn't pretty, and his breast looks different, but it's nothing to be ashamed of. Plenty of our friends who were in the war have scars and bullet wounds. His scar doesn't look any worse than theirs. I don't think it's as traumatic when a man loses a breast. Maybe I'd feel differently if it were me. Ben was okay over losing his breast.

THE CHILDREN

Ed, his son: My older brother, younger sister and I supported Dad in his decision to have a mastectomy. My children, then two and five, knew their grandpa was sick, but only my five-year-old daughter understood. We told her that her grandpa was having an operation and was going to be okay. She knew her mom and I were worried. It was pretty obvious. After his surgery, she made us take her to the hospital so that she could make sure he was okay.

My siblings and I were over at my parents more often than normal. I think we tried to do things for them, but my mom is a very take-charge kind of person. She'll let you know when she needs anything. So we ended up taking more of a backseat waiting for them to ask for help. Breast cancer was a main topic of conversation among us kids. I think it's only natural for the children to talk because of the uncertainty. My brother and I talked about our now being more at risk.

Because I was concerned about the cancer having spread to two of the lymph nodes, I started reading everything I could get my hands on to educate myself. It's amazing how much information is out there and how much is recycled. I found some frightening mortality facts which scared me. I didn't say a word to anyone, including my wife. Educating yourself is important so that you can ask the right questions. Even if the questions aren't asked or if you think there's something the person with the diagnosis doesn't know, you can tell them the questions they need to ask.

Bob, his friend: I've been close to the children since they were small.

It was hard for them to see their dad, particularly on a bad day. On those days they might say something like, "Do you see him coming out of this?" Or, "How's it going to affect him in the long-term?" All I could do was to be positive and tell them it was all part of the process of chemotherapy. I said, "He'll gradually get back to normal. Just like he gradually reacted to the effects of the chemotherapy. He didn't change overnight."

MAMMOGRAMS AND BREAST SELF-EXAMINATION

Ben: I don't think Sue changed much concerning checking herself and getting mammograms as a result of my breast cancer. But, for awhile we both went in together when it was time for her yearly checkup. I still don't think it fair they didn't give Sue and me discounted rates when we went in together for our X-rays. They would X-ray my remaining breast which wasn't painful, but it was difficult getting it into the machine. I don't do mammograms anymore. I'm also not great about remembering to do breast self-examinations unless I see "buddy check" reminder on the TV. I know it's important, but it's not uppermost on my mind. If you do have a buddy system, maybe it will make you look a little bit more. Do my children do BSE? I don't know, but I probably should ask.

Sue, his wife: When I told the children, "Everyone get a mammogram" after Ben's diagnosis, my daughter's gynecologist said to her, "No way, you're only twenty-eight." Right after that, the young LPGA golfer Heather Farr died. A parent can only push so hard. The boys know they need to pay attention to their bodies. Do I worry about my children getting breast cancer? It doesn't rule my life, but like a typical parent, I worry about everything having to do with my children. Getting breast cancer isn't a big fear of mine. I do check myself, but not as much as Ben.

COPING WITH LIFE AND DEATH

Ben: I suppose in the beginning I thought about dying. But I trusted my doctor, and he told me he had gotten all the cancer. I also did all the treatment he recommended. It got to where I felt like I had beaten the cancer, that I was not going to die so I decided to stop worrying about it. Even when I lose friends to cancer my attitude is, "It's not going to happen to me."

I'm not into support groups, but I do talk to other breast cancer survivors because I'm trying to give back. I am not out on the street preaching, but I'm not hiding it. It helps to talk to someone who's had the same problem. I show my scar when someone wants to see it, and I tell them, "This is what you don't want to get."

I am not much different today than I was before I got sick. Perhaps more mellow, but I am also older. I have gotten serious about exercising and have taken off my chemotherapy weight, plus some. Food is not as important as it was before when I would awaken in the morning wondering what was for lunch and dinner. I still love fried foods, but I've cut way back on them.

I am beyond the five-year mark. My doctor says I only need to see him once a year, but I like to get a blood test every six months. That is my security blanket.

Sue, his wife: It was emotionally draining watching Ben through chemotherapy and seeing the toll it was taking on him. There was always the fear that because it had gone to his lymph nodes, it might come back. You wish you could get rid of the fear, but even with the passage of time, it's still there. Dealing with it is an ongoing thing. When he gets an ache or pain, the reality is, "Could it possibly be?" Ben knows if something new is going on with his body. Perhaps he is a little too much in tune with his body, but I would rather he be this way than not.

Those who have been through chemotherapy understand about the association of smells. Even today, walking into Ben's oncologist's office brings up a sea of emotion for both of us, him more so than me. These visits are important to both Ben and the staff. He needs that warm welcome back, and they need to see a survivor because he represents hope. Survivors like Ben make the rest of us not so afraid, because they went through it and they're okay. We used to group the big "Cs" together. But people have to understand there are different cancers, different treatments and lots of people with cancer survive. Part of the hope is seeing the long-term survivors. A positive attitude is so important.

Ben is a wonderful "fellow sister." Because he has had the disease and is so open about it, women can talk to him even when they won't talk to anyone else. It also helps Ben. The worst thing anyone can do is not to acknowledge that someone has cancer. By saying nothing, it's like saying, "Oh no. You have the plague." We've known people who have literally turned and walked the other way when they see Ben coming. We understood that they didn't know what to say, but people who have not had the disease need to realize that those who do have cancer want to be treated normally. When your battle with cancer becomes the most important thing in your life and you're fighting for your life, you just can't ignore the fact that someone has the disease and say nothing. It's not a nice feeling when you're treated differently because you have cancer. It's a strain. Don't people realize it's just cancer? Sometimes you feel sorry for people because they don't know how to handle it. My emotions are more on the surface than Ben's, although I do not mean that he does not deal with his emotions because he does. We can laugh, which is good and we can cry, which is healthy. It's hard on him when he sees a friend who is dying of cancer. Particularly when he sees that they have given up. It brings up old fears . . . "It could have been me."

Life is much more precious since he got sick. We've come through a really scary time together and have managed to overcome something. Maybe the moral here is that cancer teaches you something about the important things in life. Just in case you've had any misgivings along the way, it always gives you back your priorities.

Ed, his son: Both of my parents are strong. One of Dad's needs is to be babied by my mom, which she does very well. We all knew Mom was scared, but we did not want to make an issue out of it. We just acknowledged that she was and did not treat her any differently than we normally did. All of us kids kept up a continuous, upbeat attitude. Almost like laughing in the face of adversity. We tried not to let things bring us down.

Even though Dad and I never had any deep philosophical discussions, we did talk while he was going through treatment. He never came right out and said, "I hope I don't die," but I did catch him being reflective a time or two which was unusual for him. Even though he didn't let on a whole lot, I knew he was concerned.

Although I have always appreciated my dad and we have always been able to say "I love you," it wasn't until I thought I might lose him that I really appreciated him. And it taught me that you can't take things for granted. If you like or appreciate someone, tell that person now because there may not be a later. We go through life fat, dumb and happy until something bad happens. For me three things happened, almost back to back, which put things into perspective. The first was saying good-bye to my dog and grieving him, which was the most important thing in my life at the moment. The second was the telephone call telling me Dad had breast cancer. Suddenly, my dad took priority. No matter how much I loved my dog, there is no comparison. The third event came about a month after Dad started chemotherapy. My daughter contracted viral encephalitis on her fifth birthday. For thirty-six hours we did not know if she was going to live or die. I cried a lot during that time. My wife and I, our marriage, our family, our values, everything, were tested. It was a very bad, scary time. You think you control your destiny, but you do not even come close. You have no control. It hurts to see those you love hurting. And I have now seen it as a child and as a parent. You'd almost rather that it was happening to you. My father and my daughter are both fine today. Thank God. It's the rainy days though that make the rest of life sweeter.

Bob, his friend: This whole thing was really hard on Sue. She kept pretty much to herself and would not show her emotions too much because she didn't want Ben to see how worried she was. She has become a stronger person for it. I was never afraid that Ben would die. I always told him, "You're too stubborn to die."

It amazes me how many people are surprised that he had breast cancer. A lot of men have never heard of it. When they find out, their reaction is, "You've got to be kidding!"

Postscript, January, 2000

My oncologist and I have become good friends over the past nine years. The monthly visits that were a part of the beginning treatment have now dwindled to visits three times a year, and will continue at that rate until at least April 2001. Any aches, pains, strange feelings, tender spots and especially lumps have been reported immediately. Although that may seem as if I am apprehensive, the reality is that I am just so much more aware of my body than I was nine years ago. One has to constantly remember that an early detection is *not* a death sentence. In fact, it is quite the opposite.

Sixteen

Lolly Champion

I Didn't Set Out to Be a Political Activist

Survivor Profile:

Age at diagnosis: forty-nine (12/8/88)

Age at interview: fifty-eight (1/10/97)

Type of breast cancer: infiltrating ductal

Size tumor: 6 cm; stage III

One positive lymph node

Surgical procedure: mastectomy

Treatment: chemotherapy and radiation, tamoxifen

Reconstruction: no

Estrogen receptors: positive; Progesterone receptors: unknown

Who's Who:

John Champion, her husband

Chris Champion, her son
  (age twenty at time of diagnosis)

Craig Abell-Champion, her son
  (age nineteen at time of diagnosis)

Christine Mulder, her friend

Margaret Warnke-Shields, her friend

A COMEDY OF ERRORS:
WHO PAYS THE PRICE?

Lolly: I did not set out to be a political activist. It happened because I was angry that Cheryl died. Who was Cheryl? She was my roommate in the hospital where I had my mastectomy. Both of us were misdiagnosed. She was told she was too young to have breast cancer, and died only twenty months after her diagnosis at the age of thirty-five. Something's not right about that, so I did what I had to do. Her death was very hard on me, but it also gave me great strength to go ahead and become the "pain in the neck" that I am today.

I had found my lump in early November 1986, but had forgotten about it. As a sales representative in the gift business I travel quite a bit. About a month later, while on a trip, I felt the lump again. Stopping at a pay phone to call my doctor's office I reached whom I refer to as the "I'm in charge of everyone's life" receptionist who could *manage* to squeeze me in sometime in February. To say I became unglued is an understatement. The upshot was a huge sigh followed by an appointment the following week. Today I would have insisted he see me the next day.

Oregon was one of only seven states left in the union that did not mandate insurance companies pay for mammograms. Consequently, even though I was forty-six I'd never had one, nor did my doctor prescribe one after his diagnosis of, "It is only fibrocystic disease." In March or April of the following year the lump was still there. Why I decided to take advantage of the American Cancer Society's first-time reduced cost mammograms I'll never know. About a week later the mailman rang my doorbell, and handed me a certified, registered letter informing me the mammogram was irregular, and I needed to see a doctor. Once again I had to get past the watchdog receptionist, and a week later was told, "You are overreacting and so is the American Cancer Society. There's nothing to worry about; however, if you insist I'll prescribe another mammogram."

The radiologist who examined me told me nothing really showed on the X-ray, and he did not feel the lump was anything to be concerned about. A month passed with no word from my doctor's office, so I decided to follow up. The assistant told me, "We did not get the card sent out, but you're fine." Despite my lump now feeling like two large bubbles I breathed a sigh of relief. Almost a year after first feeling the lump I returned to the same doctor for an annual Pap smear. "Those are large cysts," he said, "but there's nothing to worry about." Again relief. I wanted to believe nothing was wrong.

THE BUBBLE BURSTS

Lolly: In April of 1988 my husband, John, and I moved to Portland, Oregon. I thought about looking for a new doctor, but it was not a priority. By August I was getting very hot, terrible pains in my breast, and the lumps were considerably larger. In addition to the pain, which was now worse, there was a swelling under my arm. I thought the kind of doctor I needed to see was an ob/gyn, but when I called to schedule an appointment the practices were closed. By Thanksgiving I had become desperate. The pain had become so bad that when a woman I met suggested that I go to the woman's clinic she went to I did, and did not argue when I was told the only doctor available to see was their new associate, a recent medical school graduate. Barely touching me she became extremely concerned, "You are going for a mammogram now, and I'm making an appointment for you to see a surgeon." I felt as though I were going to vomit. When I got home John was there with our friend he'd just picked up at the airport. Both tried to reassure me that the lump was probably nothing.

Right after Thanksgiving I met with the surgeon. It was not until he said, "This does not look good," and scheduled me for a biopsy that I began to think maybe I did have a problem. Wanting a second opinion, I called the surgeon who had saved our son's life when he was sixteen, scheduled an appointment for the following afternoon, and postponed the biopsy. John and I drove back to the community we had recently moved from to meet with him. Sitting in his office I was told to put my arm straight up over my head not behind, and shockingly, there was a huge dimpling in my very small breast. He didn't say, "Gee. I think you've got something there." It was more like, "My God. What is the size of that?" He did not mince words. "You have breast cancer." It seemed pointless to have two surgeries, so I authorized him to do a modified radical mastectomy should the lump be malignant. It was. Not only did I have a 6-cm (a medium size apple) infiltrating ductal cancer in my breast, but the large swelling under my arm was an enlarged cancerous lymph node.

John, her husband: Lolly refers to us as Mr. and Mrs. Ignorant. For two years we had believed her "Harvard Graduate" doctor's reassurances. Was it that I, like most males, was as unaware of breast cancer as anyone would want to be? Or was it that we have a tendency to not want to discuss something like this? At the time breast cancer meant nothing to me.

TELLING THE CHILDREN

Lolly: The children knew nothing until the morning of my surgery. They were of course quite shocked. Getting only as far as, "Honey, I have to go in for breast cancer surgery," I gave the phone to John who had to finish both phone calls because I had broken down into tears.

John, her husband: My words to the boys were pretty matter of fact; where we were, what the diagnosis was, and what was going to take place. I was, at the time, consumed with fears of Lolly dying as I felt her surgeon had handed her a death sentence. Neither of the children really understood the ramifications of how serious her disease was. That took time to sink in.

HOW DID WE ALL COPE THEN?

Lolly: On the drive to Colorado, where we were meeting the children and some friends, I began reading my pathology report. Panicking because even I could deduce that I had been given a very poor prognosis I suddenly realized I was reading Cheryl's report. I never told her.

It was while Cheryl and I were in the hospital that we decided we wanted to do something that would educate and empower women. We began writing pamphlets. Our first, "Doctor, I Need To Know" began what I refer to as my militant road to advocacy. I left no stone unturned and sent it everywhere: my clients, the library, the newspaper, the American

Cancer Society, Oprah Winfrey, Barbara Walters, even the White House.

John, her husband: It was good that Lolly's surgery was not in a strange community because once word went out that she'd been admitted to the hospital people began reaching out to us as a couple. During the early stages of her diagnosis a couple of men I knew took me to the country club for drinks which was their way of saying, "Hey, let's relax a little bit." It was nice that people cared about me; however, most of the attention was directed toward Lolly. I am not quite sure, nor can I really put into words how I felt except that maybe I was resentful at times that she was getting all the attention. That is why it is so important for the entire family to be acknowledged, not just the patient. What I found interesting was that some people you might expect to call did not, and those you did not expect to call did.

No matter how hard I tried, Lolly refused to cancel that ski trip to Colorado only a month after her surgery. Chris, our twenty-year-old at the time lived there, and Craig, a year younger, was flying in. She had every intention of skiing, and I was both angry and concerned. What if she falls? What if her stitches open up? Then she gave me that look, and I knew she was going to do it. Picture seven adults on skis in a wedge position around Lolly, as she flew down the slopes. That was my turning point, and I think hers, too.

Chris, her son: I had not seen either of my parents for about a year because of the distance. I had gone to college for three years, then dropped out and moved to Colorado to ski. They were not pleased. My father explained the whole situation, and it scared me some just because it was the "cancer" word.

Craig, her son: During a Navy training class my senior chief called out, "Champion, you have an emergency phone call." That memory remains vivid. My first two questions to my father were "Do I need to get emergency leave?" and "Is it life-threatening?" He told me he thought she would be fine. Shook up a little, but not too badly, I put it out of my mind as I would be on leave a couple of weeks later, and would deal with it then. What was really going through my head was, *She is tough and can make it through anything.* Besides, if it were really serious my father would have told me. I knew nothing about breast cancer then.

Frankly I was taken aback at my mother's appearance when I saw her. It had only been sixteen weeks since I'd seen her last, and she now looked sick and emaciated. I did not let her know how I felt, and most likely cracked some jokes. Our family has a really good sense of humor. How I felt is a little hard to explain. It's not that I did not feel bad for her; rather, I was almost proud of her because I knew she was going to make it.

LET THE CHEMOTHERAPY BEGIN

Lolly: It was my oncologist at that first meeting who taught me the importance of understanding the positives and negatives of any medication you take. For instance although an aspirin can give you stomach problems, on the positive side it can cure a headache, thin blood for the heart, stop some joint aches and pains, even reduce a fever. Chemotherapy is no different. If the pluses outweigh the minuses, then it needs to be realistically considered as a life-saving action. Maybe it will buy some time, even save a life; therefore, it can be perceived as a friend, an asset, instead of something to fight or be terrified of. The information, which is not privileged, is readily available from any pharmacy. All one needs to do is ask.

The oncologist told me that my best chance, since I was stage III, was to attack my cancer as aggressively as possible. That would entail eight treatments of Adriamycin, Cytoxan and 5-FU, followed by six weeks of radiation since my tumor was attached to the chest wall, then tamoxifen. She wanted me to understand it and to appreciate the risks as well as the strengths of this course of action. The next day we began. Neither Neupogen, a white cell growth factor, nor Zofran, an excellent antinausea drug were yet available. Consequently, I became either violently ill after a treatment, or in tears when one was postponed because of having a low white blood count. It was a godsend when they gave me the rest of my drugs through the portacath (a venous access catheter) they surgically inserted into the lower quadrant of my breast, because my veins collapsed after the second session.

John was marvelous. I could not have survived without him. He took me for my treatments, brought me home, became chief cook and bottle washer and baby-sat me over the weekend while I recovered. Throughout this time I had sores in my mouth, yeast infections and flaky skin on my face and forehead. Chemotherapy stopped my periods immediately and permanently. Yogurt and mouthwash helped the sores; yogurt and cranberry juice eased the yeast infections. About ten days after my first treatment, while I was sitting with a client and fiddling with a pencil in my hair, a big glob of it fell onto the table to my horror and embarrassment. I'd been forewarned that I would lose it, and fortunately had already picked out a wig; nevertheless, I was shattered, and called John in tears. No one at the time, other than friends or family, knew that I had breast cancer. My customers were unaware that I had it because I did not want any sympathy buys, but maybe the issue was larger than that. Perhaps I feared they would not see me *because* I had cancer. I guess the bottom line was, I was in denial.

The boys were very attentive to their father. They called every Sunday, "We know, Mom. You have everybody calling you. We want to talk to Dad, and see how he's doing." I loved that they did that.

One day I was feeling kind of blue. I'd just gotten out of the shower and stood looking at myself in the mirror: bald, no eyebrows or eyelashes, fresh tattoos from the start of radiation, a huge scar. Frankly I was feeling sorry for myself. As I began to cry John patted me on the back. "You know what, honey? Right now I could take you down to the docks, and you could probably shoot pool with some of the guys. You'd fit right in: You're bald and have a couple of tattoos. All you need is a cigar!" That just cracked me up, and I began laughing.

It was not until I was finished with all my treatment that I went to see an endocrinologist about the high blood sugars that kept showing up in my blood work, and which had also kept me in the hospital a few extra days after my mastectomy. I was diagnosed a Type 2 diabetic.

John, her husband: Lolly's oncologist told us what would happen, how it would happen, and where Lolly was concerning her diagnosis. She did not mince words, yet did so in a positive way. Lolly did not miss a beat as far as work was concerned. Friday was chemotherapy, Monday she was on the phone, and by Tuesday back on the road.

Her hair loss, to me, was an effect of the illness rather than a vanity thing. What both of us found difficult was the anticipation of a new cycle. She'd just be starting to live a reasonable life again and it would be, "Oh God. It's only another four to five days, and I'm back at it again!" Other than a little tenderness, and some light burns she developed towards the end of treatment, radiation was a breeze in comparison to chemotherapy. Even though by now I knew much more there was still that apprehension while she was going through everything. We reacted quite differently when all her procedures were over. I felt as though things would now be okay, and that we could move on with our lives instead of thinking about what had been. To Lolly it was very traumatic because she felt it was her last shot at doing something really positive.

Chris, her son: I knew my mother was sick, but I did not realize how sick until my father called, and told me she'd been up all night vomiting. She looked so skinny in the pictures he sent me. I began calling home more frequently than my normal once a month, and my father called me more often, too.

About six weeks after chemotherapy was finished my parents and brother came to visit. I knew she was not sure how I would react to her appearance, but I thought she looked great with her short hair. My mother was just so happy to be alive; that we were all together. It was unbelievable that she had the energy to ski.

Craig, her son: My father is the one who held my mother together during chemotherapy. He might say, "It's just another step. Take it, and get over it" when she was upset because it was time for another treatment. He was the one who kept a sense of humor. Like the time they went to a support group meeting, and he surprised her with one of those wigs that has a bright red mohawk on it, and said, "Anytime you get down just put this on, and look in the mirror." They'd been talking about what gets you down the most about chemotherapy.

Since I expected her to lose her hair it did not phase me in the slightest when she did. Nothing about the whole experience shocked me. I knew treatment would be long, that she would be sick, but I also knew that she would make it. The biggest surprise would have been if she had died. That just never entered into my equation. Those were very taxing, stressful times for my father.

TAMOXIFEN—LET'S WEIGH THE PROS AND CONS

Lolly: Tamoxifen, which I've taken for six years, has created problems for me as it has for many other women: vaginal dryness which is lousy for your sex life, hot flashes and night sweats. I'm sure John wanted to belt me sometimes when I threw the covers off, pulled them on, etc., etc. He said, "If you do that one more time . . ." I finally got through that one!

I have just met with my oncologist, and I am staying on tamoxifen indefinitely. In my case it makes no sense to arbitrarily stop taking something that I respond well to. If I develop a problem in the future we will address it then. Taking estrogen is out of the question for me; therefore, tamoxifen is the only protection I have for my heart, as well as for helping to prevent osteoporosis. Although I follow a strict exercise regime, osteoporosis runs in my family, and it is a major concern of mine. Maybe it's helping to prevent a recurrence. This whole issue gets back to the fact that cancer is a thinking person's disease, and there are no clear-cut answers. It's a double-edged sword.

SOMEONE'S GOT TO BE FIRST

Lolly: One day, while on the telephone with my mother, I said, "I'm going through chemotherapy, feel horrible, and don't know if I'm going to live through this. I'm asking you to get a mammogram, and you're denying me that?" She can be difficult at times even though she really is a sweetheart. She went, "Oh, boo hoo hoo. Are you ever putting me on a guilt trip." I didn't know she went for one, but my birthday passed and I didn't hear from her. The following day my brother called to tell me she had gone for a mammogram. It was unclear, and they suggested that she come back in six months. Apparently my mother said, "Nope. I've been through this already with my daughter, and I want you to do something today." The long and the short of it is that the doctor finally threw his hands in the air, and that night she had her breast removed. She had infiltrating ductal cancer throughout her breast. Once her drains were removed she never returned to her doctor, never went on tamoxifen, nor has she had another mammogram. That is just the way she is.

RECONSTRUCTION

Lolly: Most recurrences are on the scar line, or somewhere in the basic chest area. No way would I ever consider having reconstruction as it might hinder early detection if there were a recurrence. Because I have a job where it is important for me to look as normal as possible I wear a prosthesis. Other than wearing it to work, and maybe to parties, I don't wear it at all.

John, her husband: Losing a breast was of no consequence to me; it was something that had to be done. It took Lolly a couple of weeks to show me, and I looked at it from the standpoint of what it was. We both accepted it. My feeling is if you marry someone for their breasts, then you should not be married in the first place. There is so much more to a relationship than just the physical aspect of it.

POLITICAL ACTIVISM—LET'S GET SERIOUS

Lolly: In 1991 I read a book called *The Race Is Run One Step at a Time: Every Woman's Guide to Taking Charge of Breast Cancer and My Personal Story.* I called the Susan G. Komen Breast Cancer Foundation headquartered in Dallas, Texas, and told them I thought Portland, where I now lived, should have their own Race for the Cure. Two other women and I began working to make it happen, and the following October had one of the biggest races they've ever had—initially sixty-two hundred women. Sponsorship was incredible. From that has stemmed things I believe in strongly: an education program, a low-cost mammogram program and money donated for research.

Funding has been incredibly successful toward finding a cure for AIDS because gay men came forward and spoke to the issue. Women now are doing the same thing with breast cancer. I have been to Washington, D.C. three times to sit on the Department of Defense (DOD) Peer Reviews as well as participate in Project LEAD which is facilitated by the NBCC (National Breast Cancer Coalition). The NBCC's purpose is to bring survivors to scientific tables so they can then go out into their communities and be able to participate at the decision-making tables at our hospitals and research facilities. That has led to some other interesting projects I have become involved in: being a consumer reader for the FDA on what goes on the Internet, and participating as the one layperson on the Professional Committee for the State of Oregon for Physicians. Its purpose is to change and upgrade standards for all physicians in the state. It is our intention that all physicians will refer a woman to a specialist when she has an abnormal breast finding. We have also put together a booklet which is to be given to all women at time of diagnosis to aid in the decision-making process.

Education is a passion of mine. I teach many classes such as: breast self-examination, how to be assertive in your healthcare, how to get a referral, and how to survive your HMO. I also certify others to teach BSE. We've really worked in the medically underserved African-American, Latino, and the Tribes of Oregon communities. Now my biggest desire is to get into the workplace.

In 1993 we passed the Mammogram Bill. We were told it would never get passed. My comment was, "You have never seen a lot of women who have been intensely upset about something." We did what women do best. We networked, and in less than two weeks had gotten over forty-eight hundred signatures. John and I and about ten friends double copied, and then Scotch taped all those signatures together on sheets until we had huge rolls about two and one-half feet in diameter. Our governor, a female at the time, presented those rolls to both the Speaker of the House and President of the Senate. From that day forward we were on the move. Every time we left any kind of update, appeal, etc. to anyone on the legislature we left a candy kiss. Something to make the medicine go down a little easier. They tried holding us up in committee and pulled all kinds of shenanigans. That is when I called every newspaper in the state, and we began a calling campaign. The media put pressure on the government, a well-known political reporter did an exposé which caused a big furor, and it ended up going to the floor where the bill was unanimously passed. What a great victory!

With funding from Komen National and the Oregon Breast and Cervical Cancer Coalition a lifelong dream of mine was fulfilled. People from five states attended the Northwest Leadership Summit on Breast and Cervical Cancer. We ran three simultaneous courses: one for physicians and healthcare providers which qualified them for continuing education credits, one for community outreach folks, and one for corporate business. Currently I'm working on the national petition drive to get over 2.6 million signatures to Congress to confirm long-term funding for breast cancer research.

Although I have been the driving force behind much of this, it is a team effort. But it all happened because Cheryl died. What makes me feel good is that a few people can do a lot when their hearts are doing it for the right reason. Whenever anyone questions what we're doing or why, I always feel as though we are a bunch of Joan of Arcs. We are not doing it for ourselves, we are doing it for future generations, and for those women who don't know what they need to do. Ninety-nine percent of us who work so actively cannot take back what we have lost. I tell people, "We can choose to practice safe sex, or not; we can smoke, or not; we can eat a high-fat, or low-fat diet, but we still get breast cancer. We have no choices here. It is something that comes and it gets us. Until we have some choices, we are not going to stop fighting until we have eradicated it. We will continue our fight to educate women, so that they get the earliest and best detection they can. And we are going to continue to do that." Our single greatest ability is to get things done.

John, her husband: My concern with Lolly is that she's doing too much, but that's how she is. Her illness did not change that; it only redirected her focus, which then became "What can I do?" She does not know how to say no. If she could, she would work twenty-four hours a day although she is beginning to slow down a bit. Her frustration comes from wanting to do everything, which she just cannot do. My involvement was strictly support.

The mammogram issue is one of my proudest moments for Lolly. She went to Salem, our capital, and banged on doors. It took her almost a year to get that bill passed. Most people have no idea what Lolly does, or that her typical work day is from six A.M. until ten P.M. She has this boundless energy and is able to successfully juggle her career, with all this activism. I'll jump in only when I think she needs to slow down a bit. Sometimes she listens, other times not. She is great at getting the ball rolling, doing what needs to be done, yet is wise enough with her ego well-defined enough to be able to hand over the reins and say, "I've done it now. You guys take over." That does not mean her fingers are not still in the pie. They probably always will be.

Chris, her son: All of us have become knowledgeable because of my mother's work. I am incredibly proud of her, and have never known any-one who has worked harder, or is more impassioned. The Race for the Cure has grown tremendously; in fact, just last year, in 1995, it was the second-largest race after the Washington, D.C., Race for the Cure. My father does everything he can to support her including volunteering a lot of his time every year for the race. At one time my mother would become nervous talking about something she was unfamiliar with. Now she will speak to hundreds of people during the month. She has become much more assertive and confident. Her classes are interesting, and she and my wife, Leanne, tell me women are not dragging their husbands to these classes. The husbands are coming voluntarily.

Craig, her son: My mother doesn't talk about doing something, she just does it. Almost like tunnel vision. When she gets on the warpath there is no stopping her. She has very few inhibitions about tackling the big things; it's the little things that hang her up, such as, "What salad should I serve to my dinner company tonight?" Yet, when it comes to the things that really matter she has the best head screwed on I've ever seen.

In 1995 I did a solo installation type of show titled "Survivors" that revolved entirely around my mother's breast cancer experience. An installation is one in which the artist creates an environment within a space instead of just hanging pictures on the wall. Every aspect of the space becomes part of the piece. At times it's interactive, as was this show. She was doing a lot of speaking, and I had, by then, become curi-ous about the work she was doing. In addition, I was extremely proud of her. This show would not be just a learning experience for me, but for those who saw it. My first mistake when interviewing my mother was calling survivors "victims."

With the help of my fiancée and friends we painted the entire gallery black; then proceeded to make forty-seven thousand white chalk crosses on the walls representing the number of women who die each year from breast cancer. A full-size, working, lead-lined shower I had built represented the toxicity of the disease as well as being, according to my mother, the best place for a woman to check herself because it's private and they are naked. It was very dramatic when, as part of the show, my fiancée handed me through the black curtain I had set up nine, sand-filled, hour glass dolls. Rhythmically a cadence was established like a monotone beat as she handed them to me—one at a time. Each was placed on a shelf on the wall; however, the ninth one had a slit. Sand trickled out, and the doll sagged down and disintegrated into nothing. That represented the fact that in 1995, one in nine women was diagnosed with breast cancer. About sixty people standing on one side of the room watched the show, many in tears. As the last doll was put on the shelf, I marked the last cross on the wall. It was powerful.

My mother and I co-wrote the show. She spoke at the opening, and much of the literature written by her or from the Komen Foundation was available as handouts. There was also a fake breast with a lump that people were encouraged to feel, so they would know what to look for. It wasn't until then that I found out how serious breast cancer is, and realized maybe she wouldn't survive. For me this show was a real cleansing. I wanted to be a part of my mother's life. This was a way for me to open the door and associate myself with something that was really important to her.

Margaret, her friend: Since meeting Lolly in 1992 through Race for the Cure, I have become quite active in our local Komen chapter; first as part of the race committee, later as secretary, and now as president. When Lolly needed women to testify in Salem for the Mammogram Bill issue I became sort of the poster child, and spoke of my experience as a seven-year survivor, and the importance of mammograms having had firsthand experience about their value. At the age of thirty-six I had had a baseline mammogram. When I turned forty my doctor thought I should have another one done for comparison purposes. Because it was not what the insurance company deemed medically necessary I had to pay for it myself. Only after I was diagnosed was I was reimbursed. I was a perfect example of what we were fighting for. Many people helped her, but Lolly along with one other woman is really the one who did all the hard work, because she knew the ropes.

It would be hard to be more of an advocate than Lolly. Her focus and passion is on education and early detection. In 1995 we nominated her for the Jill Ireland Volunteer Award, a national award given by the Komen Foundation for volunteerism. Many prominent women have been the recipient of this award, such as Betty Ford and Abigail Van Buren (Dear Abby). Lolly joined their ranks. The world is a better place because of her. She is a true friend to women, one not afraid to take a stand or risks.

Chris Mulder, her friend: John, like Lolly is in the gift business, and she came with him one day to my gift shop and herb nursery because of her interest in gardening and herbs. We began talking, and I told her I was also a survivor, diagnosed in 1986. My focus then and now is running a support group an oncology nurse and I began at one of our local hospitals, as well as a program I developed similar to Reach for Recovery, but geared specifically towards breast cancer. With the support of two surgeons, the oncology nurse and a social worker, we started this program at the same hospital, and it is still running successfully eight and half years later. After inviting me to her home with two other women she asked, "Do we want to get a Susan G. Komen Breast Cancer Foundation and our own Race for the Cure started in Portland?" Since then I've been involved in many of her projects.

Neither of us is actively involved in Komen at this point as we are doing other things, yet we are always available if needed. We share many similarities: owning our own businesses and working full time, and having the ability to get a program launched; then, letting someone else take over. Lolly's vision is more global; mine local. It concerns me some because she goes a mile a minute, and although she is able to accomplish wonderful things I have seen her health suffer as a result. Our husbands are tolerant, but there is a limit. In wanting to do more we tend to overextend ourselves, which in turn adds new stresses to our lives. So I have to really look at what I am adding in a clear light, and that's hard to do sometimes particularly when I get really involved. We have an ongoing joke—learn to say "no."

THE REALITY OF A LAWSUIT— SOME OF US DON'T WIN

Lolly: In 1990 I sued the doctor who had repeatedly told me, "There's nothing to be concerned about," and the trial began in early 1991. When my attorney in Portland accepted the case he told us, "Our chances of winning are nil to none, but I'd like to break their backs." We came from a town in which the medical community is the single largest employer, the residents are reluctant to seek second opinions because that would be showing a distrust to the community, and everyone backs everyone else.

During the trial I discovered that the radiologist who had read my second mammogram had written on the report that I had a 4-cm palpable mass. None of the doctors told the truth in court which was devastating for John and me. We had made it quite clear that we weren't suing for money other than our out-of-pocket expenses pertaining to the surgery. I never believed that my doctor meant to cause me harm, but I resented his arrogance in not understanding that he had done me harm. I resent the fact that he is still referring to fibrocystic cysts as a disease—it is a condition, not a disease. He kept trying to deny that I was misdiagnosed; but he finally had to admit, in a public place, that I was. Even still I lost. As a result of the lawsuit though, good things did transpire such as the passage of the Mammogram Bill.

John, her husband: I thought the lawsuit was doomed from the beginning, and I equate it to the television show *Matlock* played by Andy Griffith, the good old country boy attorney. The entire trial was like watching a replay of one of those shows. Those doctors told out-and-out lies because it's the old saying, "If one falls they all fall." Even though we lost, we felt good that we had at least played the game. Doctors need to know they are accountable. Lolly says, "In small ways I get my retribution" because, through friends, her information finds its way into the medical pipeline down there.

Chris, her son: Our family did not talk much about the misdiagnosis while my mother was going through treatment because we wanted to concentrate their positive energy on her getting well. What was tough for me about the lawsuit was the fact that I grew up with the kids of some of the doctors my parents took to court. I'm pretty angry toward her doctors for letting something like that go on for two years, and I would like to ask, "What the hell were you thinking?" The doctors were wrong, and should have lost, but they're a tight group. My parents definitely pushed some buttons, and deservedly so. Her experience has taught me to ask questions, and to be my own advocate. You have the right to question your doctor, and if you don't understand something ask them to explain it in layman's terms.

Craig, her son: It infuriated me that the medical community would not admit they made a mistake, and that the one doctor straight up lied under oath. I was really mad, and resentful of him for a long time. To be honest I wanted to go over to his house and kick his behind. Suing was very painful for my mother to do, but I'm proud of her for doing so because even though they lost, the case created awareness in the community.

WE ALL COPE DIFFERENTLY

Lolly: Our family had lived through a crisis before when Craig, sixteen at the time, almost died because of a misdiagnosis. Consequently, John and I discussed with the boys only the realities of everything, and then relied on those coping skills we had used once before, take one day at a time. We did not discuss with them our fears about me dying.

John had changed as a result of that experience; therefore, he had already learned how to handle things. He was a great resource for me, and I counted on him often. I coped quietly at first trying to come to terms with the fact that I was not always in control of my life; in addition, I was trying to figure out what role it is that I play with everyone because I am not sure myself how I feel about all of it. Then of course I became militant. I still get caught up in the day-to-day stresses like everyone else, and wonder, *How did I get to be doing* that *again?* I thought I had trained myself better, but it happens. At least I now recognize when I'm being a jerk.

I have constant bone pain in my chest and was told by my radiologist, "That's impossible. It's in your head." My oncologist though has told me that it is a very common occurrence. Now that I know that, I can live with it. I never considered having a prophylactic mastectomy because I wanted to keep all the body parts I could. If I get breast cancer in the other breast it will be okay only in the regard that I do not consider it a recurrence. Of course I would mind, but I would rather it be a new tumor than a recurrence because that is a whole different ball game. Recurrence is the fear. That is the part I do not want to deal with.

John, her husband: I cried, but not in front of Lolly. Men need to be aware that it is okay for them to do that. The first time I really broke down was when we did not know whether Craig would survive when he was so seriously ill. Women seem to have a much easier time creating and nurturing relationships, talking about emotions and themselves. Men have relationships which tend to revolve around things and subjects. Recurrence is still a concern of mine. I am not even thinking about it, and all of a sudden I get a funny feeling and try to push it aside. It is probably part of the denial process we all go through. There is still that little kernel of fear. I am sure a lot of that is the result of Lolly getting so many phone calls from women, or friends of women in all stages of their disease asking for help or advice, plus her involvement with breast cancer in general.

Our relationship is better today than it has ever been. The worst thing a person can do is to step away from any problem and leave a person floundering. It is not a matter of what they should or should not do. Common sense tells them this person is the other half of their life. They should help, protect and nurture her just as they have in the past; as they would in the future. This is only a bump in the road as far as a relationship is concerned.

Chris, her son: When I was first told about my mother's diagnosis I was afraid she was going to die; however, I am sure my father would have flown both Craig and me home if that were the case, or at least told us if she was getting really sick. Both are pretty sensitive to that. I think it was easier to deal with because I was not there. However, if I had to do it over again I would have moved home because one never knows what is going to happen. The bottom line is regardless of age, or whether there have been conflicts in the relationship, you will always be the child, and they will always be the parents.

My father used to be a definite type A personality; always very stressed. He has changed considerably and has relaxed. My mother's illness scared him because I do not think he would know what to do without her. Even today I think he is scared. At least a little bit.

Craig and I, although we have a great relationship, never hung out together because our agendas were always different. Even today we speak only once or twice a month. My friends at the time were in their early twenties, and wanted only to ski and party. What helped me was to talk to my parents more; in fact we would speak several times a week. Since then I have gotten married, moved back to Portland, am finishing up my college degree, and have an excellent job. Going over to my parents' house is always a lot of fun. I am now very interested in breast cancer, and of course my mother has a tremendous amount of knowledge, therefore dinners are lively as we all have different perspectives about medical research, etc.

What I have learned is the importance of not desensitizing myself if I am faced with this kind of situation. I have learned to become more involved, learn about it, be a good listener and ask questions. My suggestion is to talk to your parents, or whoever the person is, yet leave them alone when they want to be left alone.

I do not consider my mother's illness or misdiagnosis a blessing; however, in one sense it is because of what she has been able to accomplish by helping so many other people. In 1988 you did not hear that much about breast cancer, or if you did it was discussed quietly; not brought out into the open. She has changed that—at least in Oregon.

Craig, her son: This experience has made my father realize his own mortality. For a long time he was very strict; then, he relaxed and really started to have fun. He wanted to be supportive to my mother. She has changed, too, and now they do more than they have since I was a child; go on more camping trips, hiking excursions, visit wineries, that kind of thing. They are like this young vivacious couple even though my mother is fifty-six and he is sixty-two.

My brother and I have never really discussed my mother's situation. When we do talk about her it never goes beyond, "Oh, how's Mom doing?" "She's doing great." I can never figure him out. He has always kept quiet about things like that. I know he is concerned in his own way, but I never know what he is thinking.

Because I lived so far away, my parents treated me on a need to know basis. If I did not ask they did not tell me unless it was really important; consequently, when I asked my father how she was, and he said, "fine" then I was okay with that. Even after interviewing my mother for the installation I did not have fears about her dying, but that was when I realized, *Wow. This is a much more serious disease than I thought.* My outlook on life is that you have to live life to the fullest, and my mother does. Yes, she could die from breast cancer, but she could also be hit by a bus and die. Everyone dies, but you cannot dwell on it, and I do not. I will worry about it then, and grieve then, not now. I am very much like my parents: Get over it, and move on. It may sound selfish, and perhaps a little weird, but I am the type of person who operates in my own little microcosm; out of sight, out of mind. I do not dwell on things, but on the other hand I knew that I could be there for her. She wants me to be happy, live my own life, and to succeed. If I stressed about her that would make her feel bad, so what is the point? It would just be counterproductive.

SOME SIMPLE GUIDELINES

Lolly: When someone says to me, "I don't know what I'm looking for," I answer, "Of course you don't if you don't know what you're looking for, and you've never done it." Getting to know your breasts is just like getting to know your face. You know that face intimately, and would notice the second something changed. Get to know your breasts. Do not look for the abnormal, *the thing;* look for the normal. It will take three months doing regular breast self-examination before you will know what is normal for you. Do it once a month, from about the third to the fifth day after you have finished your period, or if you are menopausal, the first day each month. When you do BSE your arm should go straight over your head, not behind. If you stand in front of the mirror the difference becomes obvious. Notice how much more you see of the movement on your chest area by doing it like that. Stand to one side, the other side, then front. If there is a change remember that 80 percent of the time it is absolutely fine. It is that other 20 percent you cannot risk.

If a woman feels a lump I say, "Don't panic." They have to know that lump is not normal for them, and has remained through a second cycle, or second month, and that it is not mirrored in the other breast. If your doctor says any of these kinds of things: "I don't believe you have anything to be worried about," "This feels like a cyst to me," "There's no breast cancer in your family," or "Let's follow this, and wait and see" your next step is to say to your doctor, "Can you guarantee me 100 percent that I have nothing to worry about? Because, as we all know, no one can diagnose a cancer unless there is a tissue slide, or some type of fluid. You can 'assume' something, but you cannot give me a 100 percent sure answer without some type of pathology." If your doctor will not refer you for a second opinion to a breast clinic, or suggest a fine needle aspiration, say something like, "If you will not refer me then I am going to have to take this further. I want you to write, right now, why you are guaranteeing to me that this is not breast cancer, and will not refer me to another doctor." The minute you ask them to put their name to something like that you will get a referral, or some kind of action. However, the woman must do her part, too.

When you do have a breast problem go to a breast specialist. You would not go to a proctologist for a dermatology problem would you? The science of breast health, breast disease and breast cancer is a very specialized science. Do not mess around with your internist or your gynecologist. No one can be an expert in every field. When I hear an ob-gyn say, "We know how to treat breasts," I love to challenge them. "How much are you studying each week about new things that are being discovered about breast cancer and breast disease? You do not have time." Medical professionals are very caring people overall, and I am very well received by them because we are working together in partnership.

Schedule your mammogram and Pap smear around your schedule, not the facility's. The third to fifth day after you finish your period is the best time for both as that is when you have the least amount of fluid, and you get the best image. Ask to look at your X-rays. They will do this; in fact, they are anxious to please you. Demand a written report on your mammogram; your Pap only if it is irregular. If you do not understand the language ask your doctor to explain it to you.

The minute you have been diagnosed with breast cancer and get your pathology report, sit down with your oncologist or surgeon and start learning what it means. If it is broken down into bite size-pieces and is explained it becomes understandable. If your doctor sends you for a bone scan, and you are scared witless, say something to the person who is scheduling the test such as, "My physician is ordering a bone scan. I do not want to wait for the results over the weekend, nor do I want to wait a week. I am going to need to know today, or no later than tomorrow morning. When can you schedule me in order for me to get my results that quickly? I am not asking you to take me today if you cannot do that. Put me in when it is convenient for you to do that. I am not trying to be demanding; I am just saying that I have certain requirements, and we need to partner on this."

If your surgeon takes an extra twenty to thirty minutes he or she can avoid cutting nerves. By moving them and not cutting them, you can avoid having complete numbness in your arm and down your side. I am totally numb all down one side and half of my arm. I also tell newly diagnosed women to tell their surgeon they want a scar they can show someone, and say, "Dr. so-and-so did this," because you have to look at that chest the rest of your life.

You want to talk with an oncologist who treats a lot of breast cancer. You should get a second opinion, and you most definitely want a copy of your pathology report. The night before your doctor's appointment write down all your questions. Make that time count. How many of you walk out of your doctor's office and think, "Oh God. I forgot to ask . . ."

Knowledge is your greatest power. You have to be empowered to ask the questions. That is the key. If there is one thing you can do for yourself it is to understand what this disease is, and not be afraid to take charge. That is not a choice; it is mandatory. It is your body, your job. This is a scary disease—one you need to stay on top of the rest of your life. If you do not take the offensive you'll always be on the defensive.

An analogy I use when speaking to a new group is this. "One day I got invited to join a sorority I didn't want to join. The initiation was really something. Now that I am a member I do not ever want to leave. It makes me sad to see new members, and breaks my heart to lose members. It is a very strong, special sorority. One we never take for granted. Through it we have been given gifts and strengths we never knew we had."

Postscript, January 2000

I have continued my merry-go-round of activities to educate since my interview when I was a young fifty-eight. Now at sixty-one, rather than slowing down I have continued to bite off more projects and be even more zealous in my desire to reach women. Audiences include: physicians (yes, you read that right—physicians), the workplace, government and private health agencies, and community and civic groups. If there is a group get-together and I find out about it I try to get a speaking engagement.

John and I have just celebrated our fortieth wedding anniversary, and Chris and Leanne have blessed our lives with twins. After being on tamoxifen for nine and a half years I developed huge fibroids and dysplasia which resulted in emergency surgery and my having a complete hysterectomy. I am no longer on tamoxifen. I knew tamoxifen could cause these kinds of problems, and in my case it did. Other than that incident and the Type 2 diabetes I have now had for years, my overall health remains good.

My greatest achievement has been the creation of my "Beannie Boobies." They are little flannel bags filled with marbles, dried peas and lentils. I teach women with these non-threatening little bags how to do BSE. They learn through touching these lumpy, bumpy little bags that doing monthly BSE is about learning what is normal for them, so if or when there is a change in their breast tissue area they would know it. Beannie Boobies have been copied by the American Cancer Society, breast centers and other groups who teach women BSE. It has been a reward to watch women gain confidence and a healthy attitude about monthly BSE!

Seventeen

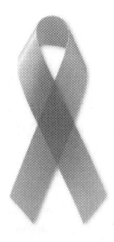

Lesley Bennett

Living with Inflammatory Breast Cancer

Survivor Profile:

Age at diagnosis: forty-nine (6/94)

Age at interview: fifty-one (9/21/96)

Type of breast cancer: inflammatory

Size of tumor: 3½ cm; stage III

No positive lymph nodes

Surgical procedure: bilateral mastectomy (one breast prophylactic)

Treatment: chemotherapy and radiation; tamoxifen until recurrence; Taxol; bone marrow transplant using stem cells followed by more radiation

Estrogen receptors: negative; Progesterone receptors: information not provided

Who's Who:

William (Bill) Bennett, her husband

Holly Dobson, her daughter (age twenty-three at time of diagnosis)

Heather Bennett, her daughter (age twenty at time of diagnosis)

Joanne Sprouse, Bill's sister

Seven friends were interviewed; to simplify, no names are being used

301

THE BEGINNING OF A LONG JOURNEY

Lesley: One morning while putting on my bra I noticed that one of my breasts was slightly red and noticeably larger than the other and thought, *How odd.* Already scheduled to see my internist in a few days I coordinated having a mammogram, so that he'd have the results by the time I saw him. The mammogram was clean; consequently, I was given antibiotics to treat the mastitis, an infection of the breast, that my doctor believed the swelling to be.

Thinking it would be a good idea to get another opinion I went to my gynecologist who was concerned enough to send me to a surgeon who *watched* it for three weeks. By now my breast was beginning to hurt, and returning to my internist I told him, "Something's wrong." He agreed, referred me to a different surgeon and within a day of that meeting I had a biopsy.

Holly, her daughter: I knew nothing until right before my mother's biopsy when my parents called saying, "Don't worry. It's not a big deal." So that's what I thought.

Heather, her daughter: Both of my parents kept telling me, "It's nothing," but when my father called I could tell from his voice that it was cancer.

HOW BAD IS INFLAMMATORY BREAST CANCER?

Lesley: To say that my husband, Bill, and I were in shock is an understatement. We both cried. Meeting with an oncologist the following day I was handed a death sentence. Worst case scenario: I had only eighteen months to live. Inflammatory is the worst kind of breast cancer to have; only 1 to 4 percent of all cases are this type. It looks like a web—stringy, and has a very high recurrence rate.

THE PROTOCOL

Lesley: Not wanting to waste any time my oncologist asked, "How soon can we can get started?" Even though it was the Fourth of July weekend in 1993, I canceled all our plans and began the first of three treatments of Adriamycin, Cytoxan and 5-FU. That would be followed by a double mastectomy; modified radical on the cancerous side, prophylactic (preventive) on the other; three more cycles of chemotherapy; and lastly six weeks of radiation to my chest wall. Heeding a friend's advice I went to a well-known cancer center only a couple of hours away for a second opinion. They, too, recommended the identical protocol adding that if I were considering reconstruction to hold off for eighteen months because of the high risk of a recurrence.

Although I was violently ill after that first treatment, each successive one became easier as my body adjusted to the drugs. Of course I lost my hair, and even though I'd walk around the house bald, not caring who saw me, in public I would wear either a scarf or wig to give the appearance of normalcy.

Bill, her husband: It was during that first meeting at the cancer center that Lesley's oncologist discussed her having a bone marrow transplant should her current treatment fail. We tape-recorded that meeting since there was so much information to absorb.

Her losing her hair made me realize the seriousness of her situation; nevertheless, I thought she looked cute. Chemotherapy was successful and Lesley proceeded with the bilateral mastectomy having chosen to remove both breasts because she was so large-breasted, and the removal of only one would have made her unbalanced.

Joanne, Bill's sister: Circumstances prevented me from lending a hand until Lesley's surgery. When Bill picked me up at the airport he forewarned me, "Don't be shocked if, when we get to the house, Lesley's walking around bald." She was, and I wasn't. My two-week stay doing whatever needed to be done helped me emotionally.

LET'S GET THROUGH THE SHOCK

Lesley: Bill has been wonderful throughout. When I was so violently ill he kept reminding me, "This is helping you. Remember, the drugs aren't poison."

When I called Texas to tell the news to my two daughters, with whom I'm very close, they went to pieces. Holly is now twenty-five and married; Heather is twenty-two and finishing up college. They wanted to come home immediately, but I asked that they wait until I was feeling better because I wanted to be able to enjoy their company. Maybe I was trying to protect them. Three weeks later they arrived. Another survivor had suggested, "Have your family pictures taken now because you never know," and I'm so glad we did even though my hair was starting to fall out.

Bill, her husband: That weekend we answered the children's many questions, and reassured them they could come home whenever they wanted to.

Holly, her daughter: It seems that our bad luck began with the fire that almost destroyed our home several months prior to my mother's diagnosis. Even though I was upset about her diagnosis, I wasn't scared because I didn't know better. I thought you just got rid of cancer and that was that—until my parents sat both my sister and me down and explained that the life expectancy with this type of cancer is only two to three years. When they played the tape they'd made at the cancer center it then became more and more horrifying to me.

Heather, her daughter: That weekend I cried a lot, and upon returning to school was torn between staying there or moving back home. Having such a fabulous support system of friends at school I decided to remain there; however, I cut my class hours so that I would have the flexibility of going home whenever I needed to.

At first I had a big problem admitting it was real. Holly, knowing how much more emotional and sensitive I am than she is, helped talk me through things. Afraid to ask my mother questions, or maybe because I thought they were stupid, I would either ask Holly or a friend whose father had gone through something similar, to explain things like: what a bone scan is; what do I expect after her first chemotherapy treatment;

how do I act when I see her bald the first time? Now I've learned the importance of asking questions, but those first few months were difficult. Whereas Holly was told everything, I wasn't, or at least not the entire truth. Finally I insisted that my mother withhold nothing even if it meant hearing, "I can't talk now because I feel sick."

To this day I won't look at her chest. Her not having breasts doesn't bother me; in fact, I agreed with her decision to remove them both. It's the scars and the way it was done.

Lesley's friends:

While reading to me one day she said, "Listen to what this book says. I'm not supposed to live beyond sixteen months." I told her it didn't matter what the book said.

Assuming a swollen breast wouldn't be breast cancer I didn't call her before the biopsy. When she called me the following morning, in tears, I cut short the conversation because I had a tennis date. The truth is, crying makes me nervous. That still doesn't ease my guilt.

I knew no one with cancer and was petrified to see her bald. Standing at her front door, heart pounding as I knocked, all I could think was, *What am I going to do when she opens the door with no hair?* I loved her bald. That's when I realized it didn't matter.

What a marvelous sense of humor Lesley has! Shortly after her hair began to fall out she visited me in California and we went shopping. When Bill picked her up at the airport she was wearing her new purchase, a hat with dreadlocks.

I had hoped never, ever to see her mastectomy scars because I was so afraid to see what they looked like. Before I knew it I was looking and feeling.

DEALING WITH A RECURRENCE

Lesley: June of the following year I was in the midst of planning Holly's wedding, was recovering from bunion surgery, and honestly believed myself cured. One night while examining my chest area, a habit I'd gotten into, I felt a tiny, pinhead-size bump on the scar line right above the skin. The next night I felt a second one. Even after being told by my doctor shortly thereafter, "I don't think they're anything," I had them biopsied. Sure enough, it had recurred. You could have blown me away. For the second time Bill and I had a meeting with an oncologist at the cancer center. That's when we decided the next logical step was a bone marrow transplant.

Before the transplant they recommended five Taxol treatments, given intravenously, over several months. Although preferring Taxol to my previous chemotherapy drugs I again lost my hair, and each time a few days afterwards, suffered flu-like symptoms. However, not only did I not have joint pain as others do, but I never needed Neupogen shots which had been necessary before to boost my blood counts. I attribute the relative ease with which I got through those months to the twice-weekly acupuncture treatments I was by then receiving. Since Bill does well as an attorney I was able to quit my job and concentrate on getting well.

Bill, her husband: Fairly certain there was still no lymph node involvement, Lesley's oncologist believed that some cancer cells had escaped into her bloodstream, hence his recommendation for a BMT. That's when it really hit us, this is real. I realized how much of a series of ups and downs cancer is. My understanding was that the Taxol would serve as a holding pattern for her until she had the BMT that was scheduled for shortly after Holly's wedding that September. Like I'd done the year before, I took Lesley for her treatments, returned to work, and then picked her up five hours later and put her to bed.

Joanne, Bill's sister: For the first time since Lesley's surgery I was visiting with her when the doctor phoned with the news that her cancer had recurred. She immediately called Bill who was home in a flash; they embraced, sobbing, while she kept repeating, "I'm so sorry."

BONE MARROW TRANSPLANT

Lesley: By enlisting the aid of my many wonderful friends my transplant now became a collaborative effort from which we all benefited. One person would coordinate the flow of visitors to the hospital; another would disperse medical information so that Bill wouldn't be bombarded with phone calls; and another would organize meals for him.

At the time of my transplant, patients were offered a choice of having either an inpatient or outpatient procedure. I chose inpatient; it felt safer. We flew the girls in for the family meeting, a mandatory meeting during which all aspects of the transplant were discussed. We had made it clear to my oncologist that the girls were to be excused when he discussed the risks, including the fact that 5 percent of those undergoing the procedure die. I did not listen when he began discussing probable complications as I wanted to maintain as positive a mental attitude as possible. Still having acupuncture treatments I additionally sought the help of a hypnotherapist hoping to cure my cancer as well as to physically prepare me for the ordeal ahead. I learned how to relax my body, and talk to my brain instructing my protectors to seek out and destroy any cancer cells encountered while leaving my intestinal tract alone. It worked because once my stem cells had been collected (a painless procedure) I had no complications from the five days of high-dose chemotherapy that bombarded my body, no mouth sores and I was barely sick to my stomach.

My friend Mary Lou, having already gone through a BMT for her breast cancer, had suggested that I bring with me soft toilet paper for the terrible diarrhea I was sure to have, and extra cotton undies and nightgowns that button down the front. I did.

Bill, her husband: Our insurance carrier declined the claim stating it was experimental treatment despite the fact that most of the renowned cancer centers disagreed. We hired an attorney who specialized in this area and we appealed, and that's when it became clear that it is all about the bottom line, not what is good for the patient. The day of her transplant we settled out of court.

During the family meeting one part of me wanted to hear everything; the other wanted to be excused along with the children. Once Lesley was admitted it made no difference emotionally whether I was home or with her at the hospital, which I was every weekend. Seeing her in such a weakened condition wasn't easy. The effort of walking only once around the nurses' station exhausted her. Some days she didn't have the energy to get out of bed; others she didn't feel like eating. To this day she doesn't remember those four to five days. That is what made me realize the seriousness of this illness she was battling.

Holly, her daughter: Just as if it were yesterday I so clearly remember hearing, "If worse comes to worse your mother can have a BMT." Heather was very up-front about not wanting to know the risks. Even though we both left the room I later listened to the tape that had been made. She didn't.

Heather, her daughter: After becoming terribly depressed, and crying continuously the week prior to my mother's BMT, I flew home and accompanied them to the hospital. Seeing where she would be and meeting the staff on her wing helped me tremendously. Once back at school I called her several times a day, afraid if I didn't something bad would happen to her. If she was unable to talk to me her friends were great at keeping me informed about her condition.

Joanne, Bill's sister: When Heather called me one evening in tears because she was having a problem coping, I told her that I was just as scared.

Lesley's friends: Never be afraid to call a friend in need because you don't know what to say. I called Lesley every day; sometimes we spoke, sometimes we didn't. It made my day when she picked up the phone and I'd hear her trademark, "Howdy."

When it became evident that her BMT would not be paid for, my husband and I decided to fund-raise. Bill's initial reaction was not to, but as time went on he changed his mind. Drawing up a list of twenty-five potential contributors we then went over the list with Bill and, with his approval, contacted them and explained the situation. It was structured so that any monies donated would be a tax deduction to the donor, and not be a tax liability to the Bennetts. Money began pouring in not only from those on the list, but others as well. Within a short period of time we had raised $150,000. When the case was settled all checks were returned along with a beautiful letter from Lesley who, at her request did not know the names of her benefactors, as well as a letter of explanation from my husband and me.

YET ANOTHER RECURRENCE

Lesley: At my three-month post BMT examination I pointed out to my oncologist two new, little bumps I had recently discovered; one on, and the other right above the scar line, but this time underneath the skin. Being uncomfortable with his, "Let's watch it," I had them biopsied. Sure enough I had recurred. It's hard to explain, but with each recurrence the devastation you feel is different, and once again I was thrown into a tailspin. On top of this, Bill had just been diagnosed with melanoma, a very serious skin cancer.

We were able to contact Holly, who was at first in shock and then kept calling asking questions, but Heather was on her way home for spring break with a friend. Thinking we'd tell her privately, Bill, who usually holds his emotions so close to the chest, blurted out the news shortly after we were all sitting together chatting in the living room. Heather just fell apart. I was so glad she had a friend she could turn to.

This time, sitting together at the cancer center overwhelmed with emotions, Bill and I waited to meet not just with my oncologist, but his. Here I was trying to support my partner, yet at the same time I was scared for myself. Not only did I wonder, *Is there any treatment left for me?* but also, *What will happen to the children?*

Bill, her husband: We had been so optimistic, and now I wondered, *Is there anymore hope?* Once again there was. Lesley was given six weeks of radiation. As for me, after the surgical removal of my two cancerous moles, I see my oncologist every three months, my dermatologist every six.

Holly, her daughter: I've never hit the wall so hard as when I got that phone call. What I hate the most is my mother's guilt, and hearing, "I'm so sorry" when she gets bad news. I'm not angry at her, but at the disease, and then feel guilty when I become angry.

Heather, her daughter: With each recurrence I've become emotionally stronger; nevertheless, I've also become more frustrated. What's been hard is seeing my mother's fear grow with each recurrence.

A friend: There was only one time I've ever heard from Lesley, "Why me?" Once composed she told me, "I'll be okay," and walking out the front door I thought, *Yes, you will.*

HOW DO MEN COPE?
AN ADULT CHILD'S PERSPECTIVE

Holly, her daughter: My father has always had difficulty expressing his emotions. His nature was to try to pretend problems didn't exist. He's become more open since my mother's BMT. Maybe he realizes that work isn't quite so important, and the "I love you's" and time together as a family are. It hurts to see him cry, but he's able to do that now with me.

It's been just as difficult on him as on my mother, but different. Had there been any more stress I truly believe he would have cracked. His saving grace was the time he had alone while my mother was in the hospital. We're very much alike in that we both conceal our feelings; therefore, I knew he was scared about both of them, and as a result Heather and I called his friends saying, "You've got to talk to him."

Heather, her daughter: I have a special bond with my father; Holly has that same bond with my mother. Because of that closeness my father could confide to me how scared he was. That's one of the reasons I wanted to go with them to the hospital. I'm able to say to him, "Cry if you need to," and even though he fights it he can. My parents are wonderfully supportive of one another; in fact, early on they made a pact that if either cried they had to tell the other why.

At first I was angry when my father was diagnosed, then the anger turned into worry. How was he going to deal with this on top of everything else? It drove me nuts when I'd ask how he was and typically hear something like this. "I'm okay, but your mom's doing great. Listen to what she went through today." Even his friends would say getting him to talk was like pulling teeth. Holly and I used to call his secretary to get the real lowdown on how he was.

HOW THE CHILDREN COPED

Holly, her daughter: I'm amazed at how I've changed. Before I was scared of bald women associating them with sick, dying people. Putting on medicine to soothe a badly burned chest would have been unthinkable. These past two and one half years have been a roller coaster; up one moment, down the next. I'm constantly playing mind games; however, my parents' openness has allowed me to be able to express my feelings. Although I think about her constantly I'm also aware there's nothing I can do to change the situation, and try not to let it ruin my day. I've learned how to deal with bad news; or at least I'm trying, but my reaction is always the same. First I'm in shock, and then I cry. Experience has taught me that if I don't cry, and keep it locked up, it's harder to deal with. It's also easier when the whole family is dealing with similar emotions at the same time. My mother may be having another recurrence now; this time in her lungs. Tests are scheduled for right before Christmas. Even though I try to pretend it's not a big deal, it is.

Getting married is supposed to be the happiest time in a girl's life, yet three weeks after I became engaged, my mother had her first recurrence. During the wedding preparations I experienced anger, worry and feelings of being cheated. *Would she even be alive to see me married?* Despite it being a beautiful wedding I was reminded constantly that life is not normal because mixed in with all the congratulations was, "How's your mom?" Even our honeymoon had a cloud hanging over it. A week after our return she was having her BMT, a procedure that could kill her.

Heather and I both feel guilty living so far from home. I'm always torn between staying where we live or moving back home with my husband Joel. I know I drive him crazy, and it's so draining. On the other hand it's easier to deal with when you can just hang up the phone and forget about it. I wish Joel knew us when we used to be a happy-go-lucky family. He probably thinks we're a bunch of crybabies, and although he's supportive and has never said to me, "Get on with your life," I bet he thinks that sometimes. There are times he wants to talk about it, but I know he won't understand because he's not in my shoes. I turn to my sister. With her I can be completely honest and know she'll be nonjudgmental. I don't have guilt telling her that I'm mad about something, and she's the same way. Although I can talk to my mother, some things I might say could unintentionally hurt her, and I don't want to do that. I suppose I should listen to the advice I recently gave a friend who's just now going through a similar situation. Being angry is normal. You can't be mad at yourself for how you feel, and you've got to stop beating yourself up for having those feelings.

Heather, her daughter: That first year, even though I'd tell myself, "Snap out it," I was unable to pull myself out of a deep depression. A doctor I'd seen at school had recognized the signs: being afraid to leave my apartment in case I missed a phone call, not caring about grades or friends, and turning to food for solace. It wasn't until after my mother's hospital admittance, when I returned to school and started taking Prozac, that my life turned around.

At times I feel as though I'm the adult, not the child. I can be weak at school, but on the phone with my parents I've often held back my tears so that I can be the strong one. My father tells me how scared he is; with my mother I often find myself saying things like, "Cry. Get it out." Then I'll call Holly and vent my emotions. We're constantly comparing notes: How did they sound? What did they say? Once I jokingly said, "I feel as though I've aged ten years in two." My mother has dealt better with my father's cancer than her own. If his had spread I don't know what we would have done.

Trying to be a normal twenty-two-year-old has not been easy because so much during the past two years has revolved around cancer. I want to talk about things other kids my age talk about like boyfriends, school, housing. What's frustrating to me is when people who haven't been through a similar situation say things like, "It's going to be okay" because they don't know that. Frankly I'd rather they say nothing. I realize people don't know how to act around me. Some have never asked me anything including how I'm doing. Others are uncomfortable complaining about everyday things because they think their problems are trivial. Others shy away from bringing up the topic of breast cancer. They need to know it's okay to do all the above.

THE JUGGLING ACT

Holly, her daughter: Holidays have become stressful. Last Thanksgiving and Christmas were understandably spent with my family. This year Joel and I had planned on spending Thanksgiving with my family, and Christmas split between his family and just the two of us. Two days before Christmas we got a command phone call, "You're coming home because this might be my last one." Needless to say we were upset. Why didn't my mother just ask us earlier? I would have understood. I do recognize that she's scared; nevertheless, even though I hope to spend many holidays together, I can't make every decision based on whether it's going to be her last this or last that.

It's not that I'm unhappy, but it seems as if I'm trying to please everyone else and don't have time to do what's right for me. I'm not even sure sometimes how I'm supposed to feel because the only person I know in the same situation is Heather. Anger and frustration turn into guilt because I'm sure I'm being selfish. Am I normal? Is this normal? When I ask these questions my therapist tells me "Yes." She also told me that I needed to go home. We did.

Heather has also been placed in this position. Although she was not planning on coming home for Thanksgiving, my mother pulled the, "What if this is my last one?" with her, so she came home. Neither of us wants to think any "what if" might be her last. Perhaps that's denial. Graduation is a few days before Christmas, and now my mother is insisting that she come home right after. Heather wants to enjoy the parties and get a chance to say good-bye to her friends. We would do anything for our mother, but sometimes she's unreasonable. Our therapist has said, "Your mother is not thinking like we would. She's almost emotionally handicapped, and you have to be sensitive to that." Caught in the middle, but even though my father might agree with us, he tends to say things like, "Do it for your mother." Sometimes the words stick in my throat, but I am able to talk to my mother, and remind her of how much Heather had sacrificed on her behalf. The end result is that Heather is coming home on Heather's terms.

Heather, her daughter: Conflicts surrounding family events were never an issue until cancer entered our lives. It would be so nice if instead of demanding by saying, "This is what I want," "I don't know how much longer I'll be alive," "This is what you're going to do," she asked. I feel as though I'm rearranging my life for her. My therapist has given me some excellent advice on how to deal with my mother such as, "I don't want you to be mad at me, but this is so important to me that it's okay if you're mad," or "I don't mind doing this, but next time don't tell me, ask." Despite my complaints to Holly or to my roommate I wouldn't change anything I've done even though I've missed out on so much during my college years. If something had happened, and I had not been there for my parents, the guilt would have been terrible.

THE BLESSINGS OF A THERAPIST

Lesley: The girls and I had been seeing the same therapist intermittently for a number of years prior to my cancer. She was the one who suggested, "Put your cancer on hold and throw yourself into the wedding." When Bill and I were both diagnosed her advice was, "Hold off telling the girls until you get more information about Bill. They're going to be overwhelmed, but remember they've gotten through it once, they'll be able to get through it again."

Heather, her daughter: My therapist was a wonderful conduit, with my permission, to get certain information back to my mother positioned so that she would understand. Not only did it help me, it helped her to understand that what I was feeling was normal.

A friend: Bill's cancer diagnosis right in the wake of Lesley's was the straw that broke the camel's back. Ten or twelve of us friends met with Lesley's therapist because we were having problems coping, and needed guidance with issues like, "What do we do?" and "How do we act?" She said, "Lesley wants you to act like this is just a normal day. Don't stay away. If you have a question, ask. If she wants to talk about it she will."

BEING MY OWN ADVOCATE

Lesley: Very quickly I learned to stand up to my doctors and ask questions. I didn't have to wait days for results on certain tests such as bone or CAT scans, and MRIs. Mary Lou taught me the importance of becoming my own advocate; how to work the system. Together we didn't feel so alone. I hope I've passed on the importance of being proactive to my children. I've told them I'm opposed to the BRCA1 and BRCA2 gene testing because not enough information is available plus if they do carry the gene they'll just live their lives in fear.

I've also learned firsthand the frustration of cancer politics. When I discovered information on the Her-2 neu oncoprotein (an overexpression of a gene present in approximately 30 percent of all breast cancers), I faxed it to Mary Lou. In addition I sent my tissues to the facility to which I'd been referred to see whether I qualified for the trial. Currently my cancer center is not participating in this trial, so they do not recommend this as a possible treatment for me.

Sometimes I was so tired of doing research that I handed the responsibility back to my doctor. That got me into serious trouble. Less than a year after my diagnosis, when my gynecologist suggested and my local oncologist agreed that I go on hormones, I did. Shortly thereafter I recurred. At the cancer center I was told, "We don't know this for a fact, but the hormones may have caused your recurrence. We feed them to breast cancer cells, and that's the only thing that gets them to grow." Needless to say I stopped taking them immediately.

ISSUES OF DEATH AND DYING

Lesley: Turning to Mary Lou when I was first diagnosed, I continued to do so until her death. Understanding perfectly my concerns, she taught me that however devastating a diagnosis or recurrence is, I could get through it. I've been determined from the onset that cancer is not going to get in the way of my life. When I recurred the first time she said to me, "Have a glass of wine tonight." When I'd blurted out, "Let me live or let me die" because I felt as though I'd been punched in the stomach after finding out I'd recurred for the second time, we talked for the first time about death and dying. Mary Lou understood when no one else could.

All of us have a tendency to procrastinate getting our affairs in order, but an excellent piece of advice given to me by my therapist was, "Get your affairs in order." I did, and that allowed me to get on with the job of living. In the beginning I talked about some of my wishes for things as well as my feelings with the children. With my second recurrence I inventoried those possessions that had either monetary or sentimental value. My grandmother had done that for me since my mother died when I was four. By my doing this the girls would have a written legacy of the heirlooms that have been in my family since the early 1800s. I have even planned my own funeral revising it each time I have had a recurrence.

Holly likes reading about near-death experiences which I can relate to because it gives an assurance of the afterlife. When Heather asks me "Why?" I have no answers for her other than to say that my system broke down. In my heart I truly believe I am cured, but my head knows otherwise. I'm somewhat prepared, but is one ever prepared? Not a day goes by that I don't think about it.

Mary Lou got tired of fighting and that was hard for me to hear because selfishly I wanted her to continue fighting. Within a week of her death I lost my twenty-seven-year-old nephew to cancer. That was so hard as they were the two people I could really talk to. When he asked me, "What do I tell my friends?" I told him that he had to take the lead and tell them he was dying because otherwise they'd be afraid to talk about it. During my last visit as he lay dying in the hospital, knowing I couldn't stay, he confided, "I'm so afraid without you." I told him, "You taught us how to live, now you're going to have to teach us to die. You're in God's arms and he's going to carry you over. Look for that light because that's what you'll see before you die, so I'm told. It's going to be wonderful, and you'll wonder why you ever wanted to stay. I'm giving you my permission to die. Don't wait for me." The day after I left he died. When my day comes I want to die at home.

Bill, her husband: I'll never forget the doctor's words, "Your life is going to change, and will never be normal again." It hasn't. That doesn't mean life has to be unpleasant, it's just different. One needs to be realistic about the situation. I've begun looking at quality rather than quantity, and wonder not *if*, but *when* it's going to come back. That's not easy to do.

Since Lesley's diagnosis my ability to concentrate has diminished because I'm always thinking about her and the future. Since my diagnosis I've become quieter and find that my thoughts tend to stray. There are times I'm depressed although I've never taken antidepressants like Lesley has. I can't remember the last time I slept through the night without tossing and turning, or waking up. I start wondering *Why?* and that's a place I don't want to go.

Holly, her daughter: Not knowing when she's going to die is the hardest part for me. Every time she has a recurrence I think, *This is the end.* Heather won't, but I've started reading books on death and dying. Because of my belief in the afterlife I know that she'll be going to a better place, but when that time does come it's not going to make it any easier for me, and it won't matter what I've read.

If the news this month is bad we'll get through it as we have before. Statistically she's beaten the odds. What an absolutely remarkable woman she is! Her attitude and faith has helped all of us. Once I overheard her on the phone telling someone she was tired of fighting and just wanted it over, yet she's never given up, and that's what gives me strength.

Heather, her daughter: My mother has been very open discussing death; in fact, she's told Holly and me that she'd like my father to remarry. We've talked about where she wants to be buried or cremated, although Holly's done most of the talking because I don't like dealing with those kinds of issues. I've wondered, *Will she see me married?* If she dies Holly and I are moving back to be near my father. We don't want him to be alone. I'm not sure my mother knows that Holly and I are aware that she wrote us letters before her BMT. In fact, I started reading one, but had to put it down because it was too upsetting; nevertheless, it gave me comfort just knowing it was there.

A friend: I've learned that it's better to stumble, but be there and be yourself. I mean, if you were to say I would *die* if that happened . . . Oh my God. I've said the "D" word!

Postscript from Bill, December 1999

Lesley passed away on July 27, 1998. She had been in the hospital for ten days with breathing complications. While there it was discovered that the cancer had spread to her brain and bones.

Her loss was a sense of emptiness, but with the support of Heather and Holly we have all grown and have learned to memorialize Lesley. She prepared me, her daughters and her friends for her death. Although it was difficult talking with Lesley about her imminent death we now thank her for it and remember those discussions often. On the anniversary of Lesley's death we invited many close friends to a memorial service. About thirty friends joined me and my daughters for prayer and testimony about the impact that Lesley left behind. The service was wonderful and a part of the closure.

I am getting remarried this February. Becky was a mutual friend of ours and attended Lesley's memorial service. The fact that Becky knew Lesley has been helpful in allowing me to freely discuss my loneliness and the sense of missing her. She has taken the position with my children of not intending to take the place of their mother, but to be their friend and be someone they can come to as a friend.

Postscript from Joanne, January 2000

I was with Lesley and her family when she died. Though I was always there to support them, it was Lesley who was always supporting us. Isn't that how it works when love is at work? Eighteen months after her death I continue to marvel at how much Lesley taught Bill, her daughters and all her friends about her death and their lives after she died. She gave many books to her family to read about death and cancer while she was living. She called many family meetings to talk about what could happen, hospice care, etc. and she expressed her wishes to her family. I was in on a number of those meetings, and they were real, painful and healing for all.

Lesley chose to live as the cancer was killing her. She never quit smiling, expressing her love and thanking each person who was assisting her when she could no longer care for all of her own needs. When she needed help getting on and off the potty beside her bed in the hospital I remember her turning to the person helping her and in the most normal manner saying to her, "Thank you for wiping my bottom."

She had a strong faith which was evident in the way that she lived. Her family grieved when she died, and they knew that it was okay to grieve because Lesley had given them permission to grieve and then to move on with their lives. And they are moving on with their lives. Holly and her husband have moved back to be near Bill, are happily settled in their new home and are expecting their first child. I know that Lesley is rejoicing somewhere about that good news. She so wanted to live to see Heather marry and to have grandchildren, though as her cancer progressed she knew that those were only wishes. Heather is also now living near her father and beginning a new job that she is excited about. The family is intact and supportive of one another.

The important thing that Lesley taught all of us was what we had always been told: Live each day and celebrate the living. Lesley lived each day; the cancer just happened to kill her body. Her spirit remains with everyone who knew her.

PART I

Anecdotal Stories of Breast Cancer Survivors and Their Families

Eighteen

Dara Kaye

One Woman's Determination to Cure Herself Using Holistic Medicine

Survivor Profile:

Age at diagnosis: forty-two (6/94)

Age at interview: forty-five (11/15/96)

Type of breast cancer: infiltrating ductal

Size tumor: 3½ cm; stage II

Positive lymph nodes: unknown

Surgical procedure: lumpectomy; mastectomy

Treatment: alternative medicine in lieu of chemotherapy or radiation

Reconstruction: no

Estrogen receptors: positive; Progesterone receptors: unknown

Who's Who:

Marlene Bjornsrud, her friend

Dana Keaton, N.M.D., her doctor

A LITTLE BACKGROUND

Dara: My parents had been in a very unhappy relationship for years, and I believe, on an unconscious level, my mother had been looking for a disease to end her life. Consequently, when she discovered a lump in her breast, even though it had become painful, not only did she ignore it, but she told no one for a year. One day she confided to me that she was in pain, but did not disclose the reason why. After I hounded her she finally confessed.

From a very early age I had been my mother's caregiver; now I became the general in her medical care and insisted that she have a biopsy. It was breast cancer, and she was stage III. At that point of my life, having only recently begun my spiritual journey, I went along with all the recommendations being made by her doctors and told my mother, "You will do everything they tell you to do." She recovered from the mastectomy, chemotherapy and radiation treatment she had, but died five years later from aplastic anemia, a suppression of the immune system, caused, I believe, by the radiation and chemotherapy she had received years earlier. Her death, and how she died has been a big influence not only in the choices I've made, but in my life as well.

I believe that the seed for my own breast cancer was planted the day my mother's surgeon said to me, "You need to know that your risk has now gone from one in eleven to one in four." At the time I was thirty-five years old.

When I was diagnosed in June of 1994 at the age of forty-two, I'd had my lump for five years. Mammograms showed only that I had dense breasts. My gynecologist, although familiar with my family history, dismissed the lump we could both feel as being nothing to be concerned about. In fact, he'd say things like, "If this were cancer you'd be dead," or "I don't think we need to do anything." At that point I had complete trust in medical professionals, and took no real responsibility for my own health because I didn't know that I needed to. It wasn't until my lump began growing and became painful that my gynecologist finally suggested that I have a biopsy.

A CONVOLUTED TURN OF EVENTS

Dara: Two months prior to the biopsy my divorce from a nineteen-year loveless marriage became final. To save my own life I had left my husband and twelve-year-old adopted daughter, who was in a treatment center for alcoholism and behavioral problems, seven months earlier. The stress had become too much. When my husband told me he had absolutely no interest in dealing with either emotional issues or spirituality I knew it was time to leave. That was a difficult decision; one I had wrestled with for a long time. My husband was very much like my father was; unable to give or receive love, emotionally cold. I left with only the clothes on my back, my antique furniture, my dog, one-quarter of the debt, and a promise that he would pay me $125 a month. Even though he is a dentist, circumstances had left us deeply in debt.

Who I was then is a world apart from who I am today. The old Dara held a very responsible job in the corporate world with excellent health insurance benefits. By the time I left my husband the new Dara had become not only a licensed massage therapist, but certified in trauma touch as well, a type of therapy in which touch releases a physical or emotional trauma held onto by the body. Insurance, which I had taken for granted, became problematic. Because I had fibrocystic breasts they were now excluded from coverage under my husband's policy.

Marlene, her friend: Dara and I have managed, in our twenty-four year friendship, to stay in touch regardless of how busy our lives are. Her telling me that she had breast cancer was the bridge that connected us on a far deeper level, and I committed to being a part of her journey wherever that led. She was the first of anyone I knew who had the big "C." Having preconceived ideas that breast cancer automatically meant mastectomy, chemotherapy and radiation, it was a huge awakening for me to hear her perspective.

HEALER, HEAL THYSELF

Dara: I knew I was a healer, and that's what my life's work was to be. This work is not just on the physical body, but on the emotional and spiritual ones as well. So when I heard I had cancer the first thing that came to mind was, *Oh, that's why you're doing this work. To heal yourself.* Yet I also knew that I would seek the assistance of others to help facilitate my healing.

My surgeon wanted me to have a mastectomy, chemotherapy and radiation. Even though I felt panic I still had the presence of mind to tell him that I needed some time to think things through. Too often women find themselves in the position of not being given an opportunity to evaluate their options. An example of this was my ex-sister-in-law who had her biopsy on a Friday and a mastectomy the following Monday. Intuitively I knew that conventional medicine was not the path I would follow.

Marlene, her friend: In typical Dara fashion she threw herself into researching every alternative avenue there was, and she began sharing with me what she was reading and who she was talking to. My turning point came when she said to me one day, "I'm not dying of cancer, I'm living with cancer" because I had wrongly assumed that cancer was a death sentence. How profound that simple statement was. That's when I committed to assisting with her fund-raising endeavors.

Around this time Dara, my roommate and I and another friend went out to lunch. We'd not shared much time together recently as a foursome because one friend lived out of state. As we talked about Dara's situation a heaviness fell over me, and excusing myself I literally ran to the bathroom, bursting into tears before I even reached it. When I returned to the table my friends were also in tears. Dara was deep in conversation with my roommate and I overheard, "I worry about how Marlene's handling this. What is she going to do without you?" Dara was amazing as she reassured not only them, but me, "It's okay. You need to grieve. Get it out, and walk away from today feeling life." She allowed the three of us to cry together in the middle of a busy restaurant. Those were the early days of my journey with Dara; days of feeling and having to deal with emotions of grief and death.

IN SEARCH OF A CURE

Dara: Having literally gone from riches to rags my challenge became one of creating the funds in order to treat my disease with nontraditional medicine. Many people I approached for financial assistance thought I was nuts for not having the lump removed, but I felt strongly that I had to follow a different path. Deepak Chopra had a week-long program I was interested in: an Ayurvedic approach which emphasized cleansing the body of all toxins by working on the mind/body/soul connection using many modalities including foods such as rice and beans, yoga and massage therapy. Much of the work focused on how powerful the mind is. What it creates, it can uncreate.

Perhaps I was guided there not so much for the program itself, but to meet the psychologist in charge of the program who, to this day, has been responsible for the focus of my journey by asking me two key questions: "Do you really love yourself?" and "Do you really want to live?" At the time I really had no answer to either one of those questions. Part of me felt as though it would be a good opportunity to die, but by the time I left there I had made the decision to proceed with the lumpectomy.

BUCKING THE SYSTEM

Dara: My doctor, who happened to be chief of surgery at a very large hospital, was still trying to persuade me to have a mastectomy. Refusing not only that, but a lymph node dissection as well, he proceeded, that October, to remove 9 cm of tissue, about the size of an orange, even though the tumor was only 3½ cm, half dollar size. That left me with almost no breast. When the pathology report came back the margins weren't clear, and once again he urged me to have a mastectomy, which I'd almost had anyway, chemotherapy and radiation because the tumor was attached to my chest wall.

To please him I met with a radiation oncologist. Sitting in her waiting room in total fear as I watched the parade of gray-colored people streaming in and out, the memory of my mother's experience came rushing back. Every fiber of my being wanted to run as fast and far away as I could, but I managed to contain my fear and met with the oncologist who was a very caring person. Once discovering that I had no insurance she offered to treat me for free—something she had done only once before in her ten years of practice. Knowing my choices were not coming from a logical place, but believing that it made no sense to "cure the cancer" by tearing down the immune system, my decision was made. I was not proceeding with conventional medicine and would continue my search for alternative therapies.

WORKING WITH A
NATUROPATHIC PHYSICIAN

Dara: Research had shown me that my body could heal itself, but I knew that I needed a professional to be my quarterback because I was almost on overload from all the information being thrown at me, conventional and holistic. I wanted a plan to build my immune system, and Dr. Dana Keaton seemed to be the right person; a naturopathic physician who, during our initial fact-finding meeting, delved not only into what was going on in my physical body, but in my emotional and spiritual self as well. For the first time it felt as though someone were paying attention to me. Our work began as a team effort, and has continued as such ever since. Even though we didn't always agree on treatment, and there were times she'd say to me, "I probably would not do that if I were you," she'd add, "but I'm hearing you and if that's what you want to do, okay." That was the kind of thing that made me feel so responsible for myself.

It is important to recognize that a disease is not only a physical problem, but an emotional one as well and that needs to be dealt with. Fear, which is always present, must be addressed, but so, too, does the *why* of it happening in the first place. Only then can one begin creating a new lifestyle for oneself. Dealing with my emotions has been the toughest part to change, and Dana has offered gentle reminders to help me look at that aspect. She asked, "What's going on emotionally?" "How are you handling this or that?" or "How do you feel about how you're handling it?"

Dr. Dana Keaton: Allopathic (conventional) practitioners believe cancer is a local disorder; holistic practitioners believe it is a systemic disorder. This is one of the main differences between the two, and both sides will state this clearly. I'm thinking, *This person has cancer;* they're thinking, *There's a cancer that needs to be removed.*

My approach is that the whole system has to be shifted, that the whole body needs to be treated. When you treat cancer locally all you do is chase it around the body until the person dies. I've seen it time and time again. There will always be people who choose to have their cancer treated in this fashion, but they should at least know that will be the pattern until they change what's happening in the body. There are ways to accomplish that, and they should know they have a choice for either method.

Mine is a general practice, and I work with many breast cancer patients in all stages of their disease. Many, who have not yet decided on a course of treatment, will come to me for a consultation to discuss what their options are. When patients are afraid they have a difficult time making reasonable choices, and too often their medical doctors do not give them a chance to think through their options. If I feel their judgment is clouded, I might suggest they postpone having a procedure done, even surgery, for a week or two to give them the time they need to really think things through. If they do have cancer it is already there, and a week or two will not make any difference. Once they get past the fear then they can get down to the basics, and get to the core of what is going on. I have lost patients who want me to make decisions for them, but I will not do that. It is their cancer experience not mine.

No two patients are treated alike. The closest I have come to a standard treatment is to almost always give a patient acupuncture after every chemotherapy treatment, and then rotate and prescribe several herb formulas for them. Even that will vary depending on what their constitution was before they began treatment. Allopathic doctors do not know how beneficial acupuncture is for those undergoing chemotherapy. Patients feel great afterwards, their white counts are not dropping and their hair is not falling out. It is the same thing with herbs. We know which herbs will not only enhance the chemotherapy, but circumvent the side effects. The trick is, we do not want to negate the effects of the chemotherapy because if they are going to take it they want it to do what it is supposed to do. We know what alternative therapies can make chemotherapy and radiation more effective, and at the same time spare the immune system. The information is readily available; they just have not taken the time to learn it. That is why it is so important to see some-one, like a naturopathic physician, who is trained in this area.

BACK TO FUND-RAISING

Dara: Having heard about the Hippocrates Health Institute, Marlene and I talked about ways of fund-raising to get me there. By October of 1995 the monies had been raised, and I was able to enroll in their three-week program. Their philosophy is that cancer is caused by what you eat, the environment and toxic relationships. Anything toxic needs to be removed from the body. Food is living; therefore, when you ingest liv-ing food, which they consider to be raw foods, you're ingesting life. That is what will heal you. Disease comes into the body as a result of blocked *chi* (energy); consequently, you need to remove the blockage, and cleanse the body which is done through the use of things such as wheat grass, enemas and high power enzymes.

The belief is that all the nutrition a body needs can be obtained from raw foods. I stopped taking vitamins and everything else I was doing and I began a regimen of eating 80 percent raw (vegetables), and 20 percent cooked (grains and some vegetables) foods. Although I had been a vege-tarian before going to Hippocrates Health Institute, I'm now vegan. I eat no dairy; nothing with a face. Those three short weeks made a major dif-ference in my life, and even though I do not adhere as strictly to their diet as I did when I was there, I will eat like this for the rest of my life.

Marlene, her friend: During the fund-raising for Dara, some people who had been in our lives for years pulled away because they thought she was making bad choices. They felt that she should have gone the conventional route. I understand that people approach things from different perspectives, and it was okay that they did not want to con-tribute, but to not be a part of her life because they disagreed with her choices was so disappointing to me.

AM I HAVING A RECURRENCE?

Dara: In February 1996 the lump had returned and felt really solid. Having made up my mind to have a mastectomy I returned to my surgeon. Because the tumor was attached to my chest wall he first wanted to shrink it using chemotherapy and radiation. We discussed my having a biopsy, but he was fairly certain it was cancer. Even though I was leaning towards having the biopsy I had to listen to that inner voice, *This is not what I want to do. What other alternative is there for me?* Several weeks later, after notifying my surgeon's office that I was not going to proceed with any treatment, I received a certified letter dismissing me from his practice.

In the meantime I had gone to see Dana, and in a panic said to her, "Oh my God. What are we going to do now?" As we had in the past we continued building my immune system. Still wrestling with one of those core issues, "Did I want to live, or did I want to die?" I thought I might find my answer in Mexico at one of those clinics that specialized in holistic therapies such as laetrile, and ozone therapy. Dana thought it also a good idea as several of her patients had gotten good results when they had gone. The fund-raising which had been successful in the past was not this time. Obviously I was not supposed to go there. What money that was raised has allowed me to do the therapy I am now doing.

Dr. Dana Keaton: I would have liked Dara to have had the biopsy as that would have confirmed whether or not the cancer had recurred, but since she had no insurance her funds were limited. Her choice then became: Does she spend the majority of what money she did have on surgery, or use it to treat the disease? As opposed to doing nothing she is treating herself as though she had gotten a positive diagnosis, and is quite comfortable with her decision not to have the biopsy. She is not overwhelmed by what she is doing; in fact, she has incorporated it into her life. Her biggest problem is money. If I knew for sure that she had cancer I might push her to try some of the newer treatments but they are costly. Her lymph nodes, which I continually monitor, are not enlarged which leads me to believe that whatever she is doing is effective and working. What I do not know is, is she doing enough? That is something I cannot know until the person dies from something else.

WHERE DO I GO FROM HERE?

Dara: Six months later I made a powerful choice: I am going to live. Now I was ready to deal with the emotional aspects of cancer: Why did I have it, and what emotionally caused it to happen? I now realize that those two questions I was asked earlier in my diagnosis, "Do you want to live?" and "Do you love yourself?" are an ongoing process. As you go through life's experiences the levels become deeper, and I am constantly having to answer those questions because that's part of what life is.

Determined to delve into whatever it was that I was holding onto, I began talk therapy to help me deal with self-worth issues which included ending a relationship with a man I had been involved with during the past eight months, as well as polarity therapy to find out what this lump is. It keeps recurring; therefore, it must be trying to tell me something. I needed to not just hear, but feel what the core issue of this cancer was. Somewhat like trauma touch, the work I had been doing, polarity therapy is also a type of bodywork therapy which incorporates several techniques, such as deep tissue massage, a rocking motion type of massage, light touch aura energy work and counseling. Its premise is that everything is made up of energy including disease and tumors which create blockages in the body. Little did I know how life-altering this work was going to be for me.

Letting go of the man I had been involved with empowered me to release what my parents, especially my mother, had taught me to be: a woman who gave herself away, allowed others to drain her energies and loved everyone except herself. I immersed myself into a lifetime of emotional pain, of being caregiver and nurturer. This time, instead of just knowing these things intellectually, I was able to feel them. The pain was deep in my heart, which is why the cancer was attached to my chest wall—the heart chakra. I would go into my separate sessions and weep.

I believe that my tumor was made up of energy and represented the many emotions of anger, hurt, distress, sadness, grief, everything I'd experienced and carried my entire lifetime. Think about it. Cancer is something that was eating me, and all those emotions were eating me up.

Around the third polarity therapy session my therapist carefully began to work on the tumor that, by now, had become achingly painful. In retrospect I know that part of the pain was related to the relationship I had just ended. Recently she told me, "I don't think there's anything in your breast; it's all soft now." What I feel, instead of a hard, massive tumor about the size of a plum, is a sponginess, and an area in the middle I believe to be old scar tissue. Perhaps what I am feeling is only the residue of fear remaining from the surgery. I believe a miracle happened. Since that time I have had very little pain other than around my period.

Trusting that this is what I am supposed to be doing right now, I have given my body to the universe. Whatever happens, happens. The work we continue to do has enabled me to get in touch with the essence of who I am. I have learned to appreciate that little girl who needs to be loved and nurtured.

When I was at Hippocrates Health Institute I had asked why they thought there was a breast cancer epidemic. This is what they had to say. "It is because of the relationships between men and women. Women have taken a subservient role for generations. They have been taught that they are supposed to take care of the man, and they are still playing that role today in many areas. Some men feel as though they are superior to women, and that attitude is clearly reflected in how they treat women. That is why there is all this resistance to women who are trying to better themselves and become equal. Furthermore, this attitude, which has been passed from generation to generation, is totally dysfunctional, and is creating disharmony between them. Only when there is harmony, instead of resistance and irritation, can healing then take place, and women will no longer have to grieve. Men need to honor women." What I have found so interesting is that so many breast lumps are on the females' left side, a physical response to what is going on emotionally.

WHAT IF MY CANCER RETURNS?

Dara: If my cancer recurs I am still not going to do traditional medicine. At least that is how I feel now. I have told my Higher Power if I die because of my decision, so be it. Hospitals, doctors, drugs, cutting and burning are not a part of who I am. To me they represent forms of torture, the taking away of your life force. However, just because conventional medicine is not my choice does not mean it is not right for someone else. I know many women who have chosen that route and have lived a full life and that is fine. It is just not how I choose to live mine.

I have not handled my cancer as most do; not just in terms of my choices, but in how I have dealt with it emotionally. Conventional medicine does not deal with the emotional aspect, and I knew that was what I needed to do in order to facilitate my healing. It has now been about two and a half years, and I am finally able to resolve many of the core issues about my cancer, the care taking, and putting myself second. Guess what I have given up for Lent for the rest of my life? Care taking! What an interesting time I have had getting to know who I am. All choices now have to be for my highest good, not someone else's. What good does it do to keep the body alive if you are not growing? What is the point of it?

Marlene, her friend: At first I was angry with God when Dara told me her cancer might have recurred. Why did he let this happen? It seemed like she was choosing the right course. Wondering sometimes what it meant that the cancer was back, I would answer, "I don't know." Was I looking for a miracle? Was I buying into the same old story where if we do all the right things then a miracle will happen? Through Dara, as well as other things in my life, I have learned that is not necessarily how life works. The miracle, if you want to call it that, is in accepting whatever comes your way every day. Going with it, and staying very much alive in your spirit and in your soul. Never, for one moment, have I felt that she has chosen the wrong path.

NOT AFRAID TO DIE

Dara: Because of the healing journey I've been on since my breast cancer diagnosis, and the fact that my daughter has been so messed up, we only see one another every couple of months. She is now sixteen and has turned her life around somewhat. When I was diagnosed I did tell her, and I think she had a lot of fear. My ex-husband has also been diagnosed with cancer: pancreatic and liver, and she is pretty much in denial about both of us having cancer, and acts like nothing is going on. It is as if she believes if she ignores it, it will not be real. Neither she nor her dad deal very well with emotions. One time she called and wanted to get together because as she told me, "I'm going to feel guilty if you die, and I don't have any type of relationship with you." The concept of motherhood has always been an issue with me. Even though I have incredible nurturing qualities I never wanted to be a mother.

Since my diagnosis my mother has come to me on four or five different occasions asking that I join her, wherever that might be. I've not had a near-death experience in terms of almost dying; nevertheless, I did experience hers. As I awakened to the sound of her death rattle, while lying in the bed next to hers in the hospital, I looked over and saw her spirit sit up in her body, and motion to me. Joining her we walked through the tunnel towards the bright light. It was exactly as I have heard it described. I know that I am walking her into her transition to the next life. A benevolent being was waiting for her as we approached the end of the tunnel. Like in real life my mother said to me, "I want you to come with me; I'm not going to let you go." As I gently removed one hand from her shoulder, and released my other hand from hers I said, "Mom, it's not my time. I can't go with you," and turning around walked back down the tunnel. Re-entering my body I looked at hers lying in the hospital bed. All that remained was the shell.

We lived such an entangled life. Hers was one of prejudice, rigidity and religion; consequently, her love for me was always conditional. In order for her to love me I had to perform, be the physician, do this, do that. It was hard for me to love myself because I was always criticized and could never live up to my mother's expectations. I believe she died so that I could live, be reborn and be who I am.

One evening during a group meditation, I was given an extraordinary gift. The Angel of Death brought my mother back to me, one last time, so that I could hold her. For the first time her love was given to me unconditionally. That was the start of my deep, deep healing.

Marlene, her friend: Some might say that Dara's choice of believing she doesn't have cancer is denial. I don't think so. That's the mystery of it, and I've learned to accept mystery and say, "I don't know." I no longer need black and white answers which is something new for me. People have to make their own choice, and then own it. Once they do, it is the right choice because it is theirs. I have watched Dara thrive in her life, in her choices, in her health. Watched her approach every day with this new sense of adventure. She has chosen to learn how to live again. She wants to know herself, not through the eyes of the evangelical church, nor through the eyes of anything but through her own soul. Because of that she can now delve into life, and not be afraid of death. She has accepted that fact, and knows that the finish line is there somewhere; therefore, she looks at life differently. Being a part of Dara's journey has been very life-giving for me in that I have been a student in the process rather than a rescuer or teacher. Dara has become the teacher because she has experienced life on a deeper level, and has so much to share. I hope if that day ever comes for me people will say to me, "I will be here for you, and I want to be a part of the process." I cannot imagine that she will ever die. Her life has such purpose. I see real life in her whereas others, with perfectly healthy bodies, have no life in their souls. So I no longer grieve.

A HIGHER POWER

Dara: I think there's an overall picture, and I have to trust that God, Higher Power, whatever you want to call "God" has this thing all laid out. I also believe that your contract is negotiable, but then Higher Power already knew that. I gave up the God of my childhood because that was a very judgmental, critical, harsh, condemning God. What I have developed is a relationship with a Higher Power, with spirit, and it takes on different forms. Sometimes it is a he/she; other times Mother Earth. Most often I use the term Higher Power or Source because I feel that is what universe is to me—a source I can draw from, very deeply.

All I ever heard growing up was that I had to have a personal relationship with God, and I had no concept what that meant. Now it just is. The closer I get to myself the closer I get to my Higher Power. I have done a lot of Higher Power work, and I see the power of a source in me constantly working—the healer. I was raised in a religion where you could not heal yourself. Now I can because God has given me that gift.

I can draw upon any abundance of the universe that I need, be it financial, friends, healing, whatever.

My mission in life is to bring people into the reality of their own soul. Soul is who we are throughout all of lifetime. I help them to stand up for themselves, and allow them to face who they are. I do that all the time. When I'm asked how I meditate I say, "My life is a meditation." At my core I'm a very spiritual being. It's how I live my life. Cancer has only brought me deeper into that journey, and made me deal with some of the things I needed to deal with.

Postscript, December 1999

In December of 1997 I had a recurrence and made the decision to have a mastectomy. The morning of surgery I instructed my surgeon he was *not* to remove my lymph nodes. I followed up with alternative medications and healing modalities instead of the chemotherapy and radiation treatment my doctor urged me to have.

It came to me after I lost my breast that I was "mal-nurtured." I had spent my entire life giving myself away to other people. Isn't that what we as women are taught to do? Now I am learning a new skill, and it is a learned skill, to love, nurture and appreciate myself in many creative ways. I have found that receiving is just as much fun as giving. I love to be loved!

In October of 1998 I met Mikhael, my beloved. Our decision to move to Sedona, Arizona, away from the stress, pollution and frenetic activity of a large city, was due in part to my health. We decided that I would take a year off from any work to heal my body completely. I found that the attention to my body finally allowed the myriad of deep emotions to surface that I had not allowed during the previous five years of my cancer journey. I believe that releasing the old emotional issues held in my body was and is paramount to the healing of my body.

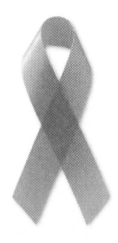

Nineteen

Cindy Shoenhair

I Have Breast Cancer
and Four Young Children

Survivor Profile:

Age at diagnosis: thirty-five (12/26/95)

Age at interview: thirty-six (7/25/96)

Type of breast cancer: infiltrating ductal and intraductal (ductal carcinoma in-situ, DCIS)

Size tumor: total size 8½ cm: 4½ cm infiltrating ductal and 4 cm intraductal (DCIS)

Five positive lymph nodes; stage III

Surgical procedure: bilateral mastectomy, one breast prophylactic

Treatment: chemotherapy as part of protocol for bone marrow transplant (using stem cells), radiation, tamoxifen

Reconstruction: no

Estrogen receptors: positive; Progesterone receptors: negative

Who's Who:

Dan Shoenhair, her husband

Judy Calvert, her mother

Jim Calvert, her father

Jordan Shoenhair, her son (age eight at time of diagnosis)

Isaac (Ike) Shoenhair, her son (age four at time of diagnosis)
Samantha and Abby Shoenhair, daughters (age two at time of
   diagnosis, not interviewed)
Cherith Bevers, her friend

A GOOD SWIFT KICK

Cindy: Abby, one of my two-year-old twins, kicked me in the chest while we were fooling around. At first I thought it was a bruise, but the swelling didn't go down and it hurt. When I went to my obstetrician/gynecologist three weeks later to have it checked out she suggested that I have a mammogram. I did—plus an ultrasound. She disagreed with the radiologist's findings which showed the swelling to be consistent with a bruise and sent me to a surgeon. He didn't think it was a bruise either and told me, "The only way to be sure is to do a biopsy." He was not concerned with the cyst I'd had in my other breast for years, but said he would biopsy it too just to be safe.

Dan, her husband: If Cindy had a lump it was not evident. However, after being kicked it went from nonexistent to the size of a ping-pong ball within a few days. That's why we thought it was a bruise. I was not concerned, but Cindy did harbor some fear and had a bad feeling about it although she did not share those concerns with me until after the mammogram. Thank God her doctor followed her instincts because we were that close to ignoring it.

IT'S SHOW TIME

Cindy: My surgeon had originally planned on doing a frozen section in which a piece of the lump would be sent to pathology for evaluation. I found out later he suspected I had breast cancer. Because of that he decided to do a needle biopsy. It would be less invasive, and he didn't want to disturb what was there. Within five minutes he received a call from pathology. His hunch was correct. My "bruise" was both infiltrating and intraductal (in-situ) cancer. I really expected it to be nothing. I was a healthy, thirty-five-year-old who had just been kicked really hard.

Two days later Dan and I returned to the surgeon's office to discuss my options. Now we wanted to know, "What do we do about it?" He recommended a bilateral mastectomy even though I had cancer in only one breast. His reasons were: my age, the fact that the lump had not shown on either the mammogram or ultrasound, and the possibility that in the future I might develop cancer in the other breast. Once I heard the diagnosis I just wanted the tumor out of my body. I liked my breasts but they certainly were not worth dying over. What my doctor said made sense; consequently, I did not get a second opinion. Surgery was scheduled for the following day. He thought the tumor was about 2½ cm.

Dan, her husband: Finding out that Cindy had cancer is something I will never, ever forget. Never have I felt like that before. It was surreal. Everything went into suspended animation. Nothing her doctor might have said would have mattered because at the time I am sure I was white as a ghost. When I went to see Cindy in the recovery room the first words out of her mouth were, "I am so sorry." As if it were her fault! I have a vivid image in my mind of me standing in the hallway of the hospital in front of a large picture window holding my cellular phone. I absolutely *had* to talk to someone. I called my sister. When I heard her voice I completely broke down and began to sob uncontrollably.

During the drive home with Cindy my fears ran rampant. *What am I going to do if she dies? I am not all that cut out to be a single father.* I could not control my thoughts about me! Later that day I told her, "Please. Take them both off. Just get the cancer out of your body." We were both on the same wave length, "Let's go after this as aggressively as we can." I then became focused. "What's the next step? What do we need to do?"

COPING

Dan, her husband: Cindy was scared. I felt so helpless. What was I supposed to say to her? What was I supposed to do? How could I help her? I just wanted to make her feel better. We had a debate about when to tell her parents. Her father, Jim had suffered a cardiac arrest several months earlier. The doctors worked for forty-five minutes to resuscitate him and a week later, when he was strong enough, he had bypass surgery.

Cindy wanted to tell her parents, but every time she picked up the phone to call she began to cry. I was the one who told them. She was on the other extension.

Judy, her mother: It was two days after Christmas, 1995, when they called. Cindy began to cry, "I'm so sorry." I asked her, "What are you sorry for? It's not your fault." I think she was apologizing for adding another crisis to our lives. Even then she was more concerned for us than for herself.

Jim, her father: When Dan told us I almost began to cry. "How can this be?" Cindy is our oldest. The boys are thirty-four and thirty-three; Jenny is twenty-eight.

So, Then What Happened?

Cindy: I was in the hospital for two days and felt a lot better than I had been led to believe I would. My surgeon had done a modified radical mastectomy on the breast with cancer; a total on the other. Other than the bandage being wrapped so tightly around me that I thought my ribs would break the surgery was a piece of cake. I was in surprisingly little pain, and other than being a little stiff the next morning I was able to lift my arms over my head and comb my hair. I have been athletic my entire life. I'm an exercise physiologist—a person who practices the application of exercise for health. I work at a community college where I teach health, wellness and physical education. Because of my profession I was very concerned about residual effects from the surgery. I repeatedly asked, "Are you going to cut any muscle?" He did not; however, he did cut some nerves. As a result I have numb spots on my elbow and numbness underneath my arm. For the most part it doesn't bother me.

Dan, her husband: I realized Cindy was probably self-conscious about her scars, and I didn't want to make her uncomfortable by asking to see them. Besides, scars make me a little queasy. So it was okay that it took about a week for her to show me. What bothered me was her not letting me help clean the drains. I felt she was being overly cautious with me.

Judy, her mother: Three days after hearing the news Jim and I were on a plane. Both of us had made arrangements with our employers to once again take an extended leave of absence. The first time was because of Jim's heart attack. When we arrived Cindy was already in the hospital. Jim and I had to shift into our parenting role as we now had four little ones to take care of. Jordan was eight, Ike five, and Samantha and Abby two. Once we got into a routine we were fine. When I became stressed Jim would say to me, "Why don't you go outside? I'll take care of . . ."

This was a very difficult time for Dan. Both of his parents are dead, and his only family is his sister. He didn't want to burden us as he felt we had enough to deal with, so he really had no one to help him through this. Consequently, he was short-tempered with the children. Cindy is very strong and very stubborn. She definitely has a first-born child personality—always looking out for every one. When I suggested she lie down she would say to me, "No. I'm fine. You do too much." I am sure she thought she was shirking her responsibility.

THE SHOE DROPS

Cindy: Five out of twenty-one lymph nodes were positive. I knew it was better to have none positive, but I wasn't quite sure what that meant. My surgeon positioned it as though it were not the end of the world, "It could be better; it could be worse." He referred me to an oncologist.

Shortly after my surgery I met Elaine Packwood, a Reach for Recovery volunteer. It felt really good to be able to talk with someone whom I thought was at least in my situation *[see chapter 8]*. I had no interest, nor did it make me feel better, talking to a woman who had had a small lump and chose lumpectomy as her treatment. People do not realize there are variations of breast cancer.

Dan, her husband: It was about a week before we received the pathology report. I almost passed out in the doctor's office that day. He did not say, "This is really bad. There is a decent chance; in fact, it is very, very likely that Cindy is not going to make it." Rather, he implied it. He went back and forth, more or less creeping up to the seriousness of Cindy's situation. "The tumor is 4½ cm." He then told us about the kind of cancer she had. Then he went back to the size, "And you also had an additional 4 cm of tissue that was involved, so the total size is

8½ cm." *[Author's note: for reference 1 inch = approximately 2½ cm.]* "You might want to consider doing a bone marrow transplant." He would then talk about some other aspect of the report working back to, "Maybe you need to think about a BMT." As he talked I felt the blood drain from my body. To me a BMT meant a person was in *really* bad shape. *How do I get to the sink that's on the opposite side of the examination table Cindy's lying on if I need to get there quickly?* I wondered. I spotted a chair in the corner near where I stood and collapsed onto it. In answer to her surgeon's, "Are you okay?" I definitely was not.

Oddly enough Cindy and I did not take negatively what the doctor told us. Rather our thoughts were more, *How do we make the most of the time she has left?* Cindy kicked into high gear and began to research her options. She wanted to know everything whereas my mind shut down and was telling me, "You need to take this a little bit a time." As a result Cindy fed me information in small pieces. Otherwise I would have gone on overload. I thought what I saw on television was real life. I quickly learned it was not. As a result I was left without a base and did not know how to deal with issues. I felt ungrounded.

At work I told only a few people about Cindy. It was the one place I could escape to where I had "Dan time" to try to come to terms with this nightmare that engulfed us. That was healthy for me. I talked with my sister and in-laws, and I have some close friends who were there if I needed them, but Cindy was the one I talked to the most. She cried; I cried; we cried together.

CLINICAL TRIALS

Cindy: I was referred to an oncologist who recommended that I do Adriamycin and Cytoxan. The only other treatment available to me, according to him, was a randomized trial that combined Taxol with those two drugs. His opinion about a well-known cancer center only two hours away was, "They are not going to tell you anything I'm not." I wondered, *How can my options be so limited? There has to be a more aggressive treatment.* That is when I began to search the Internet to learn as much as I could.

My research concerning BMT was fairly clear. I was in the gray zone. Chemotherapy is standard treatment for a person with three or less positive lymph nodes. Ten plus positive lymph nodes almost always qualifies a person for either a transplant or admittance into a study. The problem with being in a study is not having control over which arm of the study you will be assigned to. I wanted a guarantee that I would get the most aggressive treatment.

When I went to a local well-known medical facility I was the one who had to bring up the subject of BMT. They were just starting to do them. I then made an appointment at the cancer center which I had been told would be a waste of my time. They were in the midst of doing a pilot study for a clinical trial which included BMT. After meeting both the medical director and the transplant doctor I was told, "You are eligible if you are interested." This trial offered me the guarantees I was looking for. Its purpose was to either discredit or support BMT, and had been ongoing for the past two and a half years at eight different university sites across the country.

Dan, her husband: I don't know how we got through this period of time. We were repeatedly being told, "Get your affairs in order. Your wife is probably going to die." Cindy and I talked late at night after the children were in bed and told one another how scared we were. By the time we went to the cancer center I was sick and tired of hearing the same pessimistic prognosis. And then . . . someone finally offered us hope.

Cherith, her friend: I met Cindy through work and we became close friends. She became pregnant with Jordan; then six months later I became pregnant. It was difficult for both of us when I moved. Cindy isn't the type who gets close to a lot of people. By the time she called to tell me the news she had already had surgery, gotten her pathology report and was knee-deep in research. Cindy is very analytical whereas I am a combination of being both analytical and emotional. That is probably why we are such good friends. In typical Cindy fashion she said to me, "Sit down. I have something to tell you." She did not cry, but I knew she was devastated. I was numb. *How can she have cancer? She takes such incredibly good care of her body!* This was a very frustrating time for Cindy because she wanted answers and there were none.

DECISIONS, DECISIONS

Cindy: Without having a BMT my chance of recurrence was 60 percent. With it, the doctors at the cancer center felt the chances decreased to 20 to 30 percent. The risks were numerous, including a 5 percent chance of dying and long-term damage to the heart, lungs and kidneys, but Dan and I felt the benefits outweighed the risks. Finally someone was willing to step out on a ledge and take a risk. "Yes, we can help you. Maybe even cure you." They could not offer me a guarantee, but this was certainly better than anything else I had been offered.

Dan, her husband: Cindy and I were trying to figure out logistically how to temporarily move the family to be near the hospital. I was worried about that and also whether this transplant would be covered by my insurance since it was considered experimental treatment. The company I work for is large and self-insured. After I spoke with the head of human resources about our situation he twisted a few arms and told our insurance company to pay the claim. They did.

I promised Jim and Judy I would keep them apprised of what was going on. Cindy tried to protect them; therefore, her information, although truthful, was always slightly slanted. For instance, she might leave out the part about how severe her cancer was. She did not give them specifics about her survival nor did she tell them the size of the tumor for quite some time. After awhile I began to feel like the Prophet of Doom because I had to tell them all the negatives. It took a little effort to get Judy to back Cindy's decision to have the BMT. That added stress to our already stressful lives. Jim's attitude all along was, "Do what you have to do."

Judy, her mother: I was not in favor of Cindy having a BMT. About a year earlier I had seen a TV special about BMT. The women being interviewed looked like death. Most said they wished they had not done it. I said to Cindy, "Why put yourself through something so risky if you don't know whether it will help you?" She continued to send us information, and the more we read and talked to people the more comfortable we were with her decision to do it.

Jim and I told them we would come back out when she had the

transplant. That helped give her peace of mind concerning the children. Cindy asked if I wanted to stay with her in the hospital. I told her I am a person who does better cooking and cleaning. That is just my personality. It is also a good way for me to get rid of my anxiety.

Cherith, her friend: Dan talked to me openly as did Cindy about what was going on. I never gave Cindy advice. I listened. She was waiting to click with the right person, and the moment she went to the cancer center she knew: "This is it." I could tell that night she was at peace.

GETTING THE SHOW ON THE ROAD

Cindy: I passed the battery of tests that were a prerequisite for being admitted to the trial. All blood draws and chemotherapy would be done through the Hickman catheter. That required another surgery. I went back to the first oncologist I'd seen. When I told him about the study I was enrolled in he agreed to administer the drugs in accordance with the guidelines of the protocol: four cycles, every three weeks of Adriamycin and double the standard dose of Cytoxan.

I was hardly sick, had no side effects other than losing my hair and I missed only two days of work each cycle. Two days after a treatment the tiredness hit me, but it lasted only a week. Then I would be fine until the next cycle. Dan gave me shots of Neupogen (white cell growth factor) ten to fifteen days every cycle because my white blood counts dropped so low. It was not surprising that I lost ten pounds since I am not a food lover under normal circumstances. Dan took over the cooking, a chore he was no stranger to. That made him feel useful.

Clinically I think my oncologist was top notch. Personally I think he is mean spirited, depressing and a jerk. I always felt his attitude was, "I'll treat you, but why are you bothering? You are almost dead anyway." From the beginning I felt there was an underlying anger on his part toward me. Was he angry because I had found information he was unaware of, at a place he told me would be a waste of my time going to? He never offered encouragement, only worst-case scenarios. "You have done okay so far, but you could still get an infection." The final straw was when he said to me during my last cycle knowing full well I was having a transplant,

"People that have those transplants die sooner than those who do not." I vowed never to step foot in that office again, and I have not.

HOW DID THE CHILDREN COPE? AN ADULT'S PERSPECTIVE

Cindy: We tried to explain to Jordan that I had bad cells growing in my breast and I had to have an operation to get rid of them. Dan and I also explained why I was being given chemotherapy. He was old enough to understand a lot of what we told him. It upset him when I did not feel well, but he's a tough child and seemed to accept it. Ike understood only a little and also seemed to accept things pretty well although he will still say to me, "I wish you didn't get it." I tell him, "Me, too." The girls were too young. Or so I thought.

There are no secrets in our house. Children always know. Besides, keeping something a secret just makes them think it is worse than it is. We told Jordan, "If you have any questions ask us, and we'll answer as well as we can." I told Jordan's teachers at school about me. Ike was in the preschool that was part of the college where I teach so they already knew. I was really worried when my hair began to fall out because that was the first physical sign that something was wrong. Jordan wanted to shave his head, Ike initially cried, "Mom, I want your hair back," and the girls laughed hysterically. "Mommy's hair fall down. Mommy go buy new hair." I felt better once I saw that they were taking it in stride.

Dan, her husband: Cindy and I were very careful not to give Jordan any guarantees that his mother was going to live because we did not want to get caught in a situation where promises were not kept. We were very clear when he asked, "Do you think Mom is going to be okay?" and told him we did not know. He insists we told him that she was going to be okay. I suppose that is how he coped. For the longest time he could not understand the difference between cancer and the common cold. He thought cancer was short term: take some medicine and it goes away. Ike might not understand why, but he knew if his brother was upset something was wrong. So if Jordan was upset, Ike would be upset.

I believe that Cindy and I did a good job telling the children what was going on. I admit I made some personal mistakes with the children in terms of my behavior. For instance, shortly after Cindy's surgery she and I were sitting on the couch. Jordan almost jumped on her trying to give her a kiss. Without thinking I grabbed him by the shoulders and threw him across the room. Those are the things I can never forget nor change. Jordan has never said a word about that incident, but he is a child who never forgets anything. Additionally I made sharp comments to him that were well beyond what they needed to be. I have always been short-tempered and fairly strict with the children; however, I realize there needs to be some balance.

Judy, her mother: Ike concerned me the most because he holds things inside. One day he blurted out, "Mom is going to die." I told him she was not and it started. "Yes she is." "No she's not." Until finally he said, "Yes she is. I know she is. You die when you get that." I told Cindy what had transpired. He had never said anything like that to her, but apparently it was on his mind. Jordan would ask Cindy and me questions, but Ike didn't really understand even though we tried to tell him.

Jim, her father: It was hard for the children to realize that their mom couldn't do and be the same as she was before because of the surgery. They would say to her, "Show me," but of course she couldn't do that. That made it harder for them to understand.

FROM THE MOUTHS OF BABES

Jordan, her son: Mom just told us, "I have breast cancer." Then she hugged me, and I felt better. I asked, "Why did you get it?" but they did not have an answer. I did not really understand what Dad told me. I asked him if Mom was going to die. He told me no, but I was still afraid she would. I talked to my grandparents, my parents, friends and teachers about being afraid.

Usually I am a very good worker at school. My teachers asked me why I was not working like I normally do, so I told them how I felt and that I was unhappy. They understood and told me it was okay that I was not working so hard, and they made sure I was doing all right. Sometimes my teacher would tell me to sit in the back of the class so I could think about my mom if I wanted to and kind of deal with it. There were times it was easier talking to them than to my parents. I told my friends about my mom, but they didn't want to know what breast cancer was. Only one friend, who is twelve, understood because his mom had it, too. He made me feel better when he told me, "My mom can run five miles now." I did not want to tell kids I did not know that well.

Ike, her son: I told my friends about Mom. I was afraid she was going to die.

BONE MARROW TRANSPLANT

Cindy: At the mandatory family meeting my doctor laid out all the risks. This was the time for Dan and me to ask any questions we had. That was a good meeting because it put things into perspective. One of the questions I asked was, "If I get past five years, am I cured?" He said, "With some cancers, yes. Not with breast cancer. It could come back in twenty years. However, the farther out from diagnosis you are the better." There was never another negative word said after that meeting.

Once again I was given a battery of tests. Dan laughed at me because I was sure that every ache and pain I had was cancer. I passed with flying colors. Then it began. The first step was the removal of about six ounces of my bone marrow's stem cells which was done over a three-day period. It was painless. The stem cells were then frozen until they would be transplanted back into my body through the Hickman catheter.

The following week I checked into the hospital and almost panicked when I walked into my ten foot by twenty foot room. *How am I going to stand being cooped up for so long?* I wondered. For three continuous days I was given chemotherapy, twenty-four hours a day. I was fine the first day and a half; then, I passed out from one of the drugs that was apparently alcohol based. I also became badly nauseated. At first I resisted taking any medication because to me not being alert and in control was almost worse than the vomiting and nausea I was experiencing. I finally compromised, and after having an allergic reaction to Compazine, by which I became flushed and my heart began to race, I began to take Ativan which kept the nausea and vomiting at a semi-tolerable level. I never developed a fever nor did I need to take antibiotics. That was almost unheard of.

On days five, six and seven I was given back my stem cells. This, too, was part of the protocol. Normally they're given back in one day. The procedure took only a half hour a day and was no big deal. About a week later my counts bottomed out. This is the time when a person develops the worst side effects. Other than being bone tired the only condition I developed was mucousitis, in which the mucus membranes peel off from the nose down through the digestive tract into the intestines. I was lucky. It was only in my throat; however, it was *so* painful I lay in bed whimpering and crying like a baby. Dan kept saying, "Take the Demerol." Finally I stopped being so stubborn. The pain was just too great. It disappeared three to four days later when my counts began to come up.

Ten days after my stem cells were transplanted I moved into an apartment near the hospital. I was euphoric. How wonderful to feel the sun and the breeze on my face! Five days later I asked my doctor, 'When can I go home?'" He looked at my chart, at his watch, at me, and said, "Now." Twenty-two days after I had checked into the hospital I went home. I was ecstatic. The worst was over.

Dan, her husband: The hospital does not encourage overnight guests; however, neither do they forbid it. I was not going to push my luck by asking for a cot to sleep on. I made do sleeping on the window seat that was much shorter than my five-ten frame. I have always been a guy who enjoys my sleep. Not these two weeks! Besides sweating during the night I had to peel myself off the plastic cushions when I would turn over. But I told Cindy I could not have stayed home if my life depended on it. Cherith came down the third week.

Cherith, her friend: When I walked into the bone marrow ward that first day every nurse gave me a look of absolute, complete sympathy. Then Dan walked out of her room. "Boy, did you pick *the* worst day." Cindy was bald and curled into a fetal position on her bed and in extraordinary pain. I wanted to hold her. Instead I just said "Hi" and gave her a hug. This is a woman who had been in fabulous physical condition. Now she could barely walk one mile, sometimes twice a day, in the halls. Two days later she began to rally, and in typical Cindy fashion pushed herself too hard and was exhausted the next day. I tried to treat Cindy as I normally would—not as a sick person. When we checked into the apartment I was a nervous wreck driving her back and forth to the hospital so that she could be monitored and get whatever blood products she needed. *What if I get into an accident? Her immune system is wiped out.*

Jordan, her son: Dad told us what was going to happen to Mom when she was in the hospital. The first time I saw her was scary. There was a big bag of orange stuff hooked up to a big machine and tubes were going into Mom. She told me they were platelets to help her get better. I did not want to leave when it was time to go home. I was glad my grandparents stayed with us, but it would have been helpful if my parents had left a list of what they usually did with us kids.

COPING DURING AND AFTER A BONE MARROW TRANSPLANT

Cindy: I had decided from the beginning that I was going to be up-front with everyone I worked with. That has been helpful to them and to me. Because of my attitude no one feels uncomfortable talking to me. My bosses have allowed me to rearrange my schedule until I am able to come back to work full-time. Dan's boss has been equally great: "I'll pay for any kind of treatment, anywhere. Take off as much time as you need." Dan has been marvelous. He has taken over all the household responsibilities although I have begun to help out. He'll say to me, "You need to rest. You can't do so much or you'll be dead." I think he needs a break. So do I. We have grown closer. The children understand when I do not feel well and do not try to make me feel bad by saying things like, "You never do this anymore." When my daughters see me lying on the couch they cover me with a blanket. Now, Dan's first words to my parents when he calls them are, "Everything is fine."

For me the treatment was and is my focus as I am only partway through radiation which is the last part of the protocol. The only way I am able to cope is to take it one day at a time. What has been frustrating for me is trying to explain to people that there is nothing wrong with my bone marrow. They think I had the transplant *because* I had cancer in my bone marrow. I have to explain that the drugs I was given killed my bone marrow along with whatever cancer might have still been in my body at the time. That is a difficult concept for them to grasp.

Dan, her husband: Cindy and I explained to the children that we thought the BMT would be the thing to help her get better, and also told them she would be gone a long time and would not feel well for awhile. We assured them that they could visit their mother in the hospital. They seem to have sailed through this thing pretty well. Cindy, on the other hand, has some mixed emotions about being home. Happy obviously, but a little worried that the children might be a drain on her because our children are high-demand kids and demand most of the attention from their mother. This has not changed that. I believe she is less patient than she was, but that is because she does not feel well. My in-laws seem more at peace now with the treatment Cindy had, and Cindy and I have grown closer together. Oddly enough this experience was healthy for me because it became apparent to me how much Cindy counts on me, and the fact that I am an important part of her life.

I was not resentful she was getting most of the attention, and I was not happy that I had to take over all the household responsibilities, but I sure did not blame her for that. If anything I probably blame the kids for making most of the work. They make messes faster than I can clean them up! I suppose I have been resentful about that, and I have been more angry and short-tempered than normal. This has been the most grueling, difficult situation I have ever been in. Knowing what I know now, I do not think I would have the strength to go through it again. It is no wonder I have not been in a good mood these past few months. I have never been at such a low point. I used to like playing golf, and I love woodworking. Now I couldn't care less. I do not enjoy anything. Work is no longer a safe haven because there have been changes there so I have no place to escape to although things are easing somewhat at home. I am not taking care of myself physically. Nothing makes me happy. Nothing pleases me. Right now my attitude about everything, including God, is crummy. I am just a mess.

Judy, her mother: Taking care of the children was physically demanding on Jim and me. I am fifty-seven, he's a year older. The girls and I went to see Cindy once while she was in the hospital. Cindy needed to see her girls. She looked better than I thought she would although she had not yet gone through the worst. Samantha and Abby stood shyly outside her door until they saw her. Then they wanted to jump on her bed. They did get to snuggle with their mom. When it was time to go home I do not know who it was more difficult for—Cindy or the girls. I knew when she was coming home and scrubbed and sterilized the house until my hands were raw. We had just finished eating supper when I heard their car pull up in the driveway. Suddenly from behind we heard, "Hello girls." Momma was home. The girls squealed with excitement.

Jim, her father: Every night Cindy called at 6:30 to talk to the children. When the boys and I saw her the first time we visited my heart stopped. She looked as though she had come out of the death camps in Germany. The boys were also shocked. Cindy took charge. "Well, come here. Let me show you all my medicines and machines." Just as the girls did, the boys also got to snuggle with their mother. So did her dad. Ike began to cry when it came time to leave. I am sure both boys wondered as did I, *Will we ever see her again?*

Cherith, her friend: I stayed with Cindy during her transplant because she asked me to. I really respect her for asking. I know she would do the same for me.

IS IT OVER?

Cindy: I have only been home from the hospital a month. I am constantly washing my hands as I was told that is how germs are spread. I probably make the children wash their hands more frequently than I used to. They used to eat off my fork, drink from my cup, kiss me on the lips. I no longer allow them to do that because all of my immunities have been wiped out. In about a year I will begin to be re-immunized.

Radiation will be over in four weeks. So far, other than being tired, it's been a piece of cake; three one-minute blasts. I am used to being on the go constantly and it has been an adjustment not being able to do that. My muscle strength is greatly diminished, and it takes two hands to lift a gallon container of water. I have no appetite, and Dan is always after me to eat. My doctor tells me I will probably be taking tamoxifen for the rest of my life despite the findings that women should only take it for five years. He seems to feel that the two weeks of constant, excruciating headaches I suffered from were tamoxifen related. They are, according to the *Physicians Desk Reference,* which is a major pharmaceutical book that among other things lists all the side effects known about every drug. But I wonder, *Could they have been allergy or sinus related?* I don't know. As suddenly as they appeared they disappeared. I am no longer having periods, and I do have concerns about osteoporosis, although tamoxifen is somewhat protective of that.

Dan, her husband *[Author's note: Dan's interview was conducted six weeks after Cindy's interview]:* The radiation, which Cindy just completed, was more difficult than I anticipated. The fatigue was almost imperceptible and tore her down a little bit at a time. I never told her how worried I was, and the problem seems to have corrected itself, but for about three weeks she was having trouble carrying on any conversation and she began to get terrible headaches. Cindy just locked up, and I was beginning to wonder whether she had lost part of her brain function. When she wrote her master's thesis she did it in one draft. She composed it in her head, put it on paper and then made only a few corrections. She is that bright. That is why both of us were so worried. To this day she worries a little that she does not have all her brain capacity back, and says she does not remember things as well. I expected some physical inabilities, but not these kinds of things. For the most part she is flowing through this with ease as compared to the difficulties most people encounter. Even now I cannot grasp how difficult things are for her because she takes things in stride so well.

Cherith, her friend: I think Cindy has a little anger over losing about a third the capacity of her heart and lungs from all the treatment. She once said to me, "If I had not been so active my entire life, I probably would not even realize how crummy I feel." Not being able to get back into top peak performance is her fear. She thinks that just because treatment is over she should be able to do everything.

Cindy is not the same Cindy she was before this happened. I cannot quite put my finger on the change, but psychologically there is something that is different about her. Before getting cancer she probably would have said about almost anything, "Everything is fine." Now she is a little more willing to express her frustrations. I think she is tired of acting perky and cheery at work. That Ph.D. she wanted more to fulfill her own potential than to use for a job does not seem so important anymore. Now she wants to live life more than strive toward a goal.

DOING ALL THE RIGHT STUFF

Cindy: My breasts were constantly lumpy because of being pregnant and nursing babies. Although I did breast self-examination I couldn't possibly know my breasts because they were in constant change. The tumor was not so much a lump as it was a thicker spot. It did not really feel what I would imagine a lump to feel like.

I did not know my family history until several years after my diagnosis when one of my relatives sent me a family tree which showed how prevalent breast cancer is in our family. My mother's father had four sisters, two of whom had breast cancer. One of them had it twice. Once in 1973 in one breast; then in 1990 in the other. In 1987 she was diagnosed with ovarian cancer. She is still alive. One of my mother's two sisters was diagnosed twenty-two years ago at the age of twenty-eight. She is doing well. Several days before my diagnosis my mother's first cousin died from breast cancer. And there is also breast cancer on my father's side. He had an aunt who was diagnosed in her early twenties. Thirty years later she developed a secondary lung cancer which the doctors directly attributed to the radiation she had been given thirty years earlier for her breast cancer.

Judy, her mother: When Cindy first told me she had cancer I felt guilty. "This isn't right. It should be me." I would have switched places with her in a second. I am concerned about my daughter, Jenny although she is now being monitored closely. We know for a fact that our family carries the breast cancer gene because during a family reunion, which neither I nor the girls were able to attend, everyone was tested. When Cindy called the university that did the testing she was only told, "We recommend that those who were not tested be tested."

Cindy of course has concerns about her girls. Two problems I see with the testing are: insurance discrimination needs to be addressed, but even more disturbing, "What do I do if I do have the gene?"

THE CHILDREN'S REMAINING FEARS

Cindy: The children still ask, "Can you die?" I tell them, "Yes I can, but I don't think I'm going to." I never tell them I cannot die from breast cancer, but I also remind them why I took all the drugs. I always answer their questions as honestly as I can. Every once in a while a fear will surface. For instance, Jordan said to me one day, "If you ever get cancer again I bet you're going to die." All I could say was, "I hope I never get it again." Then he was fine and went outside to play. Another time he came home from school and said, "So-and-so's mother had breast cancer. Their dad had throat cancer." I replied, "A lot of people have cancer." I think kids talk among themselves. Samantha seems to have been affected the most. Every day she asks, "Why go hospital? I miss you." If she cannot find me in the house she becomes very upset. I do not even like to tell her I have a doctor's appointment because she panics.

Dan, her husband: Samantha has only recently stopped asking her mother about the hospital. If Abby took it hard I cannot tell.

Judy, her mother: Even though Cindy tried to prepare the children for her hospital stay Ike was convinced she was going to die. He came back smiling after he went to see her, but he still had fears. I do not think either boy will ever forget this period of their lives.

MY THOUGHTS

Cindy: I do not understand why a person does not do the most aggressive treatment to begin with. My opinion is, "Hit it as hard as you can while you're healthy." For me BMT can be a cure. I could have taken the easy road, but I did not. Too often I have met someone in a similar situation to mine who had completely different treatment because they were unaware of their options. Some oncologist had told them, "This is what you should do," and they did not question it. I felt there had to be more available than what I was being told, so I just kept looking. But I had to find it. I followed my instincts and did what I thought was right for me, not what some doctor told me was right for me. I will never be haunted thinking I could have done more.

DEATH AND DYING

Cindy: The doctors told us my father would either die or be a vegetable. They were wrong. That is what helped me through my ordeal. I will not say that I did not take my situation seriously; however, I realize that no one can predict with certainty how any one person is going to do.

I had recurring nightmares about the cancer returning when I got home from my transplant. Even though the nightmares have diminished they come back full force when it is time for my tests. I will always have a little fear that I can die from my cancer, but I have made the decision that it will not rule or ruin my life. I choose to make it a manageable part of my life.

Dan, her husband: Sometimes denial is a good thing when it comes to the topic of dying. I can vouch for that. When either Cindy or I hit a low point, we talk, which allows us to get it out of our system. Thankfully we have always hit that point at different times. We have not talked about it a lot lately. Should we? I suppose a person can over-analyze things!

Judy, her mother: My daughter is the most stubborn and has the most fight of all my children. It is a terrible thing to have to think about, but I was so worried that if the cancer were to take her life she would fight it to the very end and suffer horribly because she would not give up. I never really understood the pain a parent feels over the loss or serious illness of a child until it happened to me. For now I am optimistic about her future.

Jim, her father: Maybe Cindy will live another twenty-five years; maybe she will get only five. Who knows? I have no control over that. I prayed while she was going through treatment and I continue to pray. It is very stressful because the fear does not go away. I know two things.

My daughter will do anything she can to survive. The other is, there are no guarantees in life.

Jordan, their son: Kids need to know that it is okay to think about what their mom is going through. I pictured how it was going to be when it was all over. Now I am no longer afraid my mom is going to die.

Cherith, her friend: One of the most difficult things for me was being able to separate my needs from Cindy's needs. I needed to talk to her about my fears, "What if you die?" I needed to tell her how much I loved her. That was not what Cindy needed. She was sleeping the morning I left to go home. I wrote her a letter. In it I told her how I felt. That, I think, was more comfortable for her.

REFLECTIONS

Cindy: Dan and I have always had a good marriage and good jobs. We have four healthy children. We floated through life with no problems until I got breast cancer. I believe things happen for a reason. In the past an event I thought was rotten actually was good because it set into motion something else that would be terrific. I feel that way about this experience. Something really good is going to come of it. Maybe it is the fact that now students and people I work with come up to me and say, "I have a lump in my breast." I have become the expert. What a great example I can be if I remain healthy, particularly since my breast cancer was so advanced. No one should ever think it is too late, so why bother. I say—NEVER GIVE UP!

Dan, her husband: There is no single way to go through something like this. Nor is there a single answer or a single path that anyone of great wisdom can provide. People have to find their own path. They have to match the potential solution to their makeup: what fits them, their personality, their marriage, their spouse. The significant others need to look hard at how to be supportive. They need to put aside their own concerns and worries because the first priority, as in my case, was to make sure that Cindy's mental attitude was strong enough to fight this thing properly. You can deal with the other stuff later. That is the stage we are almost at now.

Cherith, her friend: When Cindy had a miscarriage years ago Dan told her something that Cindy shared with me which has stayed with me even to this day. "I am so sick and tired of everybody asking how you are doing. Not one person has asked me how I am doing. I lost a baby, too." That reminds me to be sensitive to Dan's needs. He is going through this, too.

Postscript, December 1999

My life has been blessedly wonderful since you interviewed me in 1996. Each year I undergo the gamut of tests and return to the cancer center for a thorough checkup. This week marks the four-year anniversary of my initial diagnosis. Thankfully I can report that I have remained healthy with no evidence of cancer. It took almost two years after my treatment to regain my full strength, but now I have more energy than I ever had. I remain on tamoxifen, but that is the only medication I take. I have not experienced any real side effects other than those in the beginning as my body adjusted to the drug.

Dan and I continue to be thankful for our life together and will celebrate our twentieth wedding anniversary in the year 2000. Our four children have grown, and the twins started kindergarten this year. Samantha tells everyone, "I saved my mommy's life." Jordan chose my having had breast cancer as the topic for a fifth-grade life event paper he had to write last year. As careful as Dan and I were to not make promises we couldn't keep he wrote, "My Mom promised me she would not die." I am still saddened by the impact this ordeal has had on my family and the loss of innocence my children have experienced at such a young age.

As for me, I have come to appreciate that facing and overcoming the fears and struggles that accompanied my diagnosis and treatment ultimately blessed and enriched my life in a way I could never have imagined. I have gained so much more than I lost. On behalf of all survivors, thanks for sharing our stories with the world.

Happy

I know it's the way she'd want me to be,
Without her here it's so hard for me.
I see the tragedy but mask the pain,
As I sit alone and wait in vain.
Wait to live or wait to die,
I often sit alone and cry.
My life is something I try not to waste,
But things are so hard in such a scary place.
Pain is something I know well,
I hide it well so it doesn't show.
I'm always told not to cry,
If I didn't then my life would be a lie.
I express through being me,
Why don't they know, why won't they see?
All I want is to be with my mom,
To play the piano or write a song.
Just to be with her is all I need
To be under a tree and just sit and read.
My life now will never be complete,
Not a night, day, when I sleep nor eat.
She was always the greatest friend,
It's not fair that it had to end.
Mentor, mother, friend and all,
She was always there to never let me fall.
I was happy when she was here,

Now she's gone and life's unclear.
Why touch and why see?
Who is "you" and who is "me"?
And of all the things that I could be,
I only wish that I were free.
Happy is how she'd want me to be,
It's just so hard without her here with me.

—Noelle Dupont, *(daughter of Wendy Dupont)*
[See Chapter 3]
Age 15, October 31, 1998
Wendy died September 2, 1997.

PART II

How Close Are We to a Cure?

Patricia A. Ganz, M.D.

Director, Division of Cancer Prevention and Control Research,
UCLA's Jonsson Comprehensive Cancer Center

INTRODUCTION

Cancer will soon become the number-one cause of death among the U.S. population surpassing cardiovascular disease and stroke. This has occurred because of the important decline in the incidence (number of new cases) of cardiovascular disease during the past three decades, as well as advances in the treatment of people who develop serious and potentially fatal heart disease. The major decline in death from cardiovascular disease is attributed primarily to the prevention of disease through the control of well-defined risk factors, especially lifestyle changes (diet, exercise, tobacco control) and medications (e.g., blood pressure medications, cholesterol-lowering drugs, and drugs that prevent blood clotting). As a result, fewer people are developing heart disease and if they do, these same strategies are effective for secondary prevention of complications and death from the disease.

With fewer people dying from cardiovascular disease, life expectancy has increased significantly, and we are seeing an expansion of the oldest segments of the population (greater than eighty years). As the Baby Boom generation passes into the Medicare years, we will see an increasing number of new cancer cases, simply because of the increasing number of older individuals. More than half of all cancers now occur in people over age sixty-five years, and as the population continues to age, a disproportionate number of cancers will occur in the older age population. Breast cancer accounts for about one third of all the cancers that occur in women, and currently about half of all breast cancers occur in women over age sixty. Because of the expanding elderly population, we are likely to see an absolute increase in the number of new breast cancer cases each year.

Why does cancer strike the elderly disproportionately? Cancer, in general, is the result of what we call "gene-environment interactions" over a lifetime. That is to say that the genetic material or DNA in the cells of our body are there to regulate and control the growth of our cells, so that we can repair injury to a cell (e.g., healing of a wound), but not have an overgrowth of cells (e.g., a keloid scar). As we live our everyday lives, our cells are continuously being bombarded with environmental exposures (e.g., ultraviolet rays from sunlight, minimal radiation from airplane travel or dental X-rays) or our body's own hormones (e.g., monthly menstrual cycles), that stimulate or injure the DNA and mark it in such a way that the injured cell has a growth advantage over its neighbors. We call these changes in the DNA "mutations," and it may take as many as five or six mutations in a single cell before it begins growing out of control and is the first cell of a malignant tumor. It may take many more years thereafter, depending on how fast that single cell can grow and divide, to have a tumor that can either be seen on a mammogram or be detected on clinical examination. In any case, the generation of the first cancer cell occurs over a very long period of time. As you can now expect, the longer one lives, the longer one has had to be exposed to various internal or external factors that can cause mutations and ultimately cancer.

While all cancer is genetic, and the result of acquired mutations, only a small number of cancer cases can be attributed to inherited genetic mutations that can be passed on by either a mother or father to a daughter or son. It is estimated that only about 5 to 10 percent of breast cancer cases are the result of an inherited genetic mutation in either the BRCA1 or BRCA2 genes (BRCA; Breast Cancer Gene #1 and Gene #2). Individuals who have inherited either of these genes carry this mutation in all of the cells of their body, and they need to acquire the additional mutations from exposures over the lifetime to ultimately develop a cancer. That is why we can find individuals who are gene carriers for these mutations who have lived into later life without developing cancer—they have not acquired the other necessary mutations to produce a cancer cell. Nevertheless, BRCA1 and BRCA2 mutation carriers may pass the single gene mutation on to their offspring, even if they did not develop the disease (a good example of this is men, who may never develop a cancer but still pass on the susceptibility to the disease to their daughters).

Now the title of this chapter is How Close Are We to a Cure? This provocative question suggests that the major way we will defeat breast cancer is through "a cure" or several cures. We are fortunate in that cancer, unlike heart disease, diabetes, arthritis or many other chronic diseases can, in fact, be cured when diagnosed. When detected very early, breast cancer and many other cancers are cured, because they have not had time to spread outside the initial location of the tumor to other parts of the body, or because they are very susceptible to specific treatments (e.g., chemotherapy or radiation). However, the breast cancer may come back in the future, because a small number of cells may have broken off from the breast tumor long before it was detected and removed. These silent metastatic cells can lie dormant for years, when by chance, they are stimulated to start growing again and will begin to cause symptoms in a distant organ (e.g., liver, lung, bones). Although adjuvant therapy after breast cancer surgery is aimed at eliminating these cells in the months and years following diagnosis, our current therapies are still inadequate. Therefore, while we can expect to see advances on the treatment front for breast cancer (to follow), some of the biggest gains against this disease may lie in prevention and early detection, just like the story for cardiovascular disease.

In this chapter, I will spend time discussing the variability of breast cancer behavior, the role of hormones and other factors that put women at risk for the disease, how we learn whether treatments are effective, some information about "breakthroughs" and incremental advances, and finally what the future may have in store. The areas of breast cancer prevention and treatment are in constant flux, and our strategies are in constant evolution. Thus, whatever would be written here could easily become out of date between the time of this writing and the book's publication. Therefore, I will focus on general principles with examples, rather than catalog all that is known or will soon be available.

BREAST CANCER
IS A CAPRICIOUS DISEASE

Just as two women may have entirely different reactions to the diagnosis of breast cancer, tumors that look very similar to the pathologist while viewed under the microscope can have extremely divergent clinical behaviors. Factors such as tumor size, the histologic grade (how well- or poorly-behaved the tumor cells look under the microscope), and the number of lymph nodes under the arm that contain tumor, are all critical prognostic variables for breast cancer treatment outcome and survival. Nevertheless, most breast cancer clinicians have seen patients with extensive disease at diagnosis who experience long-term disease-free survival, and rare patients with small tumors who succumb to the disease in less than two years. How can this be?

There are many other factors that can influence the patient's outcome, including her age, menopausal status, the hormone receptor status of the tumor, the presence or absence of overexpression of the Her-2-neu oncoprotein, and others.

For example, the hormone receptor characteristics of the tumor are important in determining prognosis as well as the type of treatment after breast cancer. The majority of breast cancers contain hormone receptors for estrogen and progesterone. These receptors determine whether these two important hormones can get into the cancer cell and stimulate its growth. (Normal breast cells also contain these receptors, but in lower quantity). When these receptors are present in a tumor, it means the tumor is better behaved, and usually slower growing, leading to a better overall prognosis independent of the size and extent of nodal involvement. In addition, when these receptors are present in a tumor, it means that the drug tamoxifen will usually be prescribed to prevent a breast cancer recurrence. As for Her-2-neu oncoprotein, this is a growth receptor protein on the surface of some breast cancer cells (it is increased in about 25 percent of newly diagnosed breast tumors), that when increased in those cells, leads to very rapid growth of the cancer. Those women whose tumors over-express Her-2-neu have a significantly poorer prognosis and are generally given more intensive treatments after diagnosis. Experimental studies are underway to see if use of an anti-body to the Her-2-neu protein can decrease the risk of breast cancer recurrence when given soon after diagnosis.

Thus, the patient and her treating physicians will have a lot of additional information on which to make treatment and prognostic decisions. Even so, the influence of all these factors working together in an individual patient is unique, and clinicians are hard pressed to provide any assurance about an individual patient's prognosis. Instead, we can provide general statistical information about women who are like the patient, based on summaries from research studies that have been done. This kind of information will always be a best guess. On the horizon however, are specialized tests associated with "chip technology" (use of a computer microchip to detect specific genes), in which individual tumors can be analyzed to determine which genes are turned on in the tumor and what the likely outcome will be with a specific pattern of genetic mutations. This will permit individualized treatment and eliminate the over- or under-treatment of individual women, as well as lead to more targeted therapies against specific proteins that are causing the cancer's growth.

Overall, though, the outlook for women diagnosed with breast cancer today is better than ever, with women with very small tumors (less than a centimeter in size) likely to have a normal life span that is unaffected by a breast cancer diagnosis. With increasing tumor size and extent of nodal involvement, the likelihood of long-term survival declines, but remains in excess of 75 percent of women at five years after diagnosis. While there can always be improvements in our current treatments, substantial advances have been made in the past two decades through the systematic use of adjuvant hormonal and chemotherapies which are given after surgical treatment. These treatments have reduced the likelihood of breast cancer recurrence by as much as 40 percent in some groups of women, and have improved overall survival as well.

THE BIOLOGY OF BREAST CANCER

Although the specific cause(s) of breast cancer are not known, a large body of evidence implicates the role of female reproductive hormones (estrogen and progesterone coming from the ovary) in the development of breast cancer. For example, a woman who has her ovaries removed in her early twenties will essentially eliminate her risk of getting breast cancer. Although such an extreme intervention would not be recommended for breast cancer prevention in the general population, some current experimental treatments are looking at reversible ways to suppress the production of ovarian hormones in young women at very high risk for breast cancer (breast cancer gene carriers) to see if this can decrease the risk of breast cancer. Other evidence for the involvement of reproductive hormones in the development of breast cancer include an increased breast cancer risk with a longer number of years of menstruation, an increased risk of breast cancer with the long-term use of replacement hormones after the menopause, and an increased risk of breast cancer associated with lifetime weight gain (a postmenopausal woman's fat converts adrenal gland hormones to estrogen).

The common final pathway among these risk factors is repeated and continuous exposure of the breast tissue to the stimulatory effects of estrogen and progesterone. On a monthly basis, in menstruating women, the breast tissue is bombarded by these hormones that stimulate the breast cells to grow and divide, preparing the breast for the remote possibility of a pregnancy. Since for most women pregnancy will occur two or three times (at most) over her lifetime, each month the cycle repeats itself without interruption. It is during the premenopausal years of life that most breast cancers are initiated (the first mutations and cellular growth advantages occur); however, these can only be sustained and nourished by continued availability of estrogen from internal sources (ovaries, fat tissue) or from hormone replacement therapy given at the menopause. Other known environmental exposures may rarely initiate breast cancer—an example being low-dose radiation to the breast during the second and third decades of life. While the search goes on for environmental carcinogens that can explain the risk for breast cancer, all of them will probably still require the ongoing stimulation of the breast tissue by female hormones as a cofactor.

So, if the major risk factor for breast cancer is just being a woman, how can we develop strategies to prevent it, or reduce the risk of getting breast cancer? There are a number of options to consider. First, although we cannot precisely predict or control the age at which menstruation starts, it is strongly affected by body weight and nutrition. Thus, the epidemic of childhood obesity (and associated lack of exercise) has gradually lowered the age at which menstruation starts, and thus the number of years the breasts are exposed to reproductive hormones. Increasing exercise and decreasing weight gain in young girls could substantially delay this process. Another known risk factor for breast cancer is delayed onset of childbearing. While we would not want to advocate teenage pregnancy, some would advocate considering of ways to enable women to have children at an earlier age, while still providing them with an opportunity for education and satisfying careers. Often, a first pregnancy is now postponed into the mid- to late thirties, leading to subtle increases in the risk of breast cancer among women in Western industrialized countries.

Other modifiable lifestyle factors that are associated with breast cancer risk include alcohol consumption, lifetime weight gain and regular exercise. Daily alcohol consumption is associated with an increased risk of breast cancer, probably through an increase in available estrogen in the body. Weight gain over the lifetime leads to excess body fat tissue, and the increased availability of internal sources of estrogen, especially in the postmenopausal years. Related to this is the protective effect of regular exercise, which probably reduces blood levels of estrogen in premenopausal women and also contributes to the prevention of weight gain over the lifetime.

The decision to use hormone replacement therapy (HRT) at the menopause is complex, and is influenced by a variety of factors including a woman's level of menopausal symptoms, as well as her perceived risk of other health threats such as heart disease and osteoporosis. In the near future, we will have definitive information on the cardiovascular disease prevention benefits of HRT coming from the Women's Health Initiative study. Estrogen can definitely stave off bone loss in postmenopausal women, however, not all women are equally at risk for this problem. Increasingly, we have become aware of the risks of long-term HRT with regard to breast cancer risk. In order to avoid this risk, some women may choose to take HRT for a short time while they are symptomatic (one to two years), and use other medications to lower their risk of osteoporosis and heart disease over the long term. Better information on the true risks and benefits of HRT will be available when the Women's Health Initiative Trials are completed, expected around 2004.

One of the most exciting findings of the past few years has been the result of the Breast Cancer Prevention Trial—a study which included over thirteen thousand healthy women aged thirty-five years and older who were at a very high risk of getting breast cancer based on their family history of breast cancer or an abnormal breast biopsy with pre-cancerous findings. This study tested whether the breast cancer fighting drug tamoxifen, a medication that has anti-estrogen properties in the breast, could decrease the risk of getting breast cancer. Half of the women were given the active medication and the other half were given a placebo (an inert pill). As was hypothesized in the design of the study, there was almost a 50 percent reduction in the risk of developing breast cancer in the women given tamoxifen. The reduction in risk was even greater in the women with precancerous changes in the breast! Thus, there is now a medication option for prevention of breast cancer in some high-risk women. These results further support the critical role estrogen plays in the development and promotion of breast cancer in women. We can expect to see an expanding set of medications (selective estrogen receptor modulators or SERMS) that can exploit these anti-estrogen properties in the breast while simultaneously helping the bones and heart.

HOW DO WE LEARN WHAT TREATMENTS WORK?

In order to evaluate whether a new treatment works or is better than an existing treatment, we must subject it to rigorous testing in a clinical study. The term used for this type of study is a "randomized clinical trial" or RCT. The RCT is the gold standard for providing evidence that a treatment works and to determine how much better it is than a comparison treatment. In an RCT, there are certain requirements for study entry, such as the stage of the tumor, the hormone receptor status, etc. In addition, women may need to meet other requirements such as having normal blood counts, liver and kidney function. All women meeting these requirements and agreeing to participate in the study are then assigned by chance to one of the treatments, e.g., treatment A, the new experimental treatment or treatment B, the standard or existing treatment. After the required number of women enter the trial and receive either treatment A or B, the results of the study are examined. Often this may occur after many years, especially in treatments of early stage breast cancer where the time to a first recurrence may take many years after diagnosis. These adjuvant therapy trials often require four thousand to five thousand women who are observed for as long as ten years, before a definitive answer can be reached. Nevertheless, once this period of time has elapsed and the results of the two treatments are compared, we can say with some certainty whether treatment A is better than treatment B, and by how much (e.g., number of extra years of life, percentage of women surviving at five years, etc.). In addition, these studies typically obtain information on side effects of treatment, including the possibility of death from treatment. Once this information becomes available, it is reported at a scientific meeting and then eventually published in the medical literature where it becomes available for everyone to learn about.

This scientific approach to gaining information about whether treatments are effective is called evidence-based medicine. We are fortunate that for breast cancer treatments, we have over three decades of RCTs that provide us with a substantial body of information about what treatments work and how much of an advantage they provide to patients who take them. All new promising treatments are subjected to this type of scrutiny, and that is what happened with the development of the antibody to the Her-2-Neu oncoprotein (herceptin), and to the use of high-dose chemotherapy in women with a high risk of recurrence or with metastatic disease. In the former studies, herceptin was found to significantly prolong the survival of patients with metastatic breast cancer whose tumors over-expressed this tumor growth factor. In contrast, several studies of high-dose chemotherapy with bone marrow or stem cell transplant support have failed to show a significant survival advantage for this very toxic and costly therapy. Unfortunately, thousands of women in the United States chose to take this experimental treatment (high-dose chemotherapy with bone marrow support) outside of the setting of an RCT because they and their doctors often believed that the new experimental treatment, although highly toxic, was going to be better than the standard treatments. As has now been shown, they were wrong, and many suffered from toxicity or had premature deaths as a result of the treatment. In addition, the failure of patients and their physicians to support the ongoing RCTs delayed our finding the scientific answer to this clinical question. Unfortunately, only about 3 percent of women diagnosed with breast cancer today participate in clinical trials, and this remains a major obstacle to obtaining answers to treatment questions in the shortest possible time. Hopefully, there will be growing support for participation in these trials by patients and their physicians over the next decade. With greater participation, these questions can be answered more quickly and we can ensure that experimental treatments are not adopted prematurely without evidence.

BREAKTHROUGH DRUGS AND INCREMENTAL ADVANCES

Patients and the media are always looking for the magic bullet. If only it were so simple! As we have seen, the development of breast cancer is complex, and its diverse and capricious behavior is often determined by individual tumor characteristics. Thus, we often apply a treatment to everyone for the few who may actually need it or benefit from the therapy. In the next decade, we will continue to see the testing of new experimental therapies, but they will likely be targeted to specific growth factors that are either expressed or over-expressed in a tumor. Good examples of current targeted therapies are the use of tamoxifen and other hormonal therapies only in women whose tumors contain the estrogen or progesterone receptor. The presence of these receptors in a tumor are evidence that changing the hormonal environment in the woman's body can manipulate the growth of the tumor cells. Similarly, the new herceptin immunotherapy uses an antibody that only works in tumors that demonstrate overproduction of the Her-2-neu oncogene protein, and it works best in cells that express the highest levels of the protein. This therapy is only applicable to the 25 to 30 percent of breast cancer patients whose tumors over express the protein.

As alluded to earlier, we can expect increasing understanding of how cancer cells grow and regulate their growth from ongoing laboratory studies. As specific growth factors are identified in this setting, strategies to inhibit tumor growth will initially be tested in cultured cells, and then in animals. Ultimately, promising agents will be tested in human beings with advanced cancer to evaluate their toxicity, correct dose, and possible benefit. Only the most promising agents will make it this far, and those that remain on the short list will require testing in RCTs to see if they really make a difference. Currently, there is much interest in the anti-angiogenesis substances, which in laboratory animals can inhibit the development of the new blood vessels that are required to bring nutrients to cancer cells. Without a source of blood, these cells will die. While we are all hopeful that the dramatic responses seen in laboratory animals will be translated to human benefit, there is no assurance that this will occur. In addition, while this looks promising for all types of cancer in animals, in humans, this may not necessarily be the case, and the substances might turn out to be helpful in only certain kinds of cancers. This was certainly the case for interferon, which more than two decades ago was heralded as the new miracle cure!

THE FUTURE—GREAT EXPECTATIONS!

During the next decade we will continue to reap the benefits of the scientific advances in molecular biology and the new knowledge that will be gained from the road map of our genes obtained from the Human Genome Project. For the first time, we will have an opportunity to understand the acquired genetic mutations that are associated with cancer, and may even be able to link these mutations to specific behaviors (e.g., smoking or other toxic exposures), hormonal exposures, or hereditary cofactors. Since breast cancer is the most common cancer occurring in women, it will be a high priority in this process, and the recent increases in research funding for breast cancer ensure that much work is already underway. Although treatment of women with advanced breast cancer will always be important, it is much more likely that these scientific findings will lead to more effective strategies for prevention and early detection, all of which will reduce the burden of breast cancer as a disease. If we are able to develop an effective "Pap smear for the breast" with implementation of preventive strategies in those who yield abnormal precancerous cells, then we can hope to eliminate the development of breast cancer in a large number of women who participate in screening. As mammography and other imaging tests improve their sensitivity to detect tumors as small as a few millimeters, women will only require simple excision of the tumor, with careful follow-up and a prevention medication prescription! Although this may seem like a fantasy, it is likely to be the future.

Patricia A. Ganz, M.D., is a medical oncologist who has spent the past twenty years doing systemic research on the quality-of-life impact of cancer and its treatment. Her research has been sponsored by the National Cancer Institute, The American Cancer Society (California Division), the Susan G. Komen Breast Cancer Foundation and the Department of Defense. She leads a clinical program for women with family histories of breast cancer in the Revlon/UCLA Breast Center, and heads the UCLA Familial Cancer Registry and Genetic Evaluation Program. In July 1999, she was named an American Cancer Society Professor of Clinical Research.

PART III

What You Can Do to Lessen Your Chance of Being Misdiagnosed

An Interview with
Janis Raynak, Malpractice Attorney

A LITTLE BACKGROUND

Out of the blue I received a phone call from the attorney Elaine Packwood *[see chapter 8]* had retained a year earlier to investigate a potential breast cancer malpractice lawsuit. He could no longer work on the case and was calling to let me know that he was referring her to me. We never really discussed the case other than his mentioning to me that he didn't feel the case had any merit. Why? I don't know, although delay in diagnosis cases are always hard to win.

What stands out in my mind from that first meeting were Elaine's incredible green eyes. Her hair was very short, just starting to grow back from the chemotherapy treatments she had recently completed. It was quite evident that she was angry about her misdiagnosis, and after talking with her for awhile I agreed to represent her. From that first meeting it was apparent that she was going to take an active role in her lawsuit. She came loaded with magazine and newspaper articles that she, and in particular her mother, had gathered. She was bold and aggressive, and I liked that about her.

LET'S SET A FEW THINGS STRAIGHT

Statistically breast cancer is more prevalent in older women than in younger women, and I'm guessing that during Elaine's family practitioner's career few young women had breast cancer. Clearly, Elaine had a lump when she went to see her family practitioner. Despite the very ominous finding that her lump was solid and not a cyst when, during the needle aspiration, he failed to get any fluid from the lump, he simply patted her on the head and told her, "Honey, it can't be breast cancer. You're only twenty-seven." Two years later she's saying, "This thing has gotten really big! Are you sure it's just a benign lump?"

There's still a mind-set that breast cancer is a postmenopausal disease, and that's not true. More young women are now being diagnosed in their twenties and thirties because of better detection methods even though their dense breast tissue, which shows up white on an X-ray, makes it difficult to pick things up. That's why sometimes even large lumps are missed although they can be detected as small as a ½ cm (1 cm is the size of a pea). They don't have a sign on them, nor do they always have a shape. Sometimes the only thing to look for is contrast. There is also a very high incidence of false/negative readings. On the bottom of every single mammography report it says, "If there's a clinically suspicious lump this negative mammogram should not preclude biopsy." Because they all say that, which is boilerplated to protect the radiologist, that warning is too often ignored. A mammogram might, if you do have a lump, help detect another lump in the same breast, or even in the other breast that you might not feel. Women are too often dismissed by their doctor, even if they have a palpable lump, because of the reassurance of a negative mammogram. I've read some studies that say 40 percent, and even one that said up to 53 percent, of premenopausal women whose lumps were malignant had their mammograms read as negative. That's a frightening statistic.

BECOMING AN ADVOCATE

I've always been an advocate for people who couldn't get representation elsewhere, for whatever reason. Being a malpractice attorney for women with breast cancer was something I evolved into after working with Elaine. Sure, all malpractice attorneys love to get those cases where the doctor operated on the wrong knee, or amputated the wrong foot.

Nobody wants a breast cancer case because they're difficult. A doctor doesn't give the patient cancer; therefore, all you're talking about is a lost chance. Take Elaine's situation. Why would a doctor who, knowing a lump was solid because he'd not been able to get fluid from it during the needle aspiration, not do a biopsy? I'm still baffled by that, and even now am still floored by the whole case; by what transpired. I keep hearing the same stories from women, and I just don't get it. How could her gynecologist whom we also sued claim as part of his defense that she had refused to let him examine her breasts when she'd allowed him to do a pelvic examination and a Pap smear?

I've found that what's good for the client is always bad for the patient. For example: the expert you find testifies that the cancer should have been caught two years earlier; clearly a malpractice. It's a good news/bad news scenario. Good news because you're going to make money from the misdiagnosis; bad news because your life's been shattered, and you might not get to enjoy the money. The end result, whether it's a settlement hearing or verdict, is a dose of reality for the client. And the sad truth is—the worse the prognosis the more the case is worth.

THE SETTLEMENT CONFERENCE

Elaine's reconstructed breasts were big, rough-looking mounds with two scars and no nipples. I felt that if she weren't given the opportunity to show her breasts and talk at the hearing I'd never be able to settle the case. I didn't want Elaine or her husband, George, to sit in on the part where I presented the worst-case scenario because of the emotional hurt I knew I'd cause, but I couldn't get them to leave.

Twelve of us, including defense lawyers, insurance representatives and one of her doctors, gathered in the judge's chambers; all men except for Elaine and me. She'd been sobbing as I was talking, and trying to hide behind George's shoulder as they huddled together on the couch listening to me. After I finished making my case I said that Elaine would like to make a statement. Twirling her hair, that was now much longer, she opened her coat-dress and exposed her bare breasts saying, "I'm just a mess. This is what these guys did to me." Showing her mutilated breasts was critical to the resolution of her lawsuit. She needed the defendants to know she had a daily reminder of the effects of their delay. Because her tumor had grown so large she had lost the chance of less radical surgery. Even though it was two to three years after her surgery and radiation, her reconstructed breasts were still pretty ugly.

Elaine spoke for about ten minutes. She said many touching things, but one that was quite poignant was, "I always thought I would grow old with George, and now I don't know." She later confided to me that, although she'd been prepared to talk and to show her breasts, it had been difficult for her to do.

After the hearing the doctor who'd attended the conference asked to speak privately with Elaine and George. He apologized to them. Elaine was literally transcended when she came out of that meeting. She'd been so angry before, but afterwards was a completely different person. That meeting meant everything to her, and she used the word "healing." She needed to know that he cared about her.

DOES WINNING HELP YOU TO COPE BETTER?

When people get cancer they feel as if they need to apologize to their children, that they've somehow done something horrible. One day, while the case was still pending, Elaine told me that she and George wanted to buy their first home. I said, "You never know what's going to happen. I wish you wouldn't think about the money; we could lose the case." She replied, "We're going to win." That was always her attitude. Elaine confided, "If something does happen to me at least I'll know that I provided a nice home for my family." When she and George did buy that home, it was wonderful knowing that I helped her to achieve her legacy.

Winning helped Elaine cope. By being able to provide a home for her family she felt that at least she had done something for them. There would be money for the children's college education. If she were to have a recurrence, the funds would be available; therefore, she wouldn't be taking money out of their pockets. She no longer had to worry whether she could have further reconstruction, or by whom, regardless of what insurance she had. In fact, she could use anyone and, if necessary, pay for it out of her own pocket.

HOW DO YOU CHECK OUT A DOCTOR?

If you're going to establish a relationship with a doctor, chances are that it's going to be long term. Therefore, it's worth five minutes of your time to make a phone call to the Board of Medical Examiners, which is listed in the phone book, to check out the doctor. They'll tell you whether any complaints have been filed against the doctor, and, if so, whether any disciplinary action has been taken. There may be a national registry, but you need to contact the state in which the doctor is licensed to check on complaints. If you do have a complaint against a doctor, and don't wish to file a lawsuit, you can file a complaint with the Board of Medical Examiners. Although that won't get you financial remuneration they will investigate your claim and issue some sort of ruling; no action, a letter of concern or disciplinary action. More importantly, that ruling will then be in the file permanently should another patient call to check him out. In Arizona, where I live, you can physically go to the BOMEX (Arizona Board of Medical Examiners) office. If a complaint has been filed, certain portions of it are public record.

It's also a good idea to check to see whether your doctor is board certified. Although that doesn't guarantee a high level of competence, it does mean that they took an examination and became certified as a specialist in their field. Most doctors are board certified. That information can be obtained by either checking with the doctor's office, or with the Board of Medical Examiners.

WHAT STEPS CAN YOU TAKE TO HELP PREVENT A MISDIAGNOSIS?

By the time we met, Elaine had become very bold with her physicians. No longer was she the kind of person who gave her doctors complete control. She had become aggressive and assertive because she felt it was her initial failure to be assertive that caused the two-year delay in her diagnosis. I liked that about her.

What can you do to help prevent your own misdiagnosis? Ask yourself these kinds of questions: What's my doctor like? Does he/she listen to me? Does he appreciate what I'm complaining about? I use the word *appreciate* in the medical sense. If you feel a lump, or know there's been a change in your breast and what you're feeling is new, are they just saying it's fibrocystic changes? Ask them to describe what they're feeling when doing the examination. What does the doctor feel? Are we talking about the same thing? Does it sound consistent with what you think you're feeling? If you're feeling something the size of a pea, and they tell you it feels like the size of a half dollar, then they're not feeling what you're feeling. Feedback is very important.

Ask them what their policy is with breast lumps. Do they take a wait and see attitude, or do they send you for a biopsy? It's not unusual for a doctor to want to follow you for six weeks; see you at different times during your menstrual cycle. That's okay. Waiting longer than six weeks is not okay. Is this lump something that might be hormone related, which is usually not cancer, versus a lump that either stays the same or increases in size? Cancer can't get smaller. If they say, "Let's recheck it in six months or a year" they've done nothing for you; in fact, that delay can drastically change your prognosis.

Ask to see your chart. Are they noting the lump's location on your breast; what quadrant it's in, where it is in relation to your areola? Measuring its size? Diagramming what it felt like to them? How do they know whether it's changed in size if they don't do this? If they don't do this they have nothing to compare it to the next time you come back. The patient is a very poor historian because when she finds a lump she is going to be feeling it a hundred times a day; consequently, she is not going to know, "Is it bigger today than it was last month?" When you don't see a child for six months you think, "My God, they've changed so much." However, when you're the mother and around them constantly, you hardly notice. Even though it's right in front of your eyes the change is gradual.

Elaine's family practitioner did a really good job in charting her lump.

In fact, he did everything right until he tried to aspirate it. That's when his mind-set kicked in, "She's too young to have breast cancer," and without any pathology mistakenly issued the verdict that her lump was nothing more than a benign fibroadenoma. Breast cancer, in its early stages, doesn't make you look pale or haggard. Elaine was a tanned, healthy, bubbly, twenty-seven-year-old woman who had been doing monthly breast self-examination, just like she was supposed to, for years. Where did it get her?

These delay stories need to be told. Physicians need to be educated. Most women, at some point in their lives, will have a breast complaint. Just because most lumps will be benign (non-cancerous) breast cancer can never be excluded as being a possibility. Women are too well-educated today about doing BSE. If they tell a doctor there's been a change, that has got to be taken seriously. A doctor, who only sees you once every six months or once a year, cannot become familiar with what's a normal lump in your breast, and what's a new finding. Many breasts are lumpy and bumpy. Even those that are smooth still have muscle and fat. Why teach BSE if when the patient comes in and reports a finding the doctor does nothing about it? Ninety-five percent of all palpable breast lumps are found by the patient themselves. How can you ignore that? How can a doctor say it's just a fibrous cystic change, or nothing to be worried about when that woman, who's been doing monthly BSE for years says, "It's a new finding."

No woman goes looking for a breast cancer diagnosis. Who wouldn't be relieved to hear their doctor say that it's nothing? How many women buy into that? Have you? The patient has to keep going until someone says, "Yes, I feel exactly what you're feeling" and describes it as she feels it, and has a follow-up plan that she is comfortable with. If that doesn't include a biopsy, then it had better include being rechecked within the next six weeks; not four weeks later when you're at the same place in your cycle, but two or six weeks. If by then that lump isn't completely resolved, or it hasn't gotten smaller, then it's potentially cancer. The only way to know for sure is to have a biopsy which is the only technique that can rule out cancer. A negative mammogram is not a sure thing, nor is a doctor saying the lump doesn't feel like cancer.

A needle biopsy (aspiration) is an in-office procedure and is really no more difficult than drawing blood. In fact, a Pap smear is more involved. There's no anesthesia, only a little pain, and it doesn't leave a scar. The doctor sticks a bore line needle into the lump, squirts a little fluid (if fluid is drawn) onto a slide, and it's done. Make sure, if there is fluid, that it gets sent out to be analyzed. If the fluid is analyzed as negative, you might be inclined to take a more conservative approach and watch the lump for two to three months. Perhaps during that time it will disappear, but if it doesn't, it needs to come out because it's possible that the tumor is both cancer and non-cancer. If the tumor is solid, further diagnostic work-up is necessary.

If your doctor doesn't want to do a needle biopsy, perhaps because of cost consideration, pay for it out of your own pocket, and fight with the insurance company later. All you've got are your own resources to rely on if your doctor won't help you. I say do it. Sometimes you've got to be adamant. It's well worth the money if it does come back as cancer. Maybe my perception is skewed, but the only women I see are those with breast cancer, and I keep hearing the same story. "I was worried about my lump, but I was reassured when the doctor said . . ." The information is there, everywhere you look. Don't let what happened to Elaine happen to you.

Even though most lumps are benign, a lump in the breast should be a lump in the bottle. In other words, the lump should be tested for pathology. It's the only way to find a malignant one. You can have a great prognosis with early diagnosis, and can survive breast cancer. If you catch it before it goes to your lymph nodes, your survival is 90-plus percent. We should be able to catch most breast cancers. Don't walk around for two years, worrying about a breast lump, like Elaine did.

PART IV

Sex and Sexuality: What You Really Want to Know That Nobody Will Talk About

fter a breast cancer diagnosis, we often think, "What am I going to be like?" "What is sex going to be like?" "Will he or she still want to touch me?" or even, "When do I tell someone?" Breasts are a part of who we are, and like it or not there has been much emphasis placed on them. But a breast cancer diagnosis is not just about a body part; it also affects our sexuality, and the physical act of sex itself.

Because of having either chemotherapy, a bone marrow transplant, or taking tamoxifen, too many women who have had breast cancer have experienced a decrease in sex drive, have no sex drive, or may even have been put into premature menopause. Too often our doctors do not address this issue, or if they do, they gloss over it. But these are issues women need to know about, want to know about and have the right to know about. Age is irrelevant, because breast cancer has no boundaries.

It is only human to have an innate curiosity about sex and sexuality. We want to know things like: "What is it like?" or "Did this happen to you?" Dare we be rude and ask those kinds of questions? As I stated in the beginning of this book, I delved into private areas. I took a deep breath before taking the plunge and asking some very personal questions. I hope this chapter addresses and answers some of the questions you may have about these very important and intimate issues.

Much of what you will read came from interviews that are not one of the nineteen stories in this book. You can try to guess who said what, but chances are you will be wrong! That is how it should be. In order to respect their privacy, no names are used.

MAKING LOVE
THE FIRST TIME AFTER

My having had breast cancer has not affected our sex life. I was not concerned about making love. The first time we did after my mastectomy it was the same as it always was. I do not remember it being a big deal. I cannot speak for my husband because he never said anything, but I do think he was a little concerned that he might hurt me.

Shortly after my bilateral mastectomy, my father said to me, "Don't be surprised if your husband is not sexually attracted to you." As soon as the drains were removed three weeks later, we made love. Sex was great! A few days later the three of us were having dinner at a restaurant. While I went to the ladies room my father and husband had another conversation about sex. When we got home, my husband told me that when the subject had come up, he had said to my father, "Your daughter and I f'd our brains out on Sunday!" My father then turned bright red, laughed, and said to my husband, "You are too much!"

The hardest part was trying to make love again, knowing that something was missing.

I was very concerned about hurting her. If she had had to get on top, or we needed to make adjustments we would have done that.

We were just friends when I was diagnosed. The first night we spent together we were kissing, and she started to take my shirt off. I began to cry because I had not been with anybody since I had lost my breast. This was a new relationship, and she knew what was going on, but it was being physically close to somebody after the fact. She was very good about that.

It is probably better for a woman to have a sexual experience with another woman because another woman can understand the loss of a breast: what it is like, what it means. When we made love her breast was not an issue. I wanted to see her scar, and I made sure that I made love to her scar as much as I made love to any other part of her body. We would talk about it, so it just became a part of who she was. Having one breast was the only way I knew her. It looked odd to me until I got used to it, and then it no longer looked odd.

He wanted to make love before I did. A couple of weeks after I got home from the hospital we did, but I did it only to please him. Making love brought up so much emotion.

I had not had sex in months, and panicked the first time we made love because I had never had sex without nipples. I was very scared. The first time was almost like, "Okay. Come get me."

CAN I FEEL ANYTHING?

Initially I was concerned about touching her in the area of her chest because I was afraid that would make her feel badly since she knew there was something wrong there. We talked about it, and she said to me, "My nerves still work. I can still feel you touching me, and it's okay." People need to know that it is okay to talk about it.

I have no nerve damage on my chest. In fact, I can feel that I am touching myself although it feels kind of distant. Where I do not have sensation is the back of my arm.

Kissing her scar is just a part of her. It is not ugly. After all, if I can kiss her "tush" I can certainly kiss her scar!

HOW DO I REALLY FEEL ABOUT MY SEXUALITY?

My sexuality, and sex drive never changed. It only got stronger. What changed was my self image.

I have never considered myself to be a very sexual person, and I do not think it has gotten any better or worse because I had breast cancer.

What is sexuality? I do not take such good care of myself, nor do I have a good identity. I do not use makeup that frequently, and when I do wear it someone will say to me, "You look so lovely!" I know the outside wrapping can be deceiving. I really want to get to the inside of the package.

Even though I am very proud of my body and of how I look, I am still struggling to regain my sexuality after having gone through breast cancer and reconstruction. That is the one thing that has not come out well from all of this. I am certainly not as sexually hungry a woman as I was fifteen years ago, but that may be partly because of my age. Now that does not mean that my husband and I do not have an affectionate life together, because we do.

Since I lost one implant and am now lopsided I always wear a nightgown or T-shirt to bed.

I think there are many parallels between being gay and having breast cancer. If you are comfortable with things such as: who you are, your sexuality, or having only one breast or no breasts, then other people are comfortable. It is unfair to ask somebody to accept you when you do not accept yourself. I have been comfortable for years with my sexuality and being gay, so for me it is a non-issue. Having breast cancer is like being gay and "coming out" all over again. I went through the same things: "When is it a good time to tell someone?" "Do I have to tell them?" "Is it an issue?" "Is it a non-issue?"

I needed to address my sexuality, or what I thought was my sexuality. I think I felt as though my sexuality was wrapped up in my breast. When I finally surrendered to having surgery, I realized that I was a lot more than my breast. I am who I am. I am not who I am because I am my breast. That was part of what I needed to learn about myself. It was a tough lesson.

I view my sexuality a little differently because I do not feel as though I am back to my old self yet. I do not know how much I will get back to my old self because of all the drugs I took.

I was a little self-conscious because of the tattoos, which look like little blackheads.

She was very sexy without pubic hair!

How Is Our Relationship

Maybe a little deeper, a little more connected, because he has been so involved in my medical care. But we always had a good relationship. We have been together fourteen years.

Her husband gives her no emotional support. There is no physical affection. They never walk up to one another and kiss or hug. I have never seen any of that in the five and a half years I have known them. They have no sex life, at least not since her cancer. I do not know what it was like before she got cancer, and how much stems from the fact that she did.

The loving, the tenderness is stronger.

The emotional support and affection is all there. Maybe knowing that we are vulnerable has made us a little more appreciative of one another.

Things were not good between us. From the beginning the whole thing kind of soured.

I do not know how much of the relationship we have today is a result of my having cancer, or just the fact that I am unhappy. We do not even cuddle.

I became involved with a man who could not accept me for what I looked like. He knew about the cancer and my lumpectomy before we became involved. After being together four months he began to say hurtful things to me such as: "I do not usually date women who look like you. I really like a much smaller, more athletic type body. You are everything I want, but I want a person with a thin body." That was very painful, and made me think, *Oh God. It's true. My body isn't good enough!* So many men want that "perfect" woman. A "conscious" man will see past the lumps, bumps and cellulite and "see" the essence of who you are. He just flushed my self-esteem right down the toilet, and I groveled for months. It was not until the relationship ended that I realized he had some deep, deep problems that had nothing to do with me or my breast.

My husband continued to look at me with lust.

Sex or the Lack of

One day over lunch she burst into tears. She wanted to talk about her husband's lack of tenderness toward her, and their almost nonexistent sex life. I specifically asked her, "Was it great before, and now it's crummy? Do you think it's because you had a mastectomy several years ago?" She told me she could count on one hand the number of times they have been intimate in one year, and then confided, "It wasn't great before. It never has been." I cannot imagine the resentment and feelings she must have had even before she got breast cancer. I thought, *Maybe he can't touch her because he can't handle the disfigurement,* which did happen with one of my friend's parents after her mother had a bilateral mastectomy. But I realized that their relationship was not that great before her mastectomy, and it has apparently gotten worse since. There is no intimacy between them, and their marriage is more like a living arrangement. I asked her once if she had ever told him how she felt, how much she missed being touched. She said, "No."

Our physical relationship has slowed down a little after she got cancer, but things change as people get older. I think her sex drive is as great as it was before, but I am not quite sure.

I think when I heard that I had breast cancer I just shut down. I am not much interested in sex, but then I was never a highly sexed person anyway.

My husband likens our sex life to the Woody Allen movie, *Annie Hall.* When the man is interviewed he says, "We never have sex. We have it only three times a week." The woman, when she is interviewed says, "We have it all the time! Three times a week." It is a matter of perspective. I feel as though I am always eating when it comes to sex, so I am never hungry. If we go a whole week without it, then I do feel hungry. My husband always counts. He knows the last time we had sex. When we were first married we had sex almost every day. He took the bar examination (he is an attorney) and I thought, "Thank God! He is stressed, and I will get a break!" Stress only increases his libido. I am the total opposite. I am stressed all the time now. No wonder!

My husband was never a breast man. We both miss my breasts, but not having them has certainly not wrecked our sex life. Now if I had nothing below the waist I would be in trouble!

I enjoy sex, but I have never had a huge sex drive. Chemotherapy and tamoxifen had little bearing on it; however, my libido went down a little bit more. I am very comfortable just hugging and kissing, but my husband has an insatiable appetite and always wants to make love.

We did not have sex very often prior to her diagnosis. Since her mastectomy, which was two years ago, we have had sex only once or twice. I do not find her unattractive; however I now see other traits and qualities I had not noticed before. I love her in a different way now—more as a mother and as a wife. The love is there. It is deeper than just the sexual part. We are emotionally closer now than we have ever been before.

We did not make love for a couple of months after my lumpectomy. It was not that I didn't want him touching me, I think we were just being careful.

We did not make love for a couple of months after my lumpectomy. It was not that I didn't want him touching me, I think we were just being careful.

Her sex drive is the same it has been since we were married forty years ago. I always initiate. Once she felt up to it, we resumed our sex life. I never pushed, and I always asked.

I just assumed people would accept me with one breast. She was very good about that, and it has been a non-issue.

My sex drive has decreased a lot in the last six months. I thought a woman's sex drive was supposed to increase around the age of thirty, so I feel deprived. I do not know if the chemotherapy I had has anything to do with this. I only know that I am tired morning and night.

I was only thirty-four and did not want to take tamoxifen because I thought it would put me into menopause. I liked having estrogen and those horny times during the month. When I did finally take it, it did not affect my cycles nor my sex drive.

My husband never made me feel less of a woman. I cannot speak for him, but making love was not scary for me. It just hurt emotionally, and I would cry because I felt as though I was a different person because I did not have breasts. I would think to myself, *What do we do?* We had to learn a different way to make love.

After my bone marrow transplant we were not supposed to have sexual relations without using a condom because my vaginal tissues were still not healed. We had never used condoms, so it was very strange for me to buy them. We made love about a month after I got home from the hospital. I think we only used the condoms twice and then I said, "The heck with it. I'll take my chances!" I had no problems. My sex drive is gone now. I feel no desire. If my husband initiates sex I can get into it, but otherwise I could go month after month without it. Sex, to me, is just blah.

I really miss my nipples. Not having them has been hard for me because they were one of my arousal points. To this day I still have a little problem with that, but at least he can now touch my breast, whereas before I would not let him. He loves for me to play with his nipples. That was a little difficult for me to do in the beginning because it aroused me, and then I felt bad because mine were gone. I had no idea men could get aroused from that! For a long time I wore a shirt to bed. I am still self-conscious when he takes it off, even though we have been together for two years.

CAN A RELATIONSHIP SURVIVE WITHOUT SEX?

To be held was more important than anything. We were constantly holding one another. A typical habit of his was to walk behind me and kiss the nape of my neck. We might not have said one word to one another all day.

Even without sex our relationship is stronger. I am sure he misses it, but I think he has learned that our relationship is deeper than just sex. Men do not see that because sex is so important to them.

All my strength now is going into healing, but I still feel really close to my husband, and he feels the same way. It is not like he is turned off by me not having breasts, or that it bothers him in any way. We hold each other a lot, and we know that we love one another.

LACK OF SEXUAL DRIVE AND DESIRE

Chemotherapy and radiation did not affect my sex drive at all.

I blamed chemotherapy for everything including: "That darn chemotherapy. My hair did not come out good!" Certainly I was wiped out the week after a treatment, and sex was not that great even though my sex drive was the same, but I do not think it had anything to do with chemotherapy. I just think we went through a sexually sluggish period, even before I got breast cancer. I would tell my husband after a treatment, "Forget it! No sex. Go away!!"

We did not have sex the entire six months she went through chemotherapy. She is sitting here right now saying to me, "You're crazy!" Well, if we did, it must have been toward the end!

By the time I was finished with radiation, I had open sores and blisters on my breast, and I told my husband, "Do not even come near me!"

because there was too much danger the blisters would pop. Other than that, our sex habits really did not change.

VAGINAL DRYNESS

My sex drive has diminished somewhat, but my family practitioner recently prescribed testosterone cream to be applied topically to that area. It has helped to lubricate me. Actually my dryness problem has improved a little over the past few years even though I am still taking tamoxifen. It seems that I was much drier a few years ago.

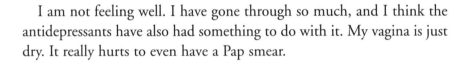

I am not feeling well. I have gone through so much, and I think the antidepressants have also had something to do with it. My vagina is just dry. It really hurts to even have a Pap smear.

My sex drive is not as good as it used to be. I am dry, and having sex is painful, which is probably from a lack of estrogen. I did try taking Mexican yam in pill form, but I stopped taking it after about a month because I saw no results. I am now using a vaginal cream.

Adriamycin stopped my period. Between that and the tamoxifen everything changed. I have not found anything that helps my vaginal dryness. My oncologist prescribed a very low dose estrogen cream that she felt would be safe for me to use, but it did not work. I felt as though I was on fire. For many women it is very effective, but not for me.

A dry vagina has been an ongoing problem and challenge for my husband and me. We have sex infrequently because it is too painful. This is a big problem, and it seems to me that we are never told this is part of the deal. It is kind of like a big surprise. I complained to my oncologist and said to her, "As good as you are, and as dedicated as you have been in my care, the one area you never broached to me was, 'You are going to have extreme vaginal dryness. It is not going to be fun.'" I never, ever knew that would happen. It came as such a shock. I thought I was doing something wrong, or that something was going on that was causing the problem. Not true!

I went to a support group meeting, and began to hear little whispers from women I had never met before. How often do you go to the grocery store, and while you are standing in line the woman in front of you turns around and says, "Say, how's your sex life? Do you have vaginal dryness?" I mean, here you are, with a complete group of strangers and suddenly everyone is talking about their vaginal dryness! It is pretty strange. Physicians need to discuss this with their patients. Will this information make us happy? No, but they told us our breasts had to come off. That did not make us happy either, but we expected it. We understood why. With this, it happens and we do not even know why it is happening, or even that it is going to happen. It always seems to happen to those women who have had chemotherapy, and who are taking tamoxifen. I would tell all women taking tamoxifen, "Sex ain't what it used to be!"

This is a very serious problem because even though my husband and I are closer today than we have ever been before, we both miss having sex. However, the alternative of not taking tamoxifen causes me to kind of make up reasons why it is okay not to have sex.

HOW I FEEL ABOUT MY RECONSTRUCTED BREASTS

Since my reconstruction I feel better about my sexuality, and much better about myself. It's not that I consciously felt bad, but maybe subconsciously I did. Having breasts has made me feel more confident about myself. When I had no breasts and would water ski in my little Speedo bathing suit, without wearing a prosthesis, men looked at me funny. That is where getting breasts back helped.

I was so excited to show him my new breasts because he had put up with me the entire time I was "imperfect." Those first few times we made love and he saw me, I felt so exposed and so self-conscious. I needed him to say, "Your breast looks great!" He was not gooey, but he said the right thing at exactly the right time.

When I got a little saline in the first expander I had, he walked up behind me, and I took his hand and placed it on my breast. "Look! I've got a boob!" and I jiggled it. He said to me, "Hey. It feels just like a boob!" I did not do that with my irradiated breast because it was hard and did not move.

My husband has never, ever touched my upper body, or felt my breasts since before my last reconstruction. I do not know whether he is afraid he will embarrass me, if he is not curious or interested to see what I look like, or does not want to make me uncomfortable. We do not talk about it. He has not even seen my new reconstructed breasts, and it has been four weeks. I know that sounds odd, but I did not want to put him on the spot by saying to him, "Hey, do you want to see?", yet at the same time he has not asked to see them. Maybe I am a little afraid to say anything because I am scared of what his reaction might be although he is really good at keeping a poker face. I do not think my breasts look too bad, and I am so pleased to have two breasts again that I see past the scars. But I do not know how someone else might feel.

I did not think that far in advance, nor did I realize that after her reconstruction her breasts would no longer be an erogenous zone for her, or that I would not enjoy them as I had her natural breasts from a sexual standpoint. For me, making love is being able to give my wife pleasure, and she no longer derives sexual pleasure from her breasts. Her nipples are cosmetically nice, and it feels good to be able to lie against her breasts, but her nipples never get hard! They are "just there." It is not a big deal, but nonetheless it was a shock. There are other places!

Frankly I would much rather have her with her breasts. To be really candid I would like to have her with her nipples. I miss the responsiveness of her nipples more than I thought I would. They are a part of the love-making process. On the other hand, they are not worth trading a life for!

She has a great body, and now her breasts fit the rest of her body, whereas before they were too small. In clothes she looks unbelievable, and she is able to wear very revealing clothing. Her breasts are perfect, but they are reconstructed breasts, not real. Unclothed I can see little ripples here and there. It was kind of a shock at first when I hugged her because she is so firm—like a twenty-year-old.

MISPLACED BLAME

She has told me I do not care about her the way I used to because she had breast cancer, and has only one breast now. She is certain that is the reason. I do not think that is true, and I tell her that. I believe there are other issues involved.

THE SCAR THAT IS VISIBLE

When I was a kid, I was in a very serious accident. As a result of that accident I have had many surgeries, and to this day I become dizzy when I think about surgery or see any scar, even if it is on television. Her having one breast never really bothered me, but the scar did a little, only because it was right there. The scar looks sort of goofy, but it is not much of a scar and it does not make my stomach turn. She thinks it does, and no matter how much I reassure her that she is wrong she thinks I am lying.

My husband touches my scar all the time.

I look like a little waif when I stand in front of the mirror. I am all bony, but I do not find myself disgusting without breasts. I do not feel sexy, which I know will come with time; however, I do feel really sexual. I do not need to have breasts in order to have sexual relations, and my husband kind of agrees. It is almost as if I need to have sex in order to feel better about myself. To affirm to myself that I am a "whole" person.

Her having a bilateral mastectomy has been very difficult for me. All I see are the scars. Obviously her body has been deformed. It is no longer a normal female body. It looks different, and that bothers me to a certain extent. Her not having breasts has changed something sexually and emotionally in our relationship. I see her naked, and I know there are no sexual feelings.

I have been quite open showing my family and friends what I look like without breasts. Anybody who knows me well enough to say to me, "I need to know what that looks like" loves me. There have been no adverse reactions.

The fact that she does not have breasts did not faze me one way or the other. The issue now is the fact that we are both still feeling stressed from everything she has been through. She does not feel well all the time, and I am just not a happy guy right now. We will have to let things take their own course. If she decides to have reconstruction, I will appreciate the visual image, but because she will not have nerves there, she will derive no sexual enjoyment from her breasts. If she does not, then I do not see how I will either. You know, I really don't care. It's funny, but I miss her hair more than I miss her breasts. She had such beautiful hair. I used to wrap myself in it, and I miss being able to do that. I do not think she will ever grow it long again.

She no longer had breasts, and she was walking around in a little, black lacy bra. I thought to myself, *She looks just like Audrey Hepburn.* She looked so remarkable, so sexy. It was a different kind of sexiness. She had had large breasts, and I have always had small breasts. I certainly love the fact that my breasts are a sensuous part of my body, but their small size makes them a less obvious part of my body. Women, regardless of whether we are sexy or sexual, are associated with breasts. If I had no breasts I am sure I would feel less of a woman. I am also sure I would be self-conscious.

When we talked about whether or not I should have the bilateral mastectomy, what it boiled down to was the fact that I would lose sensation in my nipples. It seemed a pretty good trade—my nipples, or having security for the rest of my life.

I am okay now, but in the beginning losing my breasts changed everything. I told my husband, "Let's not even go there. Do not touch my breasts!"

It took her a long time to get over losing her breasts. She did not feel sexy.

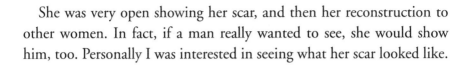

She was very open showing her scar, and then her reconstruction to other women. In fact, if a man really wanted to see, she would show him, too. Personally I was interested in seeing what her scar looked like.

SINGLES AND THE DATING GAME

I was sexually abused when I was a child and a teenager. So when I started to have sex I always had to have my shirt on. My shirt was my security blanket. After years of therapy, when I considered myself "whole," I no longer wore a shirt when I had sex.

I was recovering from a broken heart when I was diagnosed with breast cancer. I had not been with a man for nine months, and I knew the longer I put it off, the harder it was going to be to make love. I had been dating a man for a short time, and decided he was the one I would "break the ice" with. I felt safe with him because I had no romantic feelings toward him. I was twenty-nine, and he was several years younger than I was. He did not want me to take off my shirt because he was afraid of what he would see, and that his reaction might upset me. At the time I thought I had painted a really ugly picture of what I looked like because I was going through reconstruction, but in hindsight, I know I did not. I hated the way I looked! My breast was big, flat and sat very high on my chest. I slept with him several times, but always with my shirt on. When he was finally ready to "see" me, I was not ready. Maybe subconsciously I knew he was going to reject me. He called me every single day until we finally had sex again, and I took off my shirt. He never called me again. Obviously, he could not cope. My feelings were hurt. He made me start to question my appearance.

There was another man in my life at the same time, but things did not heat up between us until I had become intimate with this first man. For three months, I did not tell him I had cancer. When I did, he said to me, "Did you think I wouldn't go out with you because of that?" He also said, "This changes how your life is, but it does not change who you are. Who you are is who I like. And who you are comes through." After the other relationship was over, and we did make love, he was the most nurturing man. He never pushed me to do anything sexually with him, and he was totally comfortable with taking off my shirt, which I always tried to prevent him from doing. He finally said to me, "People will accept you once you accept it." Finally I did. Our relationship ended, but it was a very positive experience because he helped me to accept myself.

Then I began to just date, and I used different tactics to tell men that I had breast cancer. Sometimes I would blurt it out. Once, on a first date I told the man I had had a mastectomy. He never called me again. I did not feel rejected, but I was angry at him for making me feel bad. That just proved to me again how superficial men can be.

I came into the picture shortly after her prophylactic (preventive) mastectomy. She put "handcuffs" on me while we were kissing. I could not have cared less when she told me she had a mastectomy, because I really cared about her. What I thought was, *She has to be a really tough lady to have gone through that.* Here's a real person inside and out. I knew as long as we were able to talk about it, it would be all right.

He had seen my breasts, but at the time he was just a friend. Then we became romantically involved. I was not embarrassed or afraid of what his reaction would be since he had been through everything with me, but there is a line between friendship and intimacy. He always said, "Let me see," but I would wear a shirt to bed, and I would not let him touch me for two years.

I had no apprehension at all about getting into a relationship with her because she had breast cancer and a mastectomy; then later a prophylactic mastectomy and reconstruction. Her breasts were not the reason I enjoyed being with her. Breasts were not a big deal.

Dating is a challenge because it is hard to think of yourself as very marketable with a scarf on your head and no eyebrows. Telling someone I had breast cancer did not have to be the first thing out of my mouth until now, because it is obvious I am sick. Almost everyone in my life at the moment has already been in my life, and that is comfortable. But I am also a woman, so I work really hard at my looks. I am not going to accept just giving up, and I think it is important that we keep trying!

I have to look semi-glamorous when I go to work, and believe me that takes a lot of work right now. But I just do it. My eyes might be a little big from all this toxicity, so I wear my shaded glasses. I have these really cool scarves, and I put on big earrings and look like a gypsy. My entire body might be covered with a rash, but I smack a smile on my face, put on my heels and go. And no one is going to know! A woman called me after church last week, and asked, "Are you making a fashion statement, or are you back in treatment again?" I think I told her, "Both."

We are not just patients. We are people who are dateable. There is no reason I cannot fall in love even when I am in the middle of treatment. I do not have to wait. But I have to work hard at that sometimes because there are times I feel, *Geez. I guess nobody really would want to be around me right now.* All that emotion surfaces. Fear and doubt is not a good place for me to be. I can sit in it for awhile, but then I have to get out.

I am really lucky. It could have been a lot worse. I could have been single!

We had just started dating. He was kissing me, and then he kissed me "there," through my shirt. I just about shot through the ceiling. In a panic I said to him, "I have to go now. I'll see you later." Three weeks later I finally got up my courage and called him. It was easier to tell him on the telephone rather in person that I had had breast cancer, and had panicked when he kissed me on my chest area. He just listened. When I was finished he said, "Thank you for trusting me and sharing that. I know how personal this is." It was so kind the way he said it.

It was months before I was able to be intimate with him. When we did make love I wore my bra with a prosthesis. He kept trying to go under it, and touch and kiss me there and I was terrified. He would tell me how beautiful I was, and he made me feel as though my breast was not gone. Before I met him I did not feel sexy. Since I have been with him I do, and because of him my sexuality has returned.

My body has always been very important to me. It had to be perfect. I used to be very insecure about my breasts, so it is very ironic that I got breast cancer. It was not until I got breast cancer that I realized I liked my body. Even more important was the realization that I liked myself.

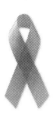# Drug Name Identification

Antacid:
Zantac (ranitidine HCL)

Antibody Therapy:
Herceptin (trastuzumab)

Antidepression/Antianxiety Drugs:
Prozac (fluoxetine HCL)
Xanax (alprazolam)
Zoloft (sertraline HCL)

Antinausea Drugs:
Compazine (prochlorperazine)
Zofran (ondansetron HCL)

Anxiety/Nausea:
Ativan (lorazepam)

Chemotherapeutic Drugs:
Adriamycin (doxorubicin)
Cytoxan (cyclophosphamide)
Doxil (doxorubicin HCL liposome injection)
5 fluorouracil (5-FU)
methotrexate
Taxol (paclitaxel)
Taxotere (docetaxel)

Growth Factor:
Neupogen (filgrastim)

Hormonal Therapy:
Armidex (anastrozole)
Catapres (clonidine)—pill
Catapres-TTS (clonidine)—patch
diethylstilbestrol (DES)
Evista (raloxifene)
Megace (megestrol acetate)
Nolvadex (tamoxifen)

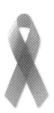

Glossary

Aneuploid: abnormal amount of DNA in a cell; can correlate with a worse cancer.

Angiogenesis: development of blood vessels.

Aspirate: to remove or withdraw fluid or tissue from a cavity by applying suction.

Atypia: change in a cell that suggests a tendency toward malignant transformation.

Atypical hyperplasia: cells that are not only abnormal but increased in number.

Axillary dissection: surgical removal of lymph nodes from the armpit. This tissue is then sent to a pathologist to determine if the breast cancer has spread.

BRCA1 and BRCA2: breast cancer genes that have been linked to familial breast cancer.

Bilateral mastectomy: surgical removal of both breasts.

Biopsy: removal of tissue. This term does not indicate how much tissue will be removed.

Bone marrow: the soft inner part of large bones that produces blood cells.

Bone scan: test to determine if there is any sign of cancer in the bones.

Calcifications: small calcium deposits in the breast tissue that can be seen by mammography.

Catheter: a tube implanted or inserted into the body to inject or withdraw fluid.

Clinical trial: a carefully designed scientific experiment for testing a new therapy or treatment approach.

Cyst: a fluid-filled benign breast lump.

Differentiated: defined. Well-differentiated cancer cells resemble normal cells more than poorly differentiated cancer cells do.

Drains: tubes or suction devices inserted after mastectomy or breast reconstruction to drain the fluids that accumulate postoperatively. Drains may be left in place for several days (or weeks) as needed.

Ductal carcinoma in-situ (DCIS): ductal cancer cells that have not grown outside of their site of origin, sometimes referred to as precancer.

Estrogen receptor: a protein in the cancer cell that binds to the hormone estrogen. A cancer cell that is estrogen receptor rich (or positive) is usually sensitive to hormones.

Expander: a polyurethane flexible implant that is placed under the tissue and is enlarged manually by inserting a fluid, usually saline. Also called tissue expander.

Fibrocystic breasts: a recurring benign condition characterized by breast tenderness, pain, swelling and the appearance of cysts or lumps.

Fine wire localization: a technique to direct a surgical biopsy to an area of the breast which is abnormal on a mammogram, but which cannot be felt. A thin wire is placed into the breast under mammographic control to guide the surgeon to the correct part of the breast to be removed.

Frozen section: freezing and slicing tissue to make a slide immediately for diagnosis.

Grade: classification of cancers according to the appearance of cancer cells under the microscope. Low-grade cancers often grow more slowly than high-grade cancers.

Halsted radical mastectomy: surgical removal of the breast, skin, pectoralis muscles (both major and minor), all axillary lymph nodes and fat for local treatment of breast cancer.

Her-2 neu oncoprotein: an oncogene that is abnormally stimulated to produce an excess of protein affecting cell division in the breast.

Holistic approach: treatment that involves the entire body, including the mind and spirit.

Hyperplasia: excessive growth of cells.

Infiltrating ductal cell carcinoma: cancer that begins in the mammary duct and spreads to areas outside the duct.

Infiltrating lobular carcinoma: cancerous cells in the breast lobule that have spread through the basement membrane into the surrounding breast tissue.

Intraductal: within the duct. Intraductal can describe a benign or malignant process.

Irradiation: a form of ionizing energy that can destroy or damage cells. Cancer cells tend to be more easily destroyed than the normal cells in the surrounding tissues. For breast cancer treatment, this therapy can be used as an adjunct to breast-conserving surgery to reduce the chance of cancer recurrence.

Invasive (infiltrating): cancers that are capable of growing beyond their site of origin and invading neighboring tissue. Invasive does not imply that the cancer is aggressive or has already spread.

Latissimus dorsi: flap of skin and muscle taken from the back and used for reconstruction after mastectomy or partial mastectomy.

Lobular carcinoma in-situ (LCIS): abnormal cells within the lobule that do not form lumps, but can serve as a marker of future cancer risk.

Lumpectomy: surgical removal of a cancerous tumor along with a small margin of surrounding tissue.

Lymphedema: a condition characterized by the collection of excess fluid in the hand and arm after lymph nodes are moved or blocked. It can be temporary or permanent, and occur immediately, or any time later.

Lymph nodes: small lima bean-shaped structures grouped at various locations along the lymph system in the body (e.g. armpits, neck, groin). They act as the main "filters" to defend against infections and may be a location to where cancer spreads. Lymph nodes under the arm are frequently removed as part of breast cancer surgery.

Margins: the area of tissue surrounding a tumor when it is removed by surgery. Positive margins indicate that this area of tissue is not clear of tumors.

Markers: blood tests that register tumor antigens.

Mastectomy: surgical removal of the breast, usually for treatment of cancer.

Metastasis: spread of cancer to another organ, usually through the bloodstream.

Microcalcifications: tiny calcifications in the breast tissue usually seen only on a mammogram. The presence of clusters may be a sign of ductal carcinoma in-situ (DCIS).

Modified radical mastectomy: surgical removal of the breast and axillary lymph nodes.

Multi-focal disease: a cancer that appears in more than one area.

Needle aspiration: diagnostic method of removing fluid or tissue from a breast tumor or cyst with a fine needle for microscopic examination.

Palpable: can be felt.

Pathology report: the pathologist's written record of the analysis of tissue.

Positive nodes: lymph nodes that have been invaded by cancer cells.

Primary care physician (PCP): a term used by insurance companies to describe the selected physician for a particular patient; usually not a specialist.

Prophylactic mastectomy: removal of high-risk breast tissue to prevent the development of a cancer. This procedure usually is combined with breast reconstruction. Also called preventive mastectomy and risk-reducing mastectomy.

Prosthesis: any artificial body part. A breast-shape form may be worn outside the body after a breast has been removed because of cancer. It fits into the woman's brassiere in a specially designed pocket. Prosthesis are made of different materials.

RCT (randomized clinical trial): an investigation of the effects of a drug administered to human subjects. The goal is to define the clinical efficiency and pharmacological effects (toxicity, side effects, interactions) of the substance. This is done by a random method of assigning subjects to experimental treatment or non-treatment groups.

Receptors: a cell component that combines with a drug, hormone, or chemical mediator to alter the function of the cell.

Recurrence: the reappearance of cancer following a period of time when there was no evidence of disease. The recurrence may be either at the original site (a local recurrence), in the adjacent lymph nodes (a regional recurrence), or elsewhere in the body (a systemic or distant recurrence).

SERM: selective estrogen receptor modulators.

Simple (or total) mastectomy: removal of the breast only; the lymph nodes and pectoralis muscle are preserved.

Staging: system for classifying cancer according to the size of the tumor, its stage of development, and the extent of its spread.

Stem cell: an immature blood cell that has the ability to generate new bone marrow.

TRAM (transverse rectus abdominis) flap: a method of breast reconstruction named for the transverse rectus abdominis muscle, the lower half of the abdomen from which the skin, muscle, and fat is taken to build a new breast. A bonus for many is the "tummy tuck" procedure that is part of it.

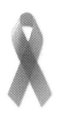

Works Cited

CHAPTER 4

Canfield, Jack et al. *Chicken Soup for the Woman's Soul.* Deerfield Beach, Fla.: Health Communications, Inc., 1996.

John-Roger, and Peter McWilliams. *You Can't Afford the Luxury of a Negative Thought.* Los Angeles, Calif.: Prelude Press, Inc., 1991.

CHAPTER 8

Chechik, Diane. *Journey to Justice: A Woman's True Story of Breast Cancer and Medical Malpractice.* Sarasota, Fla.: Catalyst, 1989.

CHAPTER 14

Anderson, Greg. *The Cancer Conqueror.* Kansas City, Mo.: Andrews McMeel, 1990.

Frahm, Anne. *The Cancer Battle Plan: Six Strategies for Beating Cancer from a Recovered "Hopeless Case."* East Rutherford, N.J.: Putnam Publishing Group, 1992.

Shaw, Eva. *What to Do When a Loved One Dies.* Irvine, Calif.: Dickens Press, 1994.

CHAPTER 16

Brinker, Nancy, with Catherine McEvily Harris. *The Race Is Run One Step at a Time: Everywoman's Guide to Taking Charge of Breast Cancer and My Personal Story.* Arlington, Tex.: Summit Publishing Group, 1995.

GLOSSARY:

Steve Austin, N.D., and Cathy Hitchcock, M.S.W., *Breast Cancer What You Should Know (But May Not Have Been Told) About Prevention, Diagnosis and Treatment.* Rocklin, CA: Prima Health, a division of Prima Publishing, 1994.

Karen Berger and John Bostwick III, M.D., *A Woman's Decision,* 3rd ed. New York: St. Martin's Griffin, 1998.

Link, John, M.D. *The Breast Cancer Survival Manual*, 2nd ed. New York: An Owl Book, Henry Holt and Company, 2000.

Love, Susan M., M.D., with Karen Lindsey. *Dr. Susan Love's Breast Book*, 2nd ed. New York: Addison-Wesley Publishing Company, 1995.

Ivo Olivotto, M.D., Karen Gelmon, M.D., and Urve Kuusk, M.D., Intelligent Patient Guide to Breast Cancer; *All You Need to Know to Take an Active Part in Your Treatment*, 2nd ed. Vancouver: Intelligent Patient Guide Ltd, 1998.

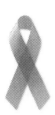

Index

Personal Journeys of Healing

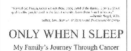
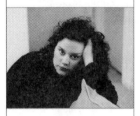
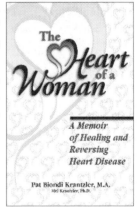

Give Your Spirit a Fresh Twist

Diary of a Modern-Day Goddess
By Cynthia Daddona

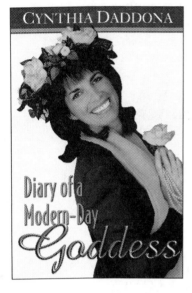

"Cynthia Daddona is a very funny lady. She got me in touch with my inner goddess, who turned out to be an old woman named Maude Frickert. I was so taken by her book on enlightenment, I leave the lights on twenty-four hours a day."
—Jonathan Winters

Code #7745
Quality Paperback • $10.95

Award-winning writer Cynthia Daddona shares her quest to become a modern-day goddess: a woman in touch with her joyful, feminine, and spiritual self. From yoga to yogurt, from finding Nirvana to finding the perfect pump at Nordstorm, to balancing her chakras, tires and checkbook for under $100 her essays and advice offer inspiration, spiritual truths and chuckles that soothe the soul. She reminds us that humor is a beautiful tool in the never-ending quest for inner wisdom and that laughter is vital to every goddess.

New Soup for the Whole Family

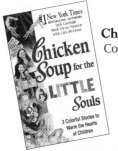

Chicken Soup for Little Souls
Code #8121• Quality Paperback • $12.95

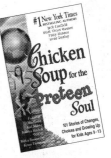

**Chicken Soup for the
Preteen Soul**
Code #8008 • Quality Paperback • $12.95

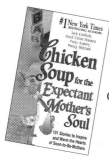

**Chicken Soup for the
Expectant Mother's Soul**
Code #7966 • Quality Paperback • $12.95

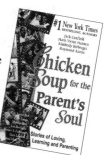

**Chicken Soup for the
Parent's Soul**
Code #7478• Quality Paperback • $12.95